BOTTOM LINE YEAR BOOK 2023

BY THE EDITORS OF

Bottom Line
PERSONAL

BottomLineInc.com

Contents

13 • CONSUMER CONCERNS

PART THREE • YOUR LIFE

14 • EMOTIONAL HELP

Preface

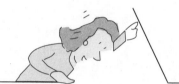

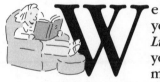We are happy to bring you our *2023 Bottom Line Yearbook*. Here you will discover numerous helpful and practical ideas for yourself and for everyone in your family.

At Bottom Line Books, it is our mission to provide all of our readers with the best information to help them gain better health, greater wealth, more wisdom, extra time, and increased happiness.

The *2023 Yearbook* represents the very best and the most useful Bottom Line articles from the past year. Whether you are looking for ways to get the most from your money or ensure the retirement of your dreams...boost your immunity or get ready for the next natural disaster...learn to love your in-laws or save on remodeling costs, you'll find it all in this book...and a whole lot more.

Over the past 40 years, we have built a network of thousands of expert sources.

When you consult the *2023 Yearbook*, you are accessing a stellar group of authorities in fields that range from natural and conventional medicine...to shopping, investing, taxes, and insurance...to house and garden care and self-improvement. Our advisers are affiliated with the premier universities, financial institutions, law firms, and hospitals. These experts are truly among the most knowledgeable people in the country.

As a reader of a Bottom Line book, you can be assured that you are receiving reliable, well-researched, and up-to-date information from a trusted source.

We are very confident that the *2023 Bottom Line Yearbook* can help you and your family have a healthier, wealthier, wiser life. Enjoy!

The Editors, *Bottom Line Personal*
Norwalk, CT

1

Health Highlights

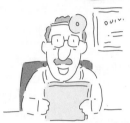

Can Exercise Trigger a Heart Attack?

Regular physical activity offers a wide range of health benefits, including protection against the development of heart disease. *But in rare cases, it appears to have the opposite effect...*

Exercise-related acute cardiovascular events—and sudden cardiac deaths—have been reported in the medical literature and the lay press. In some people with underlying heart disease, exercise-related increases in heart rate and blood pressure can cause coronary plaque rupture, thrombosis, and lethal heart rhythm irregularities. The cause of exercise-related cardiovascular events largely depends on the exerciser's age. Coronary artery disease is the most frequent autopsy finding in individuals over the age of 40. In contrast, inherited structural cardiovascular abnormalities are a major cause of fatal heart rhythms during strenuous physical activity in younger athletes.

RISK IN PERSPECTIVE

The incidence of cardiovascular events during light- to moderate-intensity activities is extremely low and similar to that expected at rest. Unaccustomed vigorous physical exertion, however, especially in people with underlying heart disease, appears to transiently increase the risk of acute cardiac events. Activities such as competitive squash/racquetball, basketball, cross-country skiing, water skiing, heavy weight-lifting, and high-intensity interval training may place undue stress on the heart and are not recommended for people with known or suspected heart disease. Arm work, straining, breath-holding, and exposure to cold and wind appear to heighten the risk of acute cardiac events as well.

Barry Franklin, PhD, director of preventive cardiology/cardiac rehabilitation at Beaumont Health in Royal Oak, Michigan. He is a member of the *Bottom Line Health* advisory board. DrBarryFranklin.com

SAFER WORKOUTS

There are several steps you can take to reduce your risk of experiencing a cardiovascular event when exercising.

• **If you are currently inactive,** always start with a walking program. An initial goal is to walk at a speed of at least 3 miles per hour on a level surface, without symptoms.

• **Warm up and cool down.** The best warm-up for any activity is performing that activity at a lower intensity.

• **Reduce the intensity of exercise** in hot, humid weather and when working at high altitudes.

• **Don't ignore symptoms** such as chest pain, dizziness, lightheadedness, heart palpitations (fast, slow, or irregular heartbeats), unusual fatigue, or shortness of breath. Many people who have experienced exercise-related cardiovascular complications had these symptoms in the days or weeks before the event. If you experience any of these symptoms while exercising or have pain or discomfort from your belly button up, stop exercise immediately and consult with your physician. Medical clearance is required before resuming your exercise regimen.

• **Exercise regularly.** The likelihood of cardiac events appears to be reduced by up to 50% in regular exercisers. For people who gradually progress to vigorous exercise, the more frequently vigorous exercise is performed, the lower the cardiac risk of each exercise bout. In other words, don't cram your vigorous exercise into just one or two bouts per week.

When it comes to extremely strenuous exercise, being a "weekend warrior" (or even less frequently) can be hazardous to your health.

Exercise Might Heal the Heart

According to a recent study, the hearts of patients with thickening of the left chamber of the heart (which makes it harder to pump blood efficiently and often is caused by high blood pressure) who participated in a high-intensity exercise group for one year became less rigid and more efficient—compared with the hearts of patients with similar heart damage who did not exercise. Researchers believe it is likely that the heart improvements would protect against future heart failure.

Bottom line: If you have any kind of heart issues, talk to your doctor before starting an exercise program.

Study of 46 patients led by researchers at Texas Health Presbyterian Hospital Dallas, published in *Circulation*.

Heart Risk Is Greater from COVID

Heart risk is greater from COVID than from the vaccine. Multiple studies have shown an elevated risk for mild-to-moderate myocarditis (inflammation of the heart muscle) among young men following mRNA vaccination against COVID-19. The risk is considerably higher from catching COVID. Plus, myocarditis is just one of several heart problems associated with COVID. Vaccination is still the safer bet.

Leslie T. Cooper, Jr., MD, chair of the department of cardiovascular medicine at Mayo Clinic in Jacksonville, Florida.

Heart Disease Risks

Beware of On-the-Job Physical Exertion

High levels of leisure-time activity are associated with reduced risks for heart problems and death.

Recent finding: Lots of physical activity at work is linked to greater risk for heart attack, stroke and death.

Possible reasons: Leisure-time exercise may be more aerobic, while occupational activity is more likely to involve repetitive resistance exercise with little recovery time. Leisure-time exercise also typically involves 30 to 60 minutes of workouts several days a week, while occupational activity is often six to eight hours a day for many days in a row.

Ten-year study of more than 104,000 adults, ages 20 to 100, by researchers at National Research Center for the Working Environment, Copenhagen, Denmark, published in *JAMA*.

HIIT and Cardiovascular Risk

HIIT may not be safe for people with heart disease.

Recent finding: High-Intensity Interval Training (HIIT) is aerobic exercise such as jogging, swimming and cycling that alternates between short bursts of high heart rate and low-heart-rate intervals. While it is generally safe for most people, even older adults, it may be dangerous for people who have or are at risk for heart disease. Check with your health-care provider.

Study of 1,500 adults led by researchers at Norwegian University of Science and Technology, Trondheim, Norway, published in *BMJ Open*.

Just One Drink Increases Risk for Atrial Fibrillation (AF)

According to a recent study, just one alcoholic drink doubled the odds of experiencing an AF event within four hours…two or more drinks tripled the odds.

If you have AF: Consider reducing or eliminating alcohol consumption. Even people without AF should be aware that drinking may be linked to increased risk for AF.

Gregory Marcus, MD, MAS, professor of medicine at University of California, San Francisco, and lead author of a study of 100 AF patients, published in *Annals of Internal Medicine*.

Why Some People Get Long COVID

For some COVID patients, symptoms—such as brain fog, fatigue and/or loss of taste and smell—last much longer than the infection, a condition known as long COVID.

Recent finding: Regardless of whether their COVID infection was mild or severe, patients who develop long COVID typically have higher levels of coronavirus RNA in their blood, indicating a high viral load…a history of Epstein-Barr virus, which young people typically get as mononucleosis…autoantibodies, which are associated with autoimmune diseases such as lupus…and type 2 diabetes. Identifying and addressing these factors early in the disease could help reduce the risk for long COVID.

Study of 200 COVID patients by researchers at Institute for Systems Biology, Seattle, published in *Cell*.

Broken Heart Syndrome

Gregory Chapman, MD, a University of Alabama at Birmingham cardiologist and professor of medicine. He is the author of *A Strong and Steady Pulse: Stories from a Cardiologist*.

We all know that severe stress is bad for our health.

In some cases, it can even cause sudden, dramatic changes in our hearts, producing chest pain, shortness of breath, and something that feels very much like a heart attack. Doctors call the condition stress cardiomyopathy.

You may know it better as "broken heart syndrome," the name often used in news stories about people who fall ill and sometimes even die in the days after the death of a loved one. It's also been suspected when deaths rise suddenly after hurricanes and earthquakes.

THE ROLE OF THE PANDEMIC

Now the condition has been tied to another big stressor: the COVID-19 pandemic. In the early months of the pandemic, researchers at the Cleveland Clinic found a clear uptick in cases among patients showing up with possible heart-attack symptoms. Before the pandemic, fewer than 2% of such patients turned out to have the disorder, but during the spring of 2020, that quadrupled. None of those patients had COVID-19 itself. Instead, researchers speculated that the stresses associated with the outbreak—everything from isolation to job loss to increased health worries—triggered the increase in stressed-out hearts.

WHAT IS STRESS CARDIOMYOPATHY?

In stress cardiomyopathy, the heart's left ventricle, the chamber responsible for pumping oxygen-rich blood to the rest of the body,

becomes enlarged and weakened. The condition develops suddenly, typically within a few days of an especially stressful event. Usually, these are upsetting events, but even a happy surprise, such as winning a lottery, can be a trigger.

A leading theory is that stress hormones, such as adrenaline, surge into the heart tissue and disrupt normal functioning. It can happen in someone with no previous heart troubles or risk factors for heart disease. Women past menopause are at the highest risk, but doctors don't know why. Some increased risk also is seen in people with anxiety, depression, and schizophrenia.

Because typical signs and symptoms include chest pain, shortness of breath, and irregular heartbeat, patients who show up in emergency rooms are rightly treated as if they might be having classic heart attacks. That kind of heart attack is technically known as a myocardial infarction and is usually caused by a clot blocking blood flow to the heart, damaging or destroying the muscle.

Someone suffering from stress cardiomyopathy will have some test findings that match those of a person suffering a myocardial infarction, such as levels of certain cardiac enzymes, but a coronary angiogram, a kind of X-ray done to look for blocked arteries, will find no blockages. Instead, tests will reveal the distinctive enlarged left ventricle.

HOW IS IT TREATED?

Once someone is diagnosed with stress cardiomyopathy, they usually spend two to three days in the hospital for observation. Many will develop no further signs of trouble and will go home without needing additional treatment. However, in studies, between 12% and 45% of hospitalized patients with stress cardiomyopathy develop acute heart failure, meaning that their hearts fail to pump enough blood through their bodies. When that happens, doctors prescribe these patients the same medications used for other heart-failure patients, such as beta-blockers, angiotensin-converting enzyme (ACE) inhibitors, and diuretics.

A smaller number of patients develop cardiogenic shock, the most severe form of heart failure. Their hearts pump so weakly that far

TAKE NOTE...

Cold, Snow and Your Heart: Are You at Risk?

Exposure to cold weather can increase your blood pressure while simultaneously constricting the arteries that feed the heart muscle, which are about the size of cooked spaghetti. In the presence of underlying heart disease, these superimposed factors can trigger a heart attack, heart rhythm irregularities, or sudden cardiac death.

Snow removal danger: We found that the people with the highest risk of cardiac complications during snow removal were older than age 45, had one or more major coronary risk factors, a history of heart problems (exertional chest pain, previous heart attack, bypass surgery, or coronary angioplasty), or had experienced symptoms that suggested a cardiac problem.

If you fit this description, don't take the risk: Paste a note to your snow shovel or electric snow thrower that reads, "Warning: Use of this instrument for snow removal may be hazardous to your health," and hire a snowplow service or neighbor to clear your driveway this winter.

Barry A. Franklin, PhD, director of preventive cardiology/cardiac rehabilitation at Beaumont Health in Royal Oak, Michigan. Dr. Franklin is a longstanding member of the *Bottom Line Health* advisory board. DrBarryFranklin.com

too little oxygen is delivered to the brain, kidneys, liver, and other organs, threatening permanent damage or death. This is the main cause of death for the 5% of patients who die from stress cardiomyopathy. Aggressive treatments, including the placement of a temporary device to help the heart pump, may be needed.

WHAT'S THE PROGNOSIS?

The good news is that 95% of patients will recover. Within two to three months, the enlarged part of the heart will return to its normal size and function. It is thought that this remodeling of the heart muscle is possible because the affected cells have been stunned, but not destroyed, by the onslaught of stress hormones. Some people will be advised to continue medications as their hearts heal, and some will suffer some lingering fatigue or other symptoms.

While survivors of broken heart syndrome can go on with their lives, they should know that they face some risk of recurrence, about 20% over 10 years, according to researchers. So, it's important to pay attention to suspicious symptoms and to always seek medical care for a possible cardiac emergency.

When Standing Is Unbearable

Cyndya Shibao MD, MSCI, FAHA, FAAS, associate professor, department of medicine, division of clinical pharmacology, Vanderbilt Autonomic Dysfunction Center, Vanderbilt University Medical Center, Nashville, Tennessee.

Like everything else, your blood is subject to the laws of gravity. When you stand up, gravity pulls blood into your abdomen and legs.

To counteract this effect, your leg muscles help pump blood back to the heart, which speeds up slightly with the help of a boost of adrenaline. A burst of norepinephrine constricts blood vessels to further guide blood

> The good news is that 95% of patients will recover. Within two to three months, the enlarged part of the heart will return to its normal size and function.

back to the heart and, in turn, the brain. If you've ever had a rush of dizziness when standing too quickly, you've experienced a momentary delay in this normally elegant system.

If you have postural orthostatic tachycardia syndrome (POTS), there's more than a delay: The mechanisms designed to avoid blood pooling into your abdomen and legs fail.

A FAULTY SYSTEM

The longer you stand, the more the blood pools. Your body still tries to correct the pooling by releasing norepinephrine and epinephrine, which cause your heart to beat faster, but the blood vessels don't constrict as they're supposed to. The pooled blood isn't returned to the heart, which creates a chain reaction where insufficient blood gets to the brain, causing symptoms such as lightheadedness, nausea, vomiting, dimmed vision, altered hearing, and fainting. The heart tries to compensate by beating faster, leading to an elevated heart rate (called *tachycardia*).

The reaction can be triggered by standing, sitting at a desk, standing in line, taking a shower, and seeing blood or gore. It can occur in people who overly restrict their salt intake or don't drink enough water—both of which help maintain healthy blood pressure by retaining fluid in blood vessels. Being overheated, scared, or anxious are triggering factors as well.

While there's not yet a cure for POTS, there are a variety of treatments and strategies that can minimize its effects on daily life.

DIETARY TIPS

Many people with POTS have low blood volume, which can often be rectified by increasing salt and fluid intake. At the Vanderbilt Autonomic Dysfunction Center, we recommend eating 6 to 9 grams of dietary salt and drinking 2 to 3 liters of water each day.

Follow a low-carbohydrate diet, and avoid large meals that divert blood flow to digestive organs. Small, frequent meals are a better option. It's also wise to avoid alcohol, which causes veins to dilate.

COMPRESSION CLOTHING

While the corsets of yore caused an epidemic of fainting spells, a modern take on abdominal compression can decrease blood pooling. Abdominal binders or back braces that can be loosened when sitting and then tightened when standing are good options. Waist-high compression stockings can also help if they have at least 30 to 40 millimeters of mercury of compression, but they can be both difficult to put on and uncomfortable to wear.

POSTURE AND MOVEMENT

When POTS symptoms strike, you may be able to move in ways that can help reduce blood pooling.

●**Stand on your toes,** cross your legs, or put one leg on a chair when standing.

●**Flex your leg and buttocks muscles.**

●**Sit in a low chair,** in a knee-chest position, or with your feet on a footstool.

●**Lean forward when sitting.**

●**Bend forward at the waist when walking** (such as when you're pushing a shopping cart).

●**Slightly elevate the head of your bed to retain fluid at night.**

●**If you feel faint,** grip one hand with the other and push your arms away while contracting your muscles for two minutes.

EXERCISE

While exercise can worsen POTS symptoms at first, a program that builds tolerance can yield dramatic benefits. Patients who could only tolerate a minute or two of activity have been able to build up to vigorous 45-minute workouts over time. The key is to start small and be patient.

Even if you are bedridden, you can start with simple exercises that can be done while reclining…

●**Put a pillow between your knees,** squeeze for 10 seconds, release, and repeat.

●**Repeat the same exercise with the pillow between your palms.**

●**Write your name in the air with your toes.** Over time, work on the whole alphabet.

●**Lie on your side,** lift your leg up sideways, and bring it back down without touching your legs together. Repeat.

●**Lie on your back,** lift your left leg up, and point your toe towards the ceiling. Switch legs and repeat.

●**Mildly stretch your whole body,** starting with your feet then moving to your legs, back, arms, and neck.

ADD CHALLENGE

For a more challenging workout, look to recumbent exercises, such as recumbent biking or rowing, that allow you to work harder without triggering the POTS response.

Swimming keeps you in a reclined position and builds strength in your legs, which itself can reduce orthostatic symptoms. Because the pressure from water helps prevent orthostatic symptoms, some people with POTS can even stand for lengthy periods in a pool.

Weight training increases strength and helps muscles more efficiently use oxygen and tolerate orthostatic stress. Start with light weights and use them in a reclined or seated position.

Tips to Avoid Triggers

●Shop at non-peak hours to avoid long lines.

●Take shorter showers and baths, and aim for a lower water temperature.

●Avoid saunas, hot tubs, and lying on a hot beach.

●Avoid standing still for prolonged periods in hot environments.

●Review all medications and supplements with your doctor or pharmacist to identify any that can worsen or cause POTS. *Niacin, codeine,* and *oxycodone* for example, can cause blood vessels to dilate and increase blood pooling upon standing. High doses of tricyclic antidepressants can also be intolerable for some people. Medications for ADHD or depression such as *atomoxetine* (Strattera) and *duloxetine* (Cymbalta) can worsen the tachycardia by increasing the release of norepinephrine.

—Dr. Cyndya Shibao

What to Eat for Good Heart Health

Dairy Fat Is Good for Your Heart

Higher dairy fat consumption correlated with lower rates of cardiovascular disease. The idea that fat reduces heart disease risk may seem counterintuitive, but our bodies don't treat all types of fat the same.

Best: Full-fat yogurt and cheese and whole milk…about three modest-sized servings per day.

Best to avoid: Butter fat.

Duane Mellor, PhD, a UK-registered dietitian and head of nutrition and evidence-based medicine at Aston Medical School in Birmingham, UK, commenting on a study published in *PLOS Medicine*.

Yogurt Helps Manage Blood Pressure

People with high blood pressure who ate a daily serving of yogurt had an average blood pressure reading seven points lower than people who never ate yogurt. Yogurt is high in calcium, magnesium and potassium—all of which help regulate blood pressure—and contains bacteria that produce proteins that have blood pressure–lowering effects.

Best: Yogurt that contains live cultures and is low in sugar.

Alexandra Wade, PhD, postdoctoral researcher at University of South Australia, Adelaide, and lead author of a study of 915 people, published in *International Dairy Journal*.

More Potassium—Not Less Sodium— Is Good for the Heart

In a review of studies examining the relationship between cardiovascular disease and the consumption of sodium and potassium, reducing sodium intake did not significantly lower risk for disease. Instead, increasing potassium consumption to achieve a lower ratio of potassium to sodium appeared key to improving outcomes.

Best food sources of potassium: Bananas, oranges, spinach, broccoli, potatoes and mushrooms.

Study by researchers at University of Porto, Portugal, published in *Nutrients*.

Focus on the muscles in your legs and abdomen. Lifting your arms over your head can aggravate symptoms.

As your fitness increases, you may be able to work up to upright activities like walking, jogging, or biking. Avoid outdoor exercise when it is hot, and always warm up and cool down. Taking the medication *propranolol* may improve your exercise capacity.

MEDICATIONS

If lifestyle strategies don't ease your symptoms, medications may help. Drugs like *fludrocortisone* and *midodrine* can increase blood volume and blood vessel contraction, which can help return blood to the heart. Beta-blockers such as *metoprolol* (Toprol-XL, Lopressor), *atenolol* (Tenormin), and propranolol (Inderal LA) can slow down the heart rate upon standing. If these medications fail, *verapamil* (Verelan, Calan SR) or *ivabradine* (Corlanor) can be added for additional heart rate control.

For patients who have symptoms such as flushing, excessive sweating, and jitters, medications such as *clonidine* (Catapres) and *guanfacine* (Intuniv) that reduce the release of or response to epinephrine and norepinephrine can help.

Exercise Could Make Up for Bad Sleep

Insufficient sleep, insomnia, snoring and daytime sleepiness increase risk for stroke, coronary heart disease and death.

Recent study: Getting the recommended amount of weekly physical activity (75 minutes vigorous/150 minutes moderate) offsets the serious health consequences of poor sleep.

Emmanuel Stamatakis, PhD, professor of physical activity and population health at University of Sydney, Australia, and leader of an 11-year study of 400,000 adults, published in *British Journal of Sports Medicine*.

Abnormal Blood Pressure During Sleep Boosts Heart Disease Risk

People whose blood pressure dropped or spiked abnormally during sleep were at significantly increased risk for cardiovascular disease events. Overnight systolic pressure (upper number) increases of 20 mmHg or more raised risk for heart disease and stroke by 18% and risk for heart failure by 25%. Blood pressure is normally about 10% to 20% lower during sleep…but overnight decreases greater than 20% were found to double risk for stroke. If you're concerned about your nighttime blood pressure level, ask your doctor about nocturnal monitoring and discuss strategies for managing blood pressure around the clock.

Kazuomi Kario, MD, professor of cardiovascular medicine, Jichi Medical University, Tochigi, Japan, and lead author of a seven-year study of 6,300 people published in *Circulation*.

Stroke: Act Fast from Onset to Rehab

Mark Tornero, MD, medical director of vascular rehabilitation at The Ohio State University Wexner Medical Center in Columbus, Ohio.

From the moment a stroke hits, the clock starts ticking, and there isn't a second to waste. Whether blood flow needs to be restored by dissolving a clot in an ischemic stroke, or a brain bleed from a hemorrhagic stroke needs to be halted, speed is the key to limiting the damage and providing the best long-term recovery.

If you recognize—or even suspect—signs of stroke in yourself or a loved one (see graphic on page 9), the most important thing you can do is immediately call an ambulance. People who take an ambulance get better care faster than those who have a family member drive them to the hospital. That care includes access

An Anti-Stroke Vaccine

Researchers reviewed more than 1 million medical records and found that people who received the first-generation shingles vaccine, zoster vaccine live (Zostavax), had a 10% to 20% lower risk of stroke. A newer vaccine, zoster vaccine recombinant, adjuvanted (Shingrix), may provide better stroke protection, as it's more effective against shingles (90% vs 50%). It's recommended for anyone over age 50, even those who have already had the Zostavax shot (which provides five years of protection) or who have already had shingles.

—Dr. Mark Tornero

to tissue plasminogen activator (tPA), a lifesaving drug that can immediately break up a clot, but only if administered within three hours of the onset of symptoms. As few as 15% of patients with ischemic stroke arrive at the hospital in time for this treatment—but those who do experience fewer poststroke impairments and better recoveries.

A growing number of cities have mobile stroke units—enhanced ambulances that are equipped to provide stroke diagnosis and care as soon as they arrive at the patient's home—saving even more precious time.

Quick tip: If you call for an ambulance from a cell phone, your address might not be available to the dispatcher like it would if you called from a landline. To make it available, register your cellphone now at Smart911.com.

A WHIRLWIND OF ACTIVITY

Once you arrive at the hospital, you'll be medically stabilized, but the race against time continues. Whether your stroke is minor or significant, the rehabilitation process will begin within just 24 to 48 hours. You may go to a rehabilitation unit in the hospital you are already in, a unit in a different hospital, a freestanding inpatient rehabilitation facility, or a skilled nursing facility. If you can care for yourself or have enough help to safely return home, you can take part in outpatient rehabilitation programs or, in some cases, receive your rehabilitation in your own home.

The setting you choose will depend upon your needs, your doctor's recommendations, your insurance, and your preferences. Carefully consider the technology available at different facilities. Generally, academic hospital programs will have the most up-to-date treatments and access to innovative technologies. The Ohio State University Wexner Medical Center, for example, has specialized walking and electrical stimulation equipment that smaller programs or community facilities may not be able to house or afford.

WHAT TO EXPECT

When you begin stroke rehabilitation, you'll first undergo a battery of evaluations and assessments by a variety of specialists to identify what you'll need to work on. Stroke can have wide-ranging effects on everything from memory to movement, so it's not uncommon to have a large team of health-care providers that includes a physical medicine and rehabilitation physician, a neurologist, a neurosurgeon, a neuropsychologist, a certified rehabilitation nurse, a physical therapist, an occupational therapist, a speech therapist, a respiratory therapist, a dietitian, and a rehabilitation engineer. Different team members will work on specific tasks.

For instance, if you have difficulty swallowing and cannot safely eat without the risk of choking, you'll work with a speech therapist to strengthen the muscles you use to swallow. If you're having trouble with things like bathing and grooming, an occupational therapist will teach you strategies to increase your independence while you rebuild your skills. Your team will also assess external factors such as your home environment, transportation concerns, social interactions, emotions, and coping skills. You're an active part of this process: Be sure to tell them about anything that you specifically want to focus on so they can include it in your care plan. Once you go home, you can expect several weekly sessions with

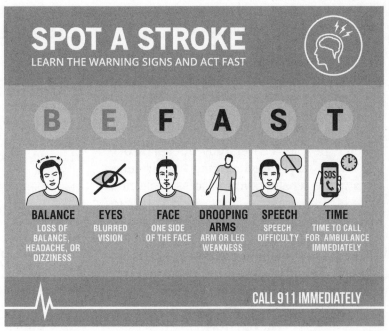

different therapists, and exercises to do on your off-days, too.

ENJOYABLE ACTIVITIES

Though stroke rehab involves lots of hard work and traditional exercise, you may be pleasantly surprised at how enjoyable some therapies can be. Activities involving art, video games, and virtual reality bring together multiple areas of the brain to perform complex activities, which can help augment core rehabilitative services.

Horseback riding has gotten a lot of attention for its healing benefits and can help with posture, muscle strengthening, and balance, but it requires a certain level of functioning, so if you're interested in that activity, ask your therapy team if it's appropriate for you.

YOUR RECOVERY TIMELINE

The complexity of the brain and the amount of damage you sustain during a stroke will factor into how well you recover and how long it takes.

The first three months after a stroke form the core foundation of your stroke rehabilitation program. That's when you'll see the quickest and most dramatic improvements. You might even experience spontaneous recovery of a lost skill or ability as your brain finds new ways to perform tasks.

After that, your recovery may slow, but you will continue to augment and expand your rehabilitation strategies to continue working on any lingering problems. You may continue to see improvements for up to a year or two after your stroke.

Some people recover fully after a stroke, but others may have lingering impairments. Even if the rehabilitation process can't eliminate all impairments, it can help you learn ways to cope and adapt to them. Even after your official rehabilitation program is finished, it's important to continue to do physical and cognitive exercises to enhance and sustain your functional levels.

FUTURE STROKE PREVENTION

Furthermore, the exercises and lifestyle strategies that you learn during rehab help lower the risk of having another stroke. (About 23% of stroke survivors have another.) Exercising, managing your blood pressure and cholesterol, eating a healthy diet, not smoking, and managing diabetes can all help lower your risk.

Antidepressants May Increase Stroke Risk

When researchers studied one million veterans with posttraumatic stress disorder, those who took a selective serotonin reuptake inhibitor (SSRI) were 45% more likely to suffer a hemorrhagic stroke. Interestingly, SSRIs were previously shown to reduce risk for ischemic stroke. Since this study concludes that serotonin-norepinephrine reuptake inhibitors (SNRIs) don't seem to carry the stroke risk, they may be a safer treatment.

Allison Gaffey, PhD, is a psychologist at Yale School of Medicine, New Haven, and VA Connecticut Healthcare System, West Haven, Connecticut, and leader of a study published in *Stroke*.

Clue That a Stroke Is Imminent

Cognitive function declines as much as 10 years before a stroke.

Recent finding: Compared with people who had not had strokes, stroke patients showed greater and faster decline in cognitive function and ability to handle activities of daily living over the previous 10 years. These may be early signs of the physiological changes that lead to stroke. Standard cognition tests may help identify those at higher stroke risk.

Alis Heshmatollah, MD, PhD candidate, is a neurology resident of Erasmus MC University Medical Center, Rotterdam, the Netherlands, and first author of a study published in *Journal of Neurology Neurosurgery & Psychiatry*.

Keeping Your Brain Sharp

Henry Mahncke, PhD, CEO of Posit Science, San Francisco, which created the Brain HQ brain-training program. Previously, he served as a science and technology advisor to the British government.

Brain fog. Senior moments. Alzheimer's disease. At nearly every stage of adult life, memory and cognition top the list of health concerns for Americans. Indeed, scientists have found that cognitive function, speed, and memory start to slowly decline at age 30.

Fortunately, researchers have good news, too: We can harness the power of neuroplasticity—the brain's ability to build new neural connections throughout the entire life span—to regain and even improve upon the mental sharpness of youth. Just as a muscle grows stronger with exercise, the brain grows stronger when challenged.

Try these three simple strategies to boost your brainpower at any age.

TRY NEW THINGS

Your brain isn't just designed to think: It's designed to learn. To fulfill its potential, it needs to encounter new challenges and novel experiences. Novelty can come in the form of taking a different route to work, or in trying a different role once you're there. It can mean learning a musical instrument or studying a new language. The idea is to do something that doesn't come easily so your brain will grow and develop new neural connections to meet the additional cognitive demand.

PLAY NEW GAMES

Crossword puzzles, sudoku, and games like poker, bridge, and chess all keep your mind busy, but it's really only when you're learning them that they change your brain. Once they become easy, you can add more challenge by seeking out more advanced puzzles or opponents, or start learning a new game to add to your repertoire.

TRAIN YOUR BRAIN

There are countless apps and computer programs that offer what's called brain games that are designed to challenge your memory and skill, but it's important to differentiate these from brain-training programs. Brain games are fun and stimulating, and you may become more adept at them the more you play, but they don't necessarily help you develop skills that translate to other tasks.

Brain-training programs can look a lot like brain games, but there's a key difference. Legitimate programs are developed by neuroscientists to improve on the building blocks of cognition in a way that yields real-world benefits. Brain-training has been used in neurorehabilitation programs to help people with brain injuries regain lost skills, but it's now also available to anyone with a phone or computer and a desire to improve daily cognitive abilities.

When scientists study cognitive function, they break it down into different domains that brain-training exercises can then target…

• **Processing speed** refers to how quickly your brain can make sense of information. For example, how quickly can you decipher a simple code?

• **Attention** refers to your ability to zero in on what you want to notice while also suppressing what you don't. Can you read this article while the radio is on in the background?

• **Executive function** is your ability to plan and organize.

• **Memory** refers to several things: Your working memory is the ability to keep information in mind in the moment, while short-term and long-term memory refer to storage and retrieval. In healthy people, these domains are all related—and all trainable.

If you practice a skill in a brain-training program and then see improvement in a similar cognitive task, it's called near transfer. For example, if you train with an exercise in which you have to remember a growing list of words and can then remember more words when your doctor tests your memory, your performance on test represents "near transfer" from the brain-training program.

UNEXPECTED BENEFITS

The more desirable—and more elusive—goal is called "far transfer." That means that the skill you learned in the game can lead to improvements in unrelated or real-world tasks.

• **Consider driving.** As we get older and our processing speed slows, our peripheral vision diminishes. This isn't a problem in the eyes: It's a change in how quickly and accurately the brain is processing information coming from the periphery. Because this is a processing issue, it's a trainable skill.

To improve it, neuroscientists at BrainHQ developed a game in which one image briefly appears in the center of the computer or phone screen while a second appears in the periphery. The player must answer questions about both of the items. Each time the player answers correctly, the exercise speeds up slightly, gently nudging the brain toward faster processing speeds. If it gets too fast and the player begins to make errors, the game slows down so the player can catch up. Over time, the training rewires how the brain processes information and provides real-world benefits: In a study of 2,800 adults, an independent team of researchers reported that people who trained with the exercise experienced a 48% reduction in at-fault car crashes.

• **Balance.** The briefest delay in transmitting visual data to the brain can mean the difference between quickly steadying oneself or experiencing an injurious tumble. After studying the effects of brain training on balance and walking in seniors, researchers from Chicago's Northwestern University and the University of Illinois Chicago suggested that improving visual speed and attention appear to improve walking speed and steadiness.

• **Hearing.** In many cases, the brain's auditory system no longer has the speed and accuracy needed to hear fast speech amidst noise. A large study at the Mayo Clinic found that using brain training to rewire the brain to make the auditory system faster and more accurate improved memory, too.

MULTIFACETED APPROACH

Brain training has been shown to improve cognitive performance in a growing body of research, but there's more you can do to enjoy a brain-healthy lifestyle. Exercising, eating a healthy diet, managing chronic health conditions, and maintaining social connections are all strongly linked to cognitive benefits.

Afternoon Naps May Boost Cognitive Ability

People over age 60 who regularly napped for five minutes to two hours after lunch scored significantly higher on tests of working memory, attention span, problem solving, verbal fluency and other cognitive measures than people who did not nap. It is possible that napping helps regulate the body's immune response, reducing the generalized inflammation that relates both to sleep disorders and cognitive decline.

Study of 2,214 residents of several large cities in China, all of whom averaged 6.5 hours of nighttime sleep, by researchers in Shanghai and elsewhere in China, published in *General Psychiatry*.

Alzheimer's Link to Early-Onset Diabetes

Type 2 diabetes at any age is associated with increased risk for Alzheimer's disease.

Recent finding: The earlier the onset, the greater the risk. For each five years earlier onset, risk for dementia increases by 24%. While association does not mean either condition causes the other, it is likely that an underlying condition is responsible for both...and new research reinforces the importance of diagnosing and treating type 2 diabetes as early as possible.

Study of more than 10,000 people, ages 35 to 55 at the start of the study, by researchers at Inserm, the French national health institute, published in *JAMA*.

You May Need More Than Lifestyle Changes to Beat Diabetes

There's no one-size-fits-all lifestyle approach for diabetes.

According to a recent study, intensive lifestyle intervention (diet and exercise) benefited most subgroups—but among those with poor glycemic control at the study start, intensive lifestyle intervention was associated with 85% higher risk for cardiovascular events. Ask your doctor about the best approach, which may include glucose-lowering drugs to improve cardiovascular risk factors and modest exercise when feasible.

Michael Bancks, PhD, assistant professor of epidemiology and prevention at Wake Forest School of Medicine, Winston-Salem, North Carolina, and leader of a 10-year study of 5,145 adults, published in Diabetes Care.

The Surprising Causes of Peripheral Neuropathy

Mary Vo, MD, an assistant professor of neurology and assistant attending neurologist at New York Presbyterian/Weill Cornell Medical College.

Diabetes isn't the only disease that can damage the nerves that lead to the hands and feet.

The pain arrives mainly at night: burning, tingling, or electric-shock stabbing that stymies sleep. Just covering your feet with a blanket can feel unbearable. If you get up in the dark, you may find yourself tripping or bumping into things, not because you can't see, but because you can't fully feel your feet. Creeping slowly from your toes upward over months or years, this pain and numbness, which can also affect your hands and arms, is perplexing and alarming.

The likely culprit? Peripheral neuropathy, which is damage to the peripheral nerves that reach throughout your body. While diabetes is the leading cause of this condition, peripheral neuropathy is surprising in both its origins and scope, with an extensive list of possible causes.

THE ROOT OF THE PROBLEM

Peripheral nerves, which carry messages to and from the brain, contain large fibers that are covered with a type of fatty insulation and small, skinny, uninsulated fibers. The small fibers report sensory information such as pain, heat, or cold, while also controlling involuntary vital functions, such as heart rate and blood pressure. The most common form of peripheral neuropathy strikes the longest nerves in the body, those leading to the skin of the hands and feet, where it can cause pain or numbness. *Small-fiber nerve damage can also trigger problems in other parts of the body...*

- **Low blood pressure** can lead to symptoms that include fainting, dizziness, or lingering fatigue.
- **Bloating, nausea, indigestion, constipation, or diarrhea** are often misdiagnosed as irritable bowel syndrome.
- **Incontinence or sexual problems,** while rare, are unquestionably distressing when they occur.
- **Heat intolerance may lead to excessive sweating,** or sufferers may lose the ability to sweat.

FINDING ANSWERS

As with many conditions, early diagnosis and treatment offer the best chance for effective symptom and damage control. But by the time many people with peripheral neuropathy seek a diagnosis, doctors find that the condition is actually worse than a patient's symptoms may suggest, so don't delay. Even if your symptoms seem vague, see your primary care doctor as soon as possible.

Your physician will review your medications and supplements, screen you for diabetes, thyroid issues and vitamin levels, and may perform a variety of tests to pinpoint peripheral neuropathy and its causes. These may include nerve conduction and electromyography to measure large-fiber damage, a skin biopsy to count small-nerve fiber endings in the skin, or a sweat test to gauge the body's ability to regulate temperature. A spinal tap may be used to examine spinal fluid for signs of infection or other dangerous conditions, while a tilt-table test may be used to monitor heart rate and blood pressure.

TAILORING TREATMENT

If your doctor can pinpoint the cause of your neuropathy, your treatment options can be tailored to address the underlying issue. For example, patients with autoimmune disease will be referred to a rheumatologist, who may prescribe immune-modifying treatments that can actually reverse nerve damage and symptoms. Diabetes patients should work with an endocrinologist to improve blood sugar control and monitor medications.

Recovery can be more challenging when peripheral neuropathy has no traceable cause, which is true in up to half of all cases. Even then, a variety of approaches can provide meaningful relief, though full nerve repair is typically elusive.

●**Medication.** Over-the-counter pain medications, such as nonsteroidal anti-inflammatory drugs, can relieve mild symptoms, as can topical treatments such as capsaicin cream.

When these aren't sufficient, there are several types of drugs to try. Some patients find relief with anti-epilepsy drugs like *gabapentin* (Gralise, Neurontin, Horizant) and *pregabalin* (Lyrica) or antidepressants like *duloxetine* (Cymbalta) and *venlafaxine* (Effexor XR). The antidepressants *amitriptyline*, *doxepin* (Silenor, Zonalon) and *nortriptyline* (Pamelor) may also help, as they interfere with the chemical processes in your brain and spinal cord that cause you to feel pain.

●**Physical and occupational therapy** can help you cope with limitations in how you walk or use your hands.

LIFESTYLE FACTORS

Some simple lifestyle changes can also improve your symptom…

●**Exercise regularly to improve blood flow to nerves.**

●**If you have diabetes, limit your sugar intake.**

●**Vitamin B12 protects nerves and may even enhance nerve regeneration.** Ensure that you get enough by eating foods like dairy, lean meat, poultry, and eggs. If you are vegetarian or vegan, talk to your doctor about taking a supplement.

●**Avoid eating fish that are high in mercury,** a toxin that can worsen neuropathy. The worst offenders are king mackerel, orange roughy, swordfish, tuna, and grouper.

●**Limit alcohol,** which is toxic to nerves and can make neuropathy symptoms worse.

●**Don't smoke.** Smoking narrows and damages peripheral blood vessels.

●**Review your medications regularly with your primary care doctor.** A variety of medications can cause reversible peripheral neuropathy—even long after you've been taking them with no problems.

Disorders of the Gut-Brain Axis

Douglas A. Drossman, MD, president emeritus and chief operating officer, Rome Foundation, Raleigh, North Carolina, professor emeritus of medicine and psychiatry, University of North Carolina at Chapel Hill; President, Center for Education and Practice of Biopsychosocial Care (DrossmanCare) and Drossman Gastroenterology; and Johannah Ruddy, MEd, executive director of the Rome Foundation and secretary-treasurer of DrossmanCare. Dr. Drossman and Ms. Ruddy are co-authors of *Gut Feelings: Disorders of Gut-Brain Interaction and the Patient-Doctor Relationship*.

If you've ever gotten diarrhea from being nervous or felt excessively anxious after a stomach bug, you've experienced a gut-brain interaction.

The brain and gut are hardwired to maintain constant communication with each other. That means that when things go awry, they can each wreak havoc on the other, causing what's called disorders of gut-brain interaction (DGBI).

SYMPTOM DIVERSITY

DGBIs, formerly called functional gastrointestinal (GI) disorders, can cause anything from difficulty swallowing to lack of control over bowel movements. The most well-known DGBI is irritable bowel syndrome, which causes pain, bloating, diarrhea or constipation, and a high risk of depression or anxiety.

These disorders don't come from structural diseases: They're not visible on an X-ray or endoscopy or identifiable in a blood test. *Rather, they relate to abnormal functioning of the GI system caused by one or more of five elements…*

●**Abnormal movement inside the bowels** (motility disturbance)

●**More intense abdominal pain than usual in response to stimuli** (visceral hypersensitivity)

●**Changes to the bowel's mucous membrane and immune response**

●**Changes to the normal microbes found in a healthy gut** (gut dysbiosis)

●**Changes in how the brain processes pain and other GI symptoms.**

Because of the communication along the gut-brain axis, the pain, nausea, or vomiting that can come from these dysfunctions can directly cause anxiety or depression. In turn, emotional distress can affect motility, causing diarrhea or nausea, and even change the way we perceive pain.

PAIN AND THE BRAIN

To understand how stress and emotions affect pain, envision a walkway with a gate. Pain signals from the gut have to pass through the gate on their way to the brain. At the same time, the brain acts as a gatekeeper, sending signals that determine how far the gate will open—and how much pain you will feel. For example, if you're running a race and sprain your ankle, the brain could send norepinephrine (similar to adrenaline) to slam the gate shut and block the pain signals. Emotional distress has the opposite effect: It causes the brain to throw the gate wide open, allowing a flood of pain signals to rush through.

When you experience gut pain, nerves in the spinal cord amplify the signals, making the same pain feel worse. That produces emotional distress, which further lowers the pain threshold, creating a vicious circle that creates hypersensitivity in both the gut and the brain, sometimes transforming acute pain into a chronic condition.

Brain scans show that chronic pain and chronic and severe stress can cause the deterioration of brain cells (neurodegeneration) in the brain's pain center, the anterior cingulate cortex. Fewer cells in that area make it harder to control pain. Fortunately, this process is reversible. Physical and mental activity, yoga, meditation, and medications called neuromodulators can promote regrowth of those cells (neurogenesis), and reduce GI pain.

TREATMENT APPROACHES

DGBI can be harder to diagnose than illnesses that show up on diagnostic tests, so if you suspect you may have one, such as irritable bowel syndrome or fecal incontinence, do a little homework before seeing your physician. Keep a diary of your symptoms. Record the time, severity, and presence of associated factors. If you identify triggers, such as specific foods—alcohol, caffeine, lactose, and fatty foods are common culprits—eliminate them from your diet. Share the diary with your doctor to help guide a treatment plan.

He or she may recommend medications that address specific symptoms, such as diarrhea or pain, and may prescribe neuromodulators like *amitriptyline*, *nortriptyline* (Pamelor), *desipramine* (Norpramin), and *duloxetine* (Cymbalta). You might recognize some of these drugs as antidepressants, but that doesn't mean that DGBIs are in your head. Just like aspirin can prevent a heart attack and tackle pain, neuromodulators have more than one function: They can treat pain, lessen emotional distress, and promote nerve-cell growth. When it comes to DGBIs, that's a particularly powerful combination. Brain-gut behavioral treatments, such as cognitive behavioral therapy, relaxation, hypnosis, and mindfulness can reduce anxiety levels, encourage health-promoting behaviors, and potentially improve pain tolerance.

TEAM UP WITH YOUR DOCTOR

The cornerstone of all of this, however, is the patient-doctor relationship. Disorders of gut-brain interaction are complicated and often chronic illnesses, so it's important to have a doctor who will be a trusted partner. You'll be working together to customize a treatment plan that works best for you. That means you need to know how each treatment works, what side effects are expected, how effective it's expected to be, and how long it will take. Be honest with your physician about any questions or concerns that you have. A doctor who is a good partner will answer your questions and pay attention to your experiences.

You might not have that experience with the first doctor that you see. DGBI can be frustrating for doctors who like to deal with concrete test results and clear answers.

If the doctor suggests that stress is entirely the problem and that you need to live with it or see a psychologist instead of a medical doctor, you may need to move on to a physician with a better understanding of DGBIs.

A neurogastroenterology pain treatment center can provide a multidisciplinary approach that addresses pain management, coping skills, and overall well-being. A comprehensive listing can be found in *Gut Feelings* at https://romedross.video/GutFeelingsWebsite.

Overcome Fatty Liver Disease

Arun J. Sanyal, MD, a professor in the division of gastroenterology, hepatology, and nutrition at the Virginia Commonwealth University School of Medicine, current chair of the Liver Study Section at the National Institutes of Health.

The liver is a three-pound, rubbery organ that sits on the right side of your abdomen, below the diaphragm and above the stomach, and it's a multitasker.

It filters blood; manufactures proteins, including those that help clot the blood; detoxifies chemicals and drugs; stores and regulates cellular fuel; produces the bile that helps digest fat; metabolizes and stores several nutrients, like iron and vitamin D; and helps respond to and destroy viruses and other germs. In other words, the liver is crucial to your health and well-being. But a lot of our livers aren't doing very well.

An astounding one out of every three Americans—more than 80 million people—have a fatty liver: Their liver cells are filled with excess fat, in the form of triglycerides. Most people with fatty liver have a relatively innocuous form that doctors call nonalcoholic fatty liver (NAFL), but about 20% to 25% have a more active form of the disease called nonalcoholic steatohepatitis (NASH). Together, they are called nonalcoholic fatty liver disease (NAFLD).

HIGH-RISK NASH

In NASH, fat-engorged liver cells weaken, balloon, and die in greater numbers than normal, leaving the liver inflamed and scarred (a condition called fibrosis). NASH increases your risk of colon cancer and death from a heart attack, heart failure, or stroke. It doubles the risk of liver cancer, and it can lead to cirrhosis, or extensive and life-threatening scarring of the liver. NASH is the fastest-growing cause of cirrhosis-related liver transplants.

And the situation is only getting worse. Research shows that by the end of this decade, more than 100 million Americans will develop NAFLD, with the number of deaths from NAFLD expected to double.

Here is perhaps the most daunting statistic of all: Nine out of 10 people who have NAFLD don't know they have the problem, because it doesn't usually cause symptoms.

RISK FACTORS

Here's how to determine if you're at risk for NAFLD and what to do about it.

• **You're more likely to have NAFLD if you are overweight or obese,** have high blood pressure, and/or have type 2 diabetes. If you have all three of those risk factors, the odds are 75% that you have NASH.

• **If you have any or all of the three main risk factors for NAFLD,** talk to your primary care physician about monitoring the health of your liver. An easy way to do that is with a measurement called Fibrosis-4, or FIB4. This uses two blood tests: a liver panel, which measures liver enzymes, and a platelet count, which is part of a standard blood test called a complete blood count (CBC) test. A formula using two liver enzymes, platelet count, and your age produces a measurement that correlates to the amount of fibrosis in the liver. (Your doctor can find a FIB4 calculator at HepatitisC.uw.edu/page/clinical-calculators/fib-4.)

• **If your score is 1.3 or lower,** there is a low probability that you have liver scarring.

• **If your score is between 1.4 and 2.5,** you may want to see a hepatologist for additional testing to determine your risk of cirrhosis, such as a special ultrasound test of your liver called Fibroscan.

• **If your score is 2.6 or higher,** there is a high probability that you have significant scarring. You should see a liver specialist (hepatologist) to determine your treatment options, with the goal of preventing cirrhosis or diagnosing cirrhosis that may already be present.

The FIB-4 test should be repeated every year. An increasing score is a strong indication that the condition of your liver is worsening and treatment is needed.

WEIGHT LOSS

The first and most important lifestyle treatment is decreasing fat in the liver—in other words, losing weight.

But you don't have to lose a lot of weight: Losing just 5% to 10% of your total body weight will generate dramatic improvement in your risk for NAFLD. For example, if you weigh 200 pounds, losing 10 pounds is significant.

Don't try to lose it all at once. First, stop weight gain, and then start to lose weight at a reasonable, achievable pace of about one pound per month. *The best way to lose weight is also the simplest…*

•**Generate a mildly negative caloric balance so you burn more calories than you consume.**

•**Limit your intake of refined carbohydrates** (such as white flour and white sugar) and other processed foods, and favor whole foods, such as lean meat, fish, low-fat dairy products, fruits, vegetables, beans, whole grains, nuts, and seeds.

•**Limit your consumption of high-fructose corn syrup,** a sweetener that has been linked to liver inflammation and fibrosis.

•**Increase your intake of omega-3 fatty acids,** which are found in fatty fish such as salmon and sardines.

•**Drink more coffee,** which may protect against fibrosis.

IMPROVE FITNESS

Any type of aerobic exercise is good for reducing the level of triglycerides in the liver. Walk, bicycle, swim, dance, or do any activity that makes your heart beat faster for 30 minutes at least five days a week. Regular resistance exercise and/or high-intensity intermittent training are also effective. Talk to your doctor before starting an exercise program.

MEDICAL TREATMENTS

There are several medications for NASH in clinical trials—such as obeticholic acid, which reduces inflammation and balances blood sugar—but none have yet been approved by the U.S. Food and Drug Administration.

In the interim, some physicians treat NASH with off-label (not FDA approved) medications.

They include the diabetes drug *pioglitazone* (Actos), which improves insulin resistance, and the weight loss drug *semaglutide* (Ozempic). There is also evidence that high-dose vitamin E (800 international units daily)—a prescriptive dose that should be used only with the approval and supervision of a physician—may help control NASH. The American Association for the Study of Liver Disease recommends both pioglitazone and vitamin E for most people with proven NASH.

Bariatric surgery for weight loss is also an important consideration for people with obesity. In one study, NASH was completely resolved in 84% of those who had the surgery. However, 10% to 20% of those who undergo bariatric surgery suffer from complications, such as abdominal hernia, nausea, heartburn, gallstones, and nutritional deficiencies.

Daily Aspirin Fights Inherited Bowel Cancer

People with a hereditary condition called Lynch syndrome are at high risk for colon cancer.

Recent finding: Lynch syndrome patients who took two full-strength aspirin a day for two years were 50% less likely to develop colon cancer over a decade than those who did not take aspirin. Lynch syndrome affects about one out of 200 people. Talk to your doctor if you have Lynch syndrome or any strong family history of cancer—the benefits of aspirin may outweigh the known risks.

Five-year study of 861 Lynch syndrome patients in 16 countries by researchers at Newcastle University, UK, published in *The Lancet*.

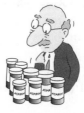

Is That Spot Dangerous?

Carolyn I. Jacob, MD, a board-certified dermatologist and founder and medical director of Chicago Cosmetic Surgery and Dermatology.

Skin irregularities can be harmless or a sign of something serious. Here's how to know the difference.

Some of us age with subtle, gradual, changes in our complexions, while others show dramatic effects from a lifetime of sun exposure and other influences. But, at some point, most of us encounter unexpected bumps and spots.

So how do you know which skin spots are harmless and which should concern you enough to check in with a doctor? Here's a quick guide to help you know.

URGENT ISSUES

The most important reason to pay attention to the marks on your skin is to detect the earliest signs of melanoma, a cancer that can develop in the cells that give skin its color. Melanoma is less common than other types of skin cancer, but more likely to spread to other parts of the body. Risk factors include having many moles, many unusual moles (large or oddly shaped), a family history of melanoma, or fair skin, though darker-skinned people can get it too. Exposure to the sun and tanning beds raises the risk, but melanomas can also grow on skin that doesn't get much exposure, such as the soles of the feet. Some melanomas develop from existing moles, while others arise as new growths.

Here are the signs that should prompt an immediate visit to a dermatologist…

• **Asymmetry.** If you draw an imaginary line down the middle of the spot, do the two sides look the same or different? Melanomas may look different on each side.

• **Border.** A melanoma may have an irregular, scalloped, or poorly defined border.

• **Color.** A melanoma may have a mixture of colors, such as tan, brown and black, or even red, white, and blue.

• **Diameter.** Typical melanomas are larger than a pencil eraser, about 6 millimeters, when diagnosed.

• **Evolving.** The most concerning sign may be if a spot on your skin is getting bigger, changing color or shape, rising up from the skin, or looking different from anything else on your skin.

A melanoma doesn't have to show all of these attributes. In some cases, it may show just one, such as rapid growth. If you have a new mole or even a bump that looks like a pimple that keeps growing, visit the dermatologist. When melanoma is caught early, the survival rates are excellent, but they drop precipitously if it spreads to other parts of the body.

LOWER-RISK SPOTS

The most common forms of skin cancer are basal and squamous cell carcinomas. They are rarely life-threatening, but they can be disfiguring, so a doctor's visit is in order if you have a spot that sounds like those described below. Anyone can develop these cancers, but they are most common in people with fair skin who have spent a lot of time in the sun.

• **Basal cell carcinomas** most often appear the face, ears, and hands. They can look like pearly, shiny bumps with tiny blood vessels. They can be the same color as your skin or a little reddish and may have a dip in the middle. They can look like a pimple, a minor injury, or a wound that won't heal. They can have a waxy, scar-like appearance. They may bleed, ooze, become scaly, or start to itch.

• **Squamous cell carcinomas** most commonly appear on the face, scalp, lips, and hands, but they can also appear in the mouth, under a nail, or even inside the anus.

The earliest sign of what could become a squamous cell carcinoma is a lesion called an actinic keratosis. Usually appearing in people ages 40 or older, these are often dry, scaly pink or red patches, but they also can be brown or white. They may feel rough, sensitive, painful, itchy, prickly, and burning. They may look and feel inflamed, and they may come and go in the same location. Left untreated, these lesions can progress to squamous cell carcinoma. They may then become a raised, red bump, or even stick out like a small horn. These skin spots are highly treatable, but shouldn't be ignored.

BENIGN SPOTS

There are many benign causes of spots, lumps, and bumps that can appear—especially as we get older…

• **Acrochordons (skin tags) tend to grow in areas where there are skin folds.** They are harmless and do not require removal, but your dermatologist can take them off if they are bothersome.

• **Warts are caused by the human papilloma virus, and they can take many forms.** They may be flat, cauliflower-shaped, or have finger-like projections. You can treat them at home with over-the-counter salicylic acid. If that fails, see your dermatologist for other options, such as laser therapy or cryotherapy.

• **Cherry angiomas.** These are small, bright red spots that are flat or slightly raised and typically appear on the trunk and extremities. They can be as small as a pinpoint and as large as a quarter inch in diameter. They most often grow on the arms, legs, or trunk, and are considered harmless.

• **Age spots (also known as lentigines).** These flat, oval spots are tan to dark brown. You are most likely to notice them on skin that has had heavy sun exposure, such as the back of your hands, shoulders and face. They can be lightened with creams and lotions or treated with lasers or chemical peels.

While these are all examples of benign conditions, when in doubt, check it out.

New Cell-Phone Health Risks

Devra Lee Davis, PhD, MPH, founder and president of Environmental Health Trust in Teton Village, Wyoming. She is author of *Disconnect: The Truth About Cell Phone Radiation, What the Industry Is Doing to Hide It, and How to Protect Your Family.* EHTrust.org

While the coming of 5G cellular service sounds exciting, the health risks of this fifth-generation wireless technology and the radiation it emits are concerning. Cell-phone companies warn shareholders that they may be sued for cancer and other health impacts from 5G and other wireless devices, while at the same time aggressively marketing these same devices to consumers.

Talking about the risks of cell-phone radiation is not new. But 5G and wireless dramatically increase the risk. These new networks rely on 4G connections and use the same wireless frequencies we have now but with new, higher frequencies. More than a million new "short" cell towers are being built, bringing microwave-radiating antennas closer than ever before and more than tripling exposure. You have no say at all about antenna location—one could be right outside your bedroom wall! And you're at risk of exposure whether or not you have a 5G phone.

One of the most ironic things about 5G is that it actually doesn't improve reception for voice calls. What it does do is create a new, faster way for wireless devices to communicate with one another, such as in a smart home. It also boosts download speeds for data, movies and video games.

HOW TO REDUCE YOUR EXPOSURE

To protect yourself and your family from radiation associated with 5G, 4G, and 3G, follow these guidelines. *These steps are more important than ever…*

• **Don't carry your cell-phone in your pocket,** bra or against your body unless it is turned off.

• **When you are not using the phone,** power it off or set it to Airplane/Flight mode. Also turn off Wi-Fi and Bluetooth.

• **When talking on the cell phone,** use speaker mode or a plug-in earpiece to keep your the phone away from your brain and body. Or, even better, send texts rather than make voice calls.

• **Don't use your cell phone when you have only one or two bars or when you are between cell towers.** A cell phone sends signals to a tower up to 900 times a minute, and each time, some of that radiation is absorbed into your body.

• **Don't sleep with your cell phone nearby.** If you use your phone as an alarm, set it to Airplane/Flight mode and turn off Wi-Fi and Bluetooth before putting it on your nightstand.

Better: Purchase a battery-powered alarm clock (plug-in digital clocks can emit EMF radiation).

• **Keep your corded-phone landline,** which is free of wireless radiation and works in an emergency. Cordless home phones emit the same type of radiation as cell towers.

• **Use a wired mouse, keyboard and printer** to avoid unnecessary radiation, and don't buy smart-home wireless devices.

• **Get engaged in your community and at the state and federal levels** to prevent cell-phone towers from being built near your home and schools.

• **Hang onto your non-5G phone as long as possible.** Newer phones usually have more antennas, and you can't always turn them off.

Vitamin B-3 (Niacin) Protects Against UV Exposure

In the lab, treating skin cells with vitamin B-3 before exposing them to ultraviolet light protected them from DNA damage caused by direct sunlight, the main risk factor for non-melanoma skin cancers. Niacin from food is not protective. Take a supplement (500 mg to 1 g) prior to sun exposure. People with a history of non-melanoma skin cancer should take B-3 daily.

Lara Camillo, PhD, and Paola Savoia, MD, PhD, University of Eastern Piedmont, Novara, Italy, are leaders of a study presented at the European Academy of Dermatology and Venereology Congress.

Unexposed Skin Still Can Be Damaged by the Sun

Genetic mutations to the skin can be caused by the body's own processes over time, as well as by exposure to UV light. When researchers compared the roles of those

different causes of skin changes in 21 adults, they took samples from the volunteers' hips, reasoning that skin in that area was unlikely to have been exposed to much direct sunlight. Still, they found that UV-related changes to skin cells were common even in sun-shielded tissue.

Study by researchers at National Institute of Environmental Health Sciences, Research Triangle Park, North Carolina, published in *PLOS Genetics*.

Smoking Marijuana Damages Lungs

Recent finding: The more marijuana someone smokes—and the longer he/she smokes it—the more likely he will develop a particular type of lung damage. The lungs will have to expand more to supply the body with enough oxygen (lung hyperinflation) and will perform less efficiently.

Warning: Quitting stops the damage from getting worse, but it is cumulative—and may be permanent.

Robert Hancox, MD, research professor of respiratory epidemiology at University of Otago, Dunedin, New Zealand, and lead author of a study of 1,000 people published in *American Journal of Respiratory and Critical Care Medicine*.

TAKE NOTE...

Another Reason Not to Vape

Vaping causes brain fog. Two new studies involving nearly one million students and adults point to an association between vaping and difficulty concentrating. Both smokers and vapers are more likely to report mental fog, and kids who start vaping before age 14 are more likely than their peers to struggle with concentrating, recall and making decisions.

Studies by researchers at University of Rochester Medical Center, New York, published in *Tobacco Induced Diseases* and *PLOS One*.

2

Medical Matters

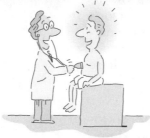

Telehealth Transformation

Before the pandemic, seeing a doctor meant being limited to health-care providers in a drivable distance, trudging to the office, and sitting for up to an hour in a germy waiting room—even after you were told to arrive 15 minutes early. But the widespread acceptance of telehealth—the use of telecommunication technologies and electronic information to deliver care—has changed everything.

With telehealth, you receive care from home, appointments are usually on time, and you can see a provider from anywhere in the country if you live in a state that has waived in-state doctor requirements. That's because the federal government responded to the overwhelming need for care and a shortage of health-care providers in any given place by easing restrictions on telehealth and providing more money for the visits.

FROM ACUTE TO CHRONIC CARE

In the simplest form of the technology, you can use a phone or computer to have a doctor's visit using a platform such as Zoom. These programs are easy to use, and most doctors' offices will walk you through getting set up. You and the doctor can see each other during the visit.

A growing number of health-care providers are going a step further and using technology to better monitor chronic health conditions to keep you well and out of the hospital. At home, you can use tools such as wireless blood pressure cuffs, pulse oximeters, and scales, a glucometer, and wearables such as Fitbits or Apple Watches to gather data and up-

David Wilcox DNP, MHA, BSN, RN-BC, LSSBB, the author of *How to Avoid Being a Victim of the American Healthcare System: A Patient's Handbook for Survival.* Dr. Wilcox has a doctorate in nurse executive leadership with a focus on using technology to improve patient care.

load it into software and services that run on the Internet (the Cloud). Your doctor's office can then monitor that data manually or with the use of artificial intelligence. When a nurse navigator (a nurse who serves as a liaison between you and your doctor) sees a trend that could suggest worsening symptoms, he or she can intervene before those symptoms become a full-blown problem.

Consider a patient with congestive heart failure (CHF). When CHF worsens, patients may have a sudden weight gain in a short time and have shortness of breath that leads to walking less due to increased retention of fluid. If a wireless scale detects a 5-pound weight gain in a few days, a pulse oximeter shows low oxygen levels, and a Fitbit shows that a person's steps have dropped dramatically, a nurse navigator can set up a telehealth appointment for the patient with the doctor to address those concerns before they worsen.

HOSPITAL AT HOME

Telehealth isn't limited to routine doctor visits: It's affecting hospitalization too. Hospital-at-home can make any room in your house into a hospital room complete with oxygen tanks, medical supplies, and almost anything else you may need. Many of these programs are linked to a 24/7 monitoring system to monitor your vital signs and other pertinent health-care data in real time. Your health-care team can go over your data and communicate with you remotely and send a nurse when you need one. Plus, you'll have a button you can press at any time for emergency help.

For people with lower-level health issues, this is the perfect combination of technology and clinical care in which patients can derive the benefit of staying at home while their chronic care is being managed or they are recovering from an illness. Patients sleep better in a quiet home, fall less often, are more mobile, and can eat whatever they want. And studies are showing that patients recover just as well at home as in the hospital.

TELEHEALTH CONSIDERATIONS

The technology that doctors are using is streamlined and quick to learn and use—even for people who don't consider themselves to

Technology and Medication

For Americans ages 65 and older, 33% to 69% of hospital admissions are due to patients not taking their medications. Another 40% of nursing home admissions occur because Americans are unable to reliably self-medicate at home. With one in four people over 65 living alone, telehealth solutions could allow them to live independently longer. If a home health nurse visits a patient once a week and loads their medication-monitoring device with a week's worth of their medications, the system can notify the patient when to take their medication by several means. It could be an alarm, text message or if the device is interfaced into Google mini or Alexa, it could be delivered verbally. These systems are also capable of alerting the home health agency, a relative, or the doctor's office when the patient doesn't take their medications.

Excerpted from *How to Avoid Being a Victim of the American Healthcare System: A Patient's Handbook for Survival.*

be tech-savvy. But access isn't equally available to everyone. People in rural areas may not have the broadband internet access that is necessary for video. A telephone call may be adequate in some cases, but not all. As such, in October 2020, the Federal Communications Commission introduced a $20 billion fund to improve broadband access in rural America.

A NEW MODEL OF CARE

Telehealth will play a key role in the transformation from fee-for-service health care (where doctors are paid according to how many tests and procedures they perform) to value-based care (where doctors earn more by keeping patients healthy and out of the hospital). Value-based care is provided by groups of health-care providers called accountable care organizations (ACO). In the model, a health-care team is paid a set amount of money for each person they treat—no matter what care that person needs.

If the group spends less than they've been given for a patient, they get to keep the difference. The best way for these groups to save money on a patient's care is to keep them healthy and out of the hospital. Technology makes it easier for patients and providers alike to stay in touch and on top of chronic health conditions, reducing the likelihood of hospitalization.

Find the Doctor Who's Right for You

R. Ruth Linden, PhD, founder and president of Tree of Life Health Advocates, where she helps clients with serious illnesses navigate the health-care system. TreeOfLifeHealthAdvocates.com

---

Finding the right primary care physician or specialist may not be easy. In fact, it's likely to be extremely difficult. The best primary care doctors often have full practices, and they may not be taking new patients. A growing number of physicians accept only direct payment, not insurance. Among those who do take insurance, you have to find one who is in your network. And then you need to find one that you both like and trust.

SMART TIPS FOR FINDING THE RIGHT DOCTOR

Taking a step-by-step approach can help you work through these challenges to find the best partner in your care.

•**Identify candidates.** Start by asking your family and friends for recommendations. Try the app Nextdoor, which offers local recommendations for a range of services. If several people on the app say they love a doctor in town, there's a higher probability that he or she is a gem. Yelp also may give you useful info, but negative reviews based on experiences such as an encounter with a surly receptionist or parking challenges may have nothing to do with the quality of the doctor's care.

•**Set up consultations.** Once you've identified doctors you want to consider, call and request a new patient consultation. The front desk staff can verify if your insurance is accepted. If so, it should cover the cost of the visit, minus the copay for which you are responsible. But don't go to the consultation thinking you'll sit in the doctor's office and interview the doctor. Rather, go to the visit with a specific problem or process, such as a concerning symptom or a refill of a prescription. Most new patient consultations last about 45 minutes, so you'll have plenty of time to see how the doctor interacts with you.

•**Ask questions.** During the visit, ask the doctor at least one specific question. Any question will likely elicit more than the response to the question itself. Because the doctor doesn't know the question in advance, you'll get a sense of how well he or she responds to the unexpected—whether they're reassuring and humorous (good) or defensive and snarky (bad).

WHAT TO LOOK FOR

The two most important elements in the doctor-patient relationship are good communication and trust. If good communication is missing, you may withhold information that is critical in formulating an effective treatment plan. If trust is missing, you may not adhere to your doctor's recommendations, or you might habitually cancel appointments.

But trust isn't always obvious. It's a feeling created by actions, not words, based on how your doctor engages with you. Signs of trustworthiness include being authentic and demonstrating integrity, compassion, kindness, and humility. Another factor that contributes to trust may be "cultural concordance." For example, you may feel more trust in a doctor who shares your gender or cultural identity, or—for non-English speakers—is fluent in your native language.

YOUR CONCERNS MATTER

Another important factor is the doctor's ability to convey that he or she takes your concerns seriously. That is, if you bring a problem to the doctor and he or she says something like, "I wouldn't worry about it," without further explanation, find another doctor. Any doctor who is unwilling to order a test to rule out a serious problem that concerns you is not the right doctor for you. Rather, the doctor might say something reassuring and respectful like, "I don't think this is anything to worry about, but I can see how concerned you are. Let's explore this further."

COMPETENCE

You want to feel confident in your doctor's level of competency, which means you want an expert diagnostician who is well-informed about the latest evidence-based treatments. But the right doctor is also willing to say, "I don't know but I will find the answer to your question and message you by the end of the week." You can't expect your doctor to know everything, but it's important that he or she honestly tells you when more digging is needed.

KNOW YOUR CRITERIA

You should also know your specific criteria. For example, maybe you tend to be anxious during a doctor visit and think of questions only once you get home. Is the physician available for post-visit calls? Does the practice offer an online portal where you can send questions or request refills?

POST-VISIT EVALUATION

After the visit, evaluate whether or not the doctor is someone you'd like to work with. *The best way to do that is to ask yourself the following questions…*

• **Did I feel listened to?**

• **Did I feel like I could trust the doctor with my body and my life?**

• **Did I get all of my questions answered?**

• **Did the doctor's recommendations make sense to me?**

• **Did I feel like the doctor gave me enough time?**

• **Did the doctor say anything that rubbed me the wrong way or put me off?**

If you answered yes to those questions (except for the last one, where the right answer is no), you have likely found a doctor who is right for you. If you feel relieved of anxiety and confident about the future—trust your instincts. On the other hand, if you don't feel right about the doctor, keep looking.

First Visit with a New Doctor? How to Make the Most of It

Tziporah E. Rosenberg, PhD, LMFT, associate professor in the departments of psychiatry and family medicine at University of Rochester Medical Center, Rochester, New York, director of the Institute for the Family's Strong Family Therapy Services, and physicians' coach in the Medical Center's Patient- and Family-Centered Care Coaching Program.

It's an uncomfortable reality—at some point, or even many points, in your lifetime, you will have to start a relationship with a new health-care provider. Perhaps your primary care doctor retires, or a health condition makes it necessary for you to see a specialist. *The prospect may fill you with anxiety, but there are key steps to help you make the most of that first visit…*

CALL MY OFFICE

Gone are the days when you could talk to a new doctor in advance by phone to get a sense of his style. But you still can call a doctor's office and ask the receptionist or office manager questions that can help set your expectations. Some offices have specific staff devoted to helping new patients become established. *Questions to ask…*

• **What is the protocol for urgent needs, and how does it differ during and after business hours?**

Also: How long might you typically wait for a call back? And how will you know whether you need to go to urgent care or the ER?

• **What is the doctor's preferred style for communication between visits—e-mails or phone calls?**

• **Can a loved one accompany you to office visits?**

• **Does the doctor tend to run on time or late for patient appointments?** Many people develop preconceived notions about a doctor based on the amount of time spent in the waiting room and then are agitated when they get into the exam room or office. What matters most is the experience you have when you're in the room with your provider and his/her presence and focus on you.

Note: If the office staff is too rushed to take the time to address your questions, that could reflect on the doctor and/or the pace of the practice.

DEFINE YOUR AGENDA

You won't know until you're in the exam room if a new provider relationship is going to work, and even then, you might not know right away. But keep in mind two things about every practitioner—a doctor isn't a mind reader, and he probably has an agenda for how he conducts office visits. *What to do to get the most out of your first office visit…*

• **Bring a list of three things that you need to get done.** Your agenda and your doctor's agenda might be different, but you can agree on what will be accomplished during the appointment. You can start off by saying something as simple as, "These are the things I am hoping we can accomplish today." The best scenario is that the practitioner will respond with what he feels is most important and say that he will also address what's on your mind.

• **Tell the doctor about yourself as a person.** Say, "Here are things I'd like you to know about me that will help you to better partner with me." You might communicate that your biggest health fear is about cancer…or that you have an analytical mind and will research everything he says…or that you really want to be given recommendations for what to do and how to make decisions.

• **Be as honest as you can be about everything.** Be straightforward when you describe your health condition or answer questions—from symptoms and how bad they are…to sex, drinking, depression and drug use.

One approach: Start small by saying, "There's something I want to talk about, but I'm scared [or embarrassed] to tell you." This provides structure to the conversation. It's even helpful for the doctor to know if you don't want to take action about what you're sharing, such as "I know I drink too much, but I don't want to stop now."

• **Review communication options with the doctor.** Rather than waiting for a follow-up visit, using a portal is a way to ask questions to optimize a care plan and share important feedback, such as drug side effects or clarifying the need for new referrals or labs. Ask if that's the doctor's preferred method or if you should call the office. Also ask about the average time frame for getting a reply.

IF THINGS AREN'T WORKING

As with any relationship, it can be difficult in the moment to recognize that it's not going well. You might feel stressed, agitated and scared but find it hard to give voice to that. Tune into yourself…do a gut check…and try to put words to what's not going well. If you can articulate what's going off the rails, you may be able to remedy the situation. *Examples…*

• **If you feel that you're not being heard** or that the practitioner is just going through the motions without making a connection with you, you might say, "Can we slow down? I'm not sure you've had a chance to review my full history, and I'd like to share things that are important."

• **If you are overwhelmed by the doctor's jargon or rapid-fire recommendations,** ask for clarification by saying, "Can you give me an example that I can better relate to?"

• **If something doesn't feel right while you're in the exam room,** you are under no obligation to proceed. Call a time-out and say, "I don't feel comfortable going forward." The doctor might be willing to alleviate your concerns, but if not, you can leave or not schedule a follow-up.

AFTER THE APPOINTMENT

What if after leaving the office, you feel the appointment went so badly that the relationship can't be recovered?

• **Ask yourself if you're making too quick a conclusion.**

• **Think about whether you can collect more data**—perhaps by trying again with a second visit or communicating with the doctor via e-mail. You might send a message saying, "I don't feel that all my questions were answered—can you tell me what to do about X until our next visit?"

If you don't like the response you get, you may not want to invest more effort trying to make it work.

The Power of Prevention

Multiple members of the United States Preventive Services Task Force.

Health screenings help healthy people stay well. Physicians use them to look for signs of potential problems before they become symptomatic and when they're easier to treat. A multitude of health-care organizations develop screening guidelines, but they don't always agree. That's where the United States Preventive Services Task Force steps in. This independent, non-governmental body digs deep into the research to compare the benefits and harms of a wide variety of preventive screenings. *Here's a look at the Task Force's recommended screenings...*

• **Abdominal aortic aneurysm.** The USPSTF recommends one-time screening for abdominal aortic aneurysm (AAA) with ultrasonography in men ages 65 to 75 years with a history of smoking. Men in this age group who have never smoked may be screened selectively taking into consideration a patient's medical history, family history, other risk factors and personal values. There is insufficient evidence to assess the balance of benefits and harms of screening for AAA with ultrasonography in women ages 65 to 75 years who have ever smoked or have a family history of AAA. Women who have never smoked should not be screened.

• **Breast cancer.** Women should have a mammogram every other year starting by age 50. Some women in their 40s may benefit from screening and should discuss what's best for them with their doctor. The current evidence is insufficient to assess the balance of benefits and harms of mammography in women ages 75 years or older.

• **Cervical cancer.** Screening is recommended every three years with the Pap test (cervical cytology) for women ages 21 to 29. Women ages 30 to 65 have three options:

screening with the Pap test alone every three years, screening with high-risk human papillomavirus (hrHPV) testing alone every five years, or with both tests every five years.

Cervical cancer screening is not recommended in women who are older than age 65 who have had adequate prior screening and are not otherwise at high risk, or for women of any age who have had a hysterectomy with removal of the cervix and no history of cervical cancer or no history of high-grade precancerous lesions.

• **Colorectal cancer.** Screening should begin at age 45 and continue until age 75. The frequency of screening depends on the test used. Stool based tests should be repeated every one to three years (depending on the specific stool test used), whereas CT colonography (the use of CT scanning to produce images of the colon) and flexible sigmoidoscopy (an endoscopic examination of the rectum and lower colon) are recommended every five years. Flexible sigmoidoscopy can occur every 10 years if stool testing with a fecal immunochemical test (FIT) occurs every year. Colonoscopy, which lets your doctor see the entire colon, should be repeated every 10 years.

The USPSTF recommends that clinicians selectively offer screening for colorectal cancer in adults ages 76 to 85.

• **Hepatitis B.** Screening is recommended for people at increased risk, including those born in countries with a high prevalence of hepatitis B, unvaccinated people born in the United States to parents from a high-risk country, current or previous users of injected drugs, men who have sex with men, people with HIV, and those with household contacts or sexual partners of hepatitis-B-positive people.

• **Hepatitis C.** Screening should be done at least one time for adults ages 18 to 79. People who continue to have risk factors, such as injected drug use, should be routinely tested.

• **Human immunodeficiency virus.** Screening should occur in everyone ages 15 to 65. Adults older than 65 should be screened if they have risk factors for HIV. Risk factors include sexually active men who have sex with men, people with an HIV-positive sex partner,

Why Screenings End in Later Life

By your mid 70s, you may be surprised to find that your physician recommends fewer screening tests. There are a few reasons for this: As people age, they are more likely to have conditions that require disease management rather than prevention. Some of the screenings are for people with ongoing risk factors (around drug use or sexual activity, for example), and people's behavior may change as they age in a way that changes their risk.

Further, screening guidelines are based on a calculation between the potential benefits and the potential harms of a given procedure, but it can be difficult to tease that out in an age group that can have wide variations in health status.

An otherwise healthy 75-year-old who develops breast cancer may be both willing and able to undergo treatment, making the benefits outweigh potential risks. But another person of the same age may have a host of other health issues that are more life threatening than breast cancer, reducing or eliminating the potential benefits of screening.

Screenings in later life, then, can be more personalized. Talk to your doctor about which individual screenings are right for you.

---

injectable drug use, commercial sex work, and having other sexually transmitted infections.

• **Hypertension.** The USPSTF recommends screening blood pressure in a clinician's office for people ages 18 or older who do not have known hypertension.

• **Lung cancer.** Screening with low-dose computed tomography (a procedure that uses a computer linked to an X-ray machine that gives off a very low dose of radiation to make a series of detailed images) is recommended for adults ages 50 to 80 years who have smoked the equivalent of a pack of cigarettes a day for 20 years and currently smoke or have quit within the past 15 years. Screening should be discontinued once a person has not smoked for 15 years.

• **Osteoporosis.** Bone measurement testing is recommended in all women ages 65 and older, and in postmenopausal women who are younger than 65 but are at risk based on a formal risk assessment. Risk factors include a parental history of hip fracture, smoking, excessive alcohol consumption and low body weight. It's unclear how often this testing should occur, but limited evidence suggests that re-testing women with normal bone mass in four to eight years offers no additional benefit.

• **Prostate cancer.** Men ages 55 to 69 should talk with their physicians about undergoing periodic PSA-based screening for prostate cancer. Patients should consider family history, race and ethnicity, and other medical conditions to determine if screening is appropriate. Men 70 and older should not be screened for prostate cancer.

• **Type 2 diabetes.** People ages 35 to 70 who have a BMI of 25 and over should be screened for prediabetes and type 2 diabetes.

When Genetic Testing Can *and Can't* Save Your Life

Gillian Hooker, PhD, ScM, LCGC, past president of the National Society of Genetic Counselors. She is an adjunct associate professor at Vanderbilt University Medical Center and vice president of clinical development at Concert Genetics, both in Nashville. Concert Genetics.com

---

Until recently, genetic testing for medical purposes has brought to mind inherited changes (mutations) in so-called BRCA genes, which increase risks for breast, ovarian and other cancers.

Now: Genetic testing is being increasingly used to give advance warning of elevated risk for dozens of potential health problems. Unlike tests that help identify an existing medical condition, predictive genetic testing is done to determine whether a person carries one or more genetic mutations that make him/ her more likely to develop a particular health problem than someone without the mutations.

An early warning of potential problems allows the patient and doctor to identify preventive measures to reduce risk for the disease. Getting a positive test result, however, does not typically mean that the person will definitely develop cancer or another condition linked to a genetic mutation that shows up through testing. There are many factors that influence health and disease, including your environment, diet and health behaviors.

WHAT THE TESTS CAN TELL YOU

Genetic testing can give an early warning if you're at elevated risk for…

•**Cardiovascular disease.** Genetic testing can identify dozens of mutations, including SCN5A and MYH7, that are linked to increased risk for a range of potentially fatal heart issues, such as an abnormal heart rhythm (arryhythmia) or cardiomyopathy, a disease of the heart muscle. Heart-related mutations are more likely to occur in families that have a history of early-onset cardiac failure and death.

•**High cholesterol.** If you're diagnosed with high cholesterol, your doctor likely will recommend lifestyle changes, such as a diet that focuses on foods high in fiber and healthy fats, weight loss and exercise. But if high cholesterol is caused by a genetic condition called familial hypercholesterolemia (FH), more aggressive treatment is needed, such as regular use of a statin drug. Increased risk for FH is linked to mutations in such genes as PCSK9 and LDLR. In families that have hypercholesterolemia, high cholesterol is typically identified at very young ages, including in children. These mutations also may be associated with a family history of heart disease and heart attacks at young ages.

•**Parkinson's and Alzheimer's diseases.** About 10% to 15% of Parkinson's cases can be attributed to mutations of GBA and LRRK2 genes, among others. With Alzheimer's, a mutation in the apolipoprotein E gene, known as APOE e4, is among those that increase risk. Your risk of developing late-onset Alzheimer's is around three times higher than the average person's if you're among the 25% of people who carry one copy of APOE e4…or 12 times higher if you inherited APOE e4 from both your parents.

•**Chronic kidney disease.** Genetic tests can identify mutations in genes such as PKD1 that are associated with increased risk for kidney failure. This testing can be a potential lifesaver, since kidney failure often goes undetected until its late stages, and transplants are frequently done with donor kidneys from relatives. Signs of genetic kidney disease include kidney failure in more than one related family member and disease at younger ages than typically observed.

•**Cancer.** Recent research has confirmed how common genetic mutations are in people who develop cancer. When more than 3,000 cancer patients were tested, one in eight were found to have an inherited genetic mutation that significantly increased their odds of developing the disease.

While most people are aware of genetic testing for BRCA mutations (mentioned earlier), it's not widely known that these mutations also can occur in men, increasing their lifetime risk not only for breast cancer, which is rare in men, but also for skin, pancreatic, digestive tract, colorectal and prostate cancers. BRCA mutations can be passed on by women or men to their daughters and sons. These mutations are commonly found in those of Ashkenazi Jewish descent.

SHOULD YOU GET TESTED?

Even though genetic testing has many benefits, it's not something that everyone needs. *Speak to your doctor or a genetic counselor about this type of testing if you have…*

•**More than one family member affected by a medical condition with a possible genetic component, such as the conditions listed above.**

•**A medical problem or symptoms that your doctors haven't been able to diagnose.** Many rare diseases have an underlying genetic cause.

•**A diagnosed medical condition that could benefit from treatment that genetic testing may identify.** This could include people with certain types of cancer, high cholesterol or kidney failure.

COSTS OF GENETIC TESTING

If your doctor orders a genetic test, it generally is covered by insurance or Medicare as long as the results could be "clinically useful," meaning that a positive result would lead to preventive measures or treatment. Check with your insurer before testing to confirm whether it will be covered. If your insurance won't pay, the out-of-pocket cost varies from hundreds of dollars for a "focused" test to thousands for an "exome" or "whole genome" test.

Warning: Testing for Parkinson's and Alzheimer's risk often is not covered, because the results of these tests do not point to a specific treatment or improve the odds of survival.

One downside of genetic testing: It could potentially make it more expensive or difficult to obtain life, disability or long-term-care (LTC) insurance. Insurers sometimes ask applicants if they have had genetic testing done and/or whether they are aware of any reason why they might be at elevated risk for medical problems uncovered by genetic testing. Unlike life, disability or LTC insurers, however, health insurance companies and employers are legally barred by federal law from asking about genetic testing.

Helpful: Genetic counselors can assist you in finding the right genetic test for your medical and family history and in interpreting the results. If your hospital or medical center does not have a genetic counselor on staff, check FindAGeneticCounselor.org. Your health insurance may cover the cost of working with a genetic counselor, but check first.

More from Gillian Hooker, PhD, SCM, LCGC...

Beware DIY Genetic Tests

If you are considering genetic testing because of a family history of a specific medical condition or some other concern, it's wise to stick with tests ordered by your physician or with the support of a genetic counselor. So-called "direct-to-consumer" tests, including those advertised by such companies as 23andMe.com and Ancestry.com, check for only a few common mutations.

Example: 23andMe's test for BRCA1/BRCA2 mutations, which are linked primarily to elevated risk for breast and ovarian cancers, looks for just three of more than 1,000 variants of these genes known to increase cancer risk.

Get the Best Online Info on Alternative Medicine

Kapil Parakh, MD, MPH, PhD, author of *Searching for Health: The Smart Way to Find Information Online and Put It to Use.* He is a cardiologist based in the Washington, DC, area, adjunct associate professor at Georgetown University, and medical lead for Google Fit, a health and fitness app. Google.com/fit

Online health advice is best used to supplement treatment from medical professions, not replace it. But perhaps you would like a holistic approach to health care that incorporates natural modalities. *Where to look...*

• **Use the end of web addresses to gauge the reliability of health information.** As a rough rule of thumb, information about health issues found on official government sites ending in *.gov*...the website of the British National Health Service, ending in *nhs.uk*...or Canadian national health services, ending in *Canada.ca/en/health-canada* tends to be very reliable. Health info from sites ending *.edu* or *.org* usually is trustworthy as well—those generally are the websites of medical schools, hospitals, medical centers and health-related professional organizations, such as the American Heart Association (Heart.org). There are trustworthy sources of health info ending in the more familiar *.com*, too—WebMD.com and Health line.com both do a solid job providing largely accurate info, for example. But proceed with caution when reading health information on unfamiliar .com websites...especially sites that seem to be selling the treatments they're recommending or community-based message board sites.

• **Stick with truly trusted sites for info about alternative medicine.** There are plenty of effective traditional and alternative treatments—the challenge is determining which ones. These treatments often are not discussed on mainstream health websites, and some have never been proven to be safe and effective in large-scale studies, though many have been "proven" by the test of time. Fortunately, there are a few websites that are very authoritative on alternative medicine, including

Better Hospital Care, Nursing and You

The hospital staffing crisis doesn't come only from nurses retiring or from not enough people entering the field, though these are certainly important issues. Hospitals have increasingly moved toward lean staffing models to save money and boost profits. If you notice that the nurses are scrambling to help all of their patients and being called away from your room because there aren't enough people to help in another room, let the hospital know by filling out the survey at the end of your hospital visit.

On the other hand, be patient: If you do find yourself in the hospital, have realistic expectations about how quickly a nurse can get to you.

"You need to give a nurse about 30 minutes to respond to a call," explained Elizabeth Gamble, RN. "It can take that long to help somebody to the bathroom and back, and you can't really hurry that up. A nurse can't be in two places at once." The more patients each nurse has, the less time she can spend with each one.

Nurses are trained to prioritize the limited time they have. "You may need to go to the bathroom, which is uncomfortable, but a patient down the hall may be having trouble breathing, which could be life-threatening," she added.

Carrie Ali, editor of *Bottom Line Health*. BottomLine Inc.com

the sites of the National Center for Complementary and Integrative Health (NCCIH.NIH. gov)...The University of Arizona's Andrew Weil Center for Integrative Medicine (Inte grativeMedicine.Arizona.edu)...the National Cancer Institute's Complementary and Alternative Medicine (Cancer.gov/about-cancer/ treatment/cam)...and the National Institutes of Health's Office of Dietary Supplements (ODS.od.nih.gov).

Find a primary care physician and a pharmacist who are open to alternative treatments, and discuss these treatments before trying them. These professionals can confirm that the treatment is well-regarded and that it won't interfere with your other prescriptions or treatments.

Many Doctor Reviews Are Fake

A growing number of medical practices, doctors, dentists, and other businesses buy and sell fake reviews that appear on sites such as Google, Yelp, and Trustpilot. The reviews come from businesses that offer reviews for pay, employees, and other business owners who trade reviews with doctors.

Medical Justice

What to Bring to the ER

When you have a medical emergency, a quick and accurate diagnosis is critical. Having a written list of certain information ready to hand to the ER physician helps ensure that happens.

Information to include: A list of illnesses, surgeries and injuries—including the dates for all...whether you are being treated for a medical problem...names and contact information for your doctors and the dates of your scheduled follow-up visits...recent diagnostic tests or imaging studies...a list of all your medications and doses...your pharmacy's phone number...your next-of-kin contact...and of course, your insurance information.

Kenneth V. Iserson, MD, professor emeritus, department of emergency medicine, The University of Arizona, Tucson, and a *Bottom Line Personal* subscriber.

Is Your Forgetfulness Normal?

The Self-Administered Gerocognitive Examination (SAGE test) gives doctors a baseline of a patient's cognitive function. Taking the test again later allows changes to be evaluated for possible signs of problems. The test was developed at Ohio State University's Wexner Medical Center, College of Medicine and

College of Public Health, and has been shown effective in identifying when mild cognitive impairment is likely to progress to dementia. The test is free and easy to take on your own. You can bring the results to your doctor, who can keep it as part of your medical record.

Download the SAGE test: WexnerMedical. osu.edu/SAGE.

NeuroscienceNews.com

How to Stay Safe in the Hospital

R. Ruth Linden, PhD, founder and president of Tree of Life Health Advocates, where she helps clients navigate the health-care system and access the best possible care. She is a former professor at the University of California, San Francisco, Stanford University, and Tufts University, and has advised the FDA on developing policy to facilitate expanded access to experimental therapies. TreeOfLifeHealthAdvocates.com

---

Every year, an estimated 20,000 Americans die unnecessarily in hospitals, according to a recent study from doctors at the Yale School of Medicine.

Prior studies suggest the death toll could be even higher. In 1999, the Institute of Medicine estimated that 44,000 to 98,000 people die from medical errors each year. A paper in the *Journal of Patient Safety* suggested that the true figure could be as high as 440,000 people per year. In 2016, Johns Hopkins University researchers released their estimate of 250,000 people. These earlier studies, however, have been subject to controversy over their methods, while the Yale study took a more conservative approach.

COMMON RISKS

When you enter a hospital, you face a variety of risks…

● **You could be misdiagnosed,** especially in the emergency room.

● **You could receive the wrong treatment** or your condition could be poorly monitored and managed.

● **You could be the victim of a surgical error.** A 2015 study from Massachusetts General

Hospital found that some sort of mistake or adverse event occurred in half of all operations.

● **You could receive the wrong drug,** the wrong dose of a drug, or the drug you need might not even be ordered.

● **The Centers for Disease Control and Prevention estimates that there are 1.7 million hospital-acquired infections a year.** You could get an infection from difficult-to-treat bacteria, such as *Clostridium difficile* or *methicillin-resistant Staphylococcus aureus* (MRSA). (See also next article.)

● **You could develop a pressure ulcer (bedsore) that becomes infected.**

● **You could fall,** usually while going from the bed to the bathroom.

● **You could develop deep-vein thrombosis,** a blood clot that typically forms in the leg, but can travel to the lungs or heart, threatening your life.

All of these possibilities increased during the pandemic, when family members, friends, and professional health advocates were rarely permitted to enter hospitals and hospital staff were often spread dangerously thin. Now, more than ever, you need to look out for yourself or have someone else looking out for you. *Here are several straightforward and commonsense strategies to do that…*

CHOOSE THE BEST HOSPITAL

If possible, choose a university-affiliated teaching hospital over a public hospital or for-profit hospital. At teaching hospitals, you'll be asked the same question about your care many times—by medical students, interns, residents, fellows, and your medical team. This type of redundancy, where everybody is checking everybody else's work, is the best way to keep a patient safe. If you don't live near a city, use tools like HospitalSafetyGrade. org to research the best hospitals near you.

CHOOSE AN EXPERIENCED SURGEON

The best way to prevent errors during elective surgery is to choose an experienced surgeon. Ask, "How many such procedures have you performed in the past 12 months?" If it's a relatively low number, find another surgeon. And always get a second opinion before any surgery. ProPublica, a nonprofit that conducts investigative journalism, publishes Medicare-based data on surgeons' procedures and complication rates at Projects.Propublica.org/surgeons/.

HAVE A DESIGNATED ADVOCATE

Arrange to have an advocate who is tasked with knowing the daily details of your condition and your treatment plan, and to maintain regular communication with nurses and physicians who are supervising and delivering your care. Your advocate can be a family member, a friend, or a paid professional.

To find a professional, visit the website Advo connection.com, which provides a free directory of independent patient advocates. Interview one or more people to find out if you have a rapport with the advocate, if they've worked with patients with a similar problem to yours, and what the process of advocacy will entail. Ask about their credentials, references, and the cost.

ASK FOR A CONSULTATION

If you have or develop a symptom that you want evaluated by a specialist rather than the hospitalist (the physician who is managing your care in the hospital), ask for a consultation. If the physician says no, insist.

DEMAND SANITIZATION

This is always important to help prevent hospital-acquired infections, but it has taken on added importance during the pandemic. If a clinician or caregiver wants to come into your room but you haven't seen them wash their hands or hit the hand sanitizer dispenser, insist they do so. If they say they have done it, insist they do it again, if only to "humor" you. Likewise, ask the nurse or doctor if they have sanitized the stethoscope before putting it on you.

PREVENT FALLS

If you're unsteady on your feet or have any question about your balance, or if you're taking a medication that has drowsiness as a side effect, always get a nurse's assistant or nurse to help you to the bathroom. About 40% of falls in hospitals occur when a patient tries to get to the bathroom unassisted. If you go to the bathroom by yourself, or otherwise move about the room, always bring your hospital call button so if you do fall, you can get help as soon as possible.

PREVENT BEDSORES

Bedsores can develop when you don't move enough and there is pressure on your skin for long periods of time. People who are frail, bed-ridden, or diabetic have the highest risk. To prevent a bedsore, you should turn and reposition yourself at least every two hours to relieve the pressure on any one part of your body. Your heels and tailbone are particularly risky spots.

If you can't move yourself, call for a nurse to help you. Ask if the hospital can provide a pressure-relieving mattress or other protective devices. If you do develop a bedsore, you will need regular wound cleaning, dressing changes, and good nutrition to speed the healing.

KNOW THE DETAILS OF ANY DRUG YOU TAKE IN THE HOSPITAL

If the nurse wants to give you a pill or injection that you're not familiar with, ask about it. Who ordered it? What is it for? What are the side effects? If the answers aren't satisfactory, demand to speak with your physician before you take the drug.

ASK ABOUT YOUR MEDICATIONS AT DISCHARGE

Medications are often added or changed while you're in the hospital.

To ensure drug safety when you are being discharged, ask the nurse, hospitalist, or hospital pharmacist the following questions: Have any medications been added, stopped, or changed while I was in the hospital, and why? What medications do I need to keep taking, and why? How do I take my medications, and for how long? How will I know if my medication is working, and what side effects do I watch for?

DISCHARGE AND BEYOND

Also ask the following questions at discharge: What is my diagnosis? What medical equipment will I need? Can the hospital order it for me? What follow-up care will I need? When and how will I receive test results? Are my records available to me through a patient portal? Whom should I call if I have a question or problem? How soon should I make a follow-up appointment?

Protect Yourself from Hospital Infections

David Sherer, MD, retired American physician, author and inventor. He is the lead author of *Hospital Survival Guide: The Patient Handbook to Getting Better and Getting Out* and *What Your Doctor Won't Tell You*. Dr. Sherer's current focuses include patient education, patient advocacy and writing. DrDavidSherer.com

Fortunately, you can influence your hospital care in a way that can keep you from becoming the one in 31 hospital patients with at least one health-care-associated infection (HAI). *Here's how…*

• **If you need a catheter, request it be removed as soon as it is safe to do so.** Using a catheter for longer than six days is a risk factor for a catheter-associated urinary tract infection (CAUTI). Ask your doctor to remove it as early as possible. Always clean your hands before and after touching your catheter, and make sure your urine bag hangs below the level of your bladder to prevent urine from flowing back into your bladder, where it could cause an infection.

• **Make sure you're receiving only necessary medications.** Antibiotics are notoriously overprescribed, fueling growth of superbugs such as MRSA, which can cause infections at surgical sites, in catheters and other places. Antibiotics also can cause *C. difficile*. Ask if your antibiotic is absolutely necessary.

Important: Whether you are in the hospital or at home, let your health-care provider know if you have three or more episodes of diarrhea within 24 hours while taking antibiotics. This could be a sign of *C. difficile*.

Narcotics are problematic, too. They make it harder for older adults, especially men, to urinate, increasing the likelihood of a catheter needing to be inserted.

• **Ask all visitors to wash their hands before entering your hospital room.** This will limit your exposure to staph and other bacteria. About 30% of people have staph living on their skin or in their nose at any given time. They may not get sick from it, but they can spread it to other people.

• **Research the hospital's infection rates—** if you can choose where you will be treated—by visiting Medicare.gov/hospitalcompare (search for hospitals, rehab facilities or nursing homes). Many will list infection rates (under "Complications & Deaths") including how they compare to national benchmarks.

Note: If you belong to a Medicare Advantage Plan, this link won't provide information about whether your care will be covered in a certain hospital, so check with your plan.

• **Address major medical risk factors to stay out of the hospital.** You won't die from an HAI if you're not in the hospital.

• **Lose weight if you are overweight or have obesity.** Being overweight makes it harder to clear your airway, and excess skin folds are a perfect hiding spot for bacteria looking to cause an infection.

• **Quit smoking.** You've heard it before—smokers are more prone to infection.

• **Get vaccinated against COVID-19.** Patients hospitalized with COVID-19 are at a much higher risk of developing a number of HAIs.

Don't Throw Away Good Medicine

Sharon Horesh Bergquist, MD, associate professor of medicine, Emory University School of Medicine, Atlanta, Georgia.

An expiration date doesn't mean that a drug goes bad, like perishable food. Rather it's the date through which the pharmaceutical company guarantees the medication's full potency. Because it's expensive to repeatedly test a drug's potency for many years, most manufacturers stop testing at one to five years and set the expiration date based on their testing time. The American Medical Association has pushed for extended expiration dates, and the FDA occasionally extends a drug's expiration if there is a shortage of that medication, but no widespread changes have taken effect yet.

THESE DRUGS ARE SAFE

How long a drug remains safe and effective past an expiration date depends on many factors, including how it was stored. If kept in a cool, dry place, many medications that are in a solid form, like tablets, could be taken for at least one year past the expiration date. That includes medications for cold and allergy symptoms and nonsteroidal anti-inflammatory drugs.

While the FDA found that certain lots of drugs like the cold medicine guaifenesin or the antibiotic ciprofloxacin lasted more than 10 years, it's important to note that in the study, the medications were stored in ideal circumstances, which can't be replicated at home.

THROW THESE AWAY

While solid-form medications generally hold up well, creams, liquids, and ointments do not. After cough syrups, nasal sprays, eye drops, and topical ointments expire, toss them to avoid bacterial contamination from expired preservatives, or changing composition from evaporation. Probiotics should also be replaced before they expire, as they contain living organisms.

Any medication that you use for a serious medical issue should also be replaced upon expiration. If a drug like nitroglycerin, albuterol, insulin, or an epinephrine pen undergoes even a small decrease in potency, it could be dangerous.

MEDICATION STORAGE

The way you store medications can affect their potency even if they're not expired. Never store medications or diagnostic strips in the bathroom, where heat and humidity can affect their performance. Avoid extreme temperatures. Most medications can safely be stored from 58 to 86 degrees unless they require refrigeration. Those temperatures can easily be exceeded if you leave medications in your car while running errands on the way home from the pharmacy or if you pack them in a checked suitcase when flying.

When storing medications, take care not to mix them up. Eye drops and ear drops look very similar, so keep them separated or clearly marked. When in doubt, look for the word ophthalmic before putting anything into your eyes and otic before putting a medication in your ears. Keep pets' medications clearly marked or stored in a separate location.

MEDICATION MISHAPS

Mixing up ear and eye drops isn't the only medical error you need to watch out for. Something as seemingly harmless as taking a prescription sleep aid while also taking an over-the-counter allergy medication can be dangerous since they can both cause sedation. Some herbs and dietary supplements can alter the effectiveness of prescriptions too. *Every time you fill a new prescription or start taking a supplement, spend a few minutes with your pharmacist to ask the following questions…*

• **Will this new medication interfere with my other medication(s)?**

• **What should I do if I miss a dose?**

• **What should I do if I accidentally take more than the recommended dose?**

• **Are there any foods, drinks, other medications, or activities I should avoid while taking this medicine?**

• **How long should I take it?**

• **What are the possible side effects?** What should I do if they occur?

• **Can I cut this pill?** Some medications are specially coated to be long-acting or to protect the stomach.

• **Can I crush this pill to take with food instead of swallowing?**

Make sure any physician you see, including specialists, has a complete list of all of your current medications and supplements along with dosages. Keep a written record of your prescriptions, or use your smartphone to take photos of the labels.

Aspirin That's Easy on the Stomach

A new form of aspirin is easier on the stomach. Millions of people take daily aspirin to prevent heart attack. While effective, it can damage the gastrointestinal tract. The FDA has approved Vazalore, a capsule containing aspirin and protective fatty substances called liposomes. In trials, the aspirin in Vazalore was absorbed five times better and worked four times faster than traditional forms of aspirin, with 71% less injury. Capsules in 81 mg and 325 mg are available at Walmart, CVS and other retailers.

Byron Cryer, MD, gastroenterologist and professor at University of Texas Southwestern Medical Center, Dallas.

New Treatment for Recurrent Pericarditis

Pericarditis is a painful condition involving inflammation of the lining around the heart. Treatment with NSAIDs, colchicine and steroids is effective but comes with side effects, and there's a 15% to 30% chance of recurrent flare-ups. The FDA has approved *rilonacept* (Arcalyst), injected weekly, a biologic that treats acute flare-ups, allowing patients to taper off other drugs while reducing recurrence risk by 96%.

Allan Klein, MD, director of Center for the Diagnosis and Treatment of Pericardial Diseases, Cleveland Clinic. ClevelandClinic.org

For Appendicitis, Surgery Still Is Best

In recent years, treatment with antibiotics has emerged as a viable alternative to surgery for people with acute uncomplicated appendicitis. But in a new study, patients who received IV antibiotics until their symptoms improved, followed by a five-day course of at-home antibiotics, did worse than those who simply had their appendices removed surgically. One-quarter of the antibiotic group had another case of acute appendicitis within one year and reported a significantly lower quality of life during follow-up than the surgery group.

Study of 186 patients by researchers at Royal College of Surgeons in Ireland, Dublin, published in Annals of Surgery.

TAKE NOTE...

The iPhone 12 May Interfere with Cardiac Implantable Electronic Devices

Reports are emerging that the strong magnets used to support wireless phone charging can interfere with and even disable implantable cardioverter defibrillators and pacemakers. There have been similar reports about fitness wristbands and e-cigarettes.

Journal of the American Heart Association

Antibiotics Are Linked to Parkinson's Risk

Filip Scheperjans, MD, PhD, adjunct professor of neurology at University of Helsinki, Finland, and leader of an analysis of Parkinson's cases from 1998 to 2014, published in *Movement Disorders*.

Doctors have long known there is a connection between the bacteria in a person's gut and Parkinson's disease (PD).

Recent finding: Extensive use of oral antibiotics that wipe out gut bacteria is strongly associated with increased risk for PD. The finding was particularly robust for *macrolides* (such as *erythromycin*) and *lincosamides* (such as *lincomycin* and *clindamycin*). People whose medical histories included five or more courses of these classes of antibiotics within a five-year period had about a 40% greater risk for PD 10 to 15 years later than the general population.

Researchers aren't sure how gut bacteria affects PD risk.

Theory: Antibiotic use leaves the gut wall susceptible to inflammation, which allows the naturally occurring protein alpha-synuclein to accumulate in the gut wall's nerve cells. Over years, the alpha-synuclein travels to the brain, where it kills dopamine-producing cells. The brain chemical dopamine is involved in many basic functions, including motor coordination. Coordination problems are a major symptom of PD.

After any course of antibiotics, rebuild your gut bacteria by consuming a healthy plant-based diet. The microbiome typically will return to its original state within three months, but in some cases, it may take up to a year or may never return.

There is no evidence that probiotic supplements can help gut bacteria return to normal, although there is some evidence that probiotics can shorten/prevent antibiotic-associated diarrhea.

Don't be afraid to take an antibiotic if your doctor says it's the best treatment for your condition, but don't pressure caregivers to prescribe antibiotics without sound medical justification.

Also: Don't panic if you have taken antibiotics extensively in the past. PD is a multifactorial disease with strong genetic and environmental components that contribute to risk.

Newly Approved HIV Treatment Can Be Given Monthly

To avoid complications, HIV-infected people must take pills daily. *Cabotegravir* (Cabenuva), an FDA-approved extended-release injection given monthly, was shown to be as effective at maintaining viral suppression in HIV-infected adults.

John Farley, MD, director of the Office of Infectious Diseases, FDA Center for Drug Evaluation and Research, Silver Spring, Maryland.

Cutting Down Chemotherapy Side Effects

Keith Block, MD, the medical and scientific director of the Block Center for Integrative Cancer Treatment in Skokie, Illinois, editor-in-chief of the medical journal *Integrative Cancer Therapies*, and author of *Life Over Cancer*. BlockMD.com

Chemotherapy saves countless lives, but it comes with a high cost of side effects, such as fatigue, nausea, diarrhea, mouth

GOOD TO KNOW...

High Blood Pressure Medication Alerts

Underused Blood Pressure Medicine Has Less Side Effects

High blood pressure can be lowered as effectively with ARBs as with ACE inhibitors—and ARBs are less likely to cause side effects. Doctors prescribe angiotensin-converting enzyme (ACE) inhibitors because they've been around longer and had been less expensive (costs are comparable now). If you're starting hypertension medication, consider asking for an angiotensin receptor blocker (ARB).

George Hripcsak, MD, Vivian Beaumont Allen professor and chair of biomedical informatics at Columbia University Vagelos College of Physicians and Surgeons, New York City, and senior author of a multinational study of nearly three million patients, published in *Hypertension*.

Fewer Blood Pressure Drugs, the Better

Increasing the dosage of blood pressure medication may be more effective than adding a second drug. While both approaches lower blood pressure, patients—especially older ones—are more likely to stick to a drug regimen with fewer medications.

Best: Personalizing treatment to bring down high blood pressure.

Lillian Min, MD, associate professor of geriatric and palliative medicine at University of Michigan, Ann Arbor, and senior author of a study published in *Annals of Internal Medicine*.

sores, nerve pain, increased susceptibility to infections, hair loss, mouth ulcers, brain fog, and muscle damage. The side effects can be so severe that about 30% of patients abandon the treatment prematurely.

Research links this type of incomplete treatment to significantly shorter survival times. In one study of more than 400 people with colon cancer, the patients who didn't complete the prescribed three rounds of chemotherapy were more than twice as likely to die during a 10-year follow-up.

The good news is that there are protocols that can reduce toxicity and side effects, improve quality of life, and allow patients to complete their chemotherapy treatment. An integrative oncologist who is open to a cancer protocol that uses both conventional treatments and natural therapeutics makes an excellent resource in this pursuit.

COUPLERS

Clinical trials show that several natural therapies can mitigate the toxicity of specific chemotherapy drugs.

• *Cisplatin.* Vitamin E appears to reduce the risk of nerve, kidney, and inner-ear damage that can come from taking this drug. One clinical trial found that taking 300 milligrams (mg) of vitamin E twice a day cut the risk of developing neurotoxic symptoms from 68% to 21%.

• *5-fluorouracil (5-FU).* Glutamine can reduce intestinal toxicity and diarrhea from 5-FU.

Common dosage: 10 to 20 grams (g) daily, sipping, swishing and swallowing throughout the day. Sucking on ice chips for five minutes before, during, and after drug infusion can reduce intestinal toxicity and inflammation of mucous membranes inside the mouth and/or gut.

• *Paclitaxel.* Alpha-lipoic acid (300 to 600 mg, once or twice daily) has been reported to minimize the neuropathy associated with paclitaxel. Glutamine (5 to 10 g) and vitamin B6 (50 mg twice daily) also may counter the weakness and numbness occurring from Taxol-induced peripheral neuropathy.

• *Doxorubicin.* Coenzyme Q10 may help protect the heart against damage from this medication.

Common dosage: 200 to 600 mg per day. An extract of the herb hawthorn (300 mg to 600 mg, twice daily) may also help protect the heart.

• *Oxaliplatin* (Eloxatin). Pre-treatment with intravenous calcium and magnesium may reduce the risk of neurotoxicity from oxaliplatin. Alpha-lipoic acid, glutamine, vitamin B6 and acetyl-L-carnitine may also help.

• **Silymarin.** An extract from milk thistle, given at a dose of 250 to 500 mg, two to three times daily, may help prevent liver damage from a large number of chemotherapies.

Appetite-Boosting Tips

• **Consider when your appetite is best—**which for many people is at breakfast—and try to get most of your nutrients and calories for the day then.

• **Exercising shortly before mealtime can also stimulate appetite.**

• **Pain and pain medications can interfere with appetite,** so schedule your meal or snack at least 30 minutes after you take the medication.

• **Rather than eat regular-size meals,** have a healthy snack every two to four hours.

• **If family members or friends offer to help cook, take them up on it—**nothing increases appetite like someone else doing the cooking.

• **Make every bite count** by choosing whole, nutrient-rich foods that provide plenty of calories and protein.

• **During meals, limit the amount of liquid you drink,** since drinking may make you feel full.

• **Herbal teas such as fennel or anise,** mixed with verbena or mint, may stimulate your appetite.

—Dr. Keith Block

CONTROLLING SIDE EFFECTS

Several nutritional and herbal protocols can help control and reverse specific chemotherapy side effects.

• **Fatigue.** Try Siberian ginseng (*Eleutherococcus senticosus*), 2 to 4 g per day or *rhodiola rosea*, 300 mg per day. Engaging in 10 to 15 minutes of gentle aerobic exercise (such as walking or stationary bicycling) right before a session of chemotherapy can cut acute toxicity by 50%.

• **Nausea.** Try ginger as a tea or supplement (500 mg, every four hours).

Caution: You should not take ginger when your platelet count falls below 50,000 low due to marrow suppression from chemotherapy, since it may have anticoagulant effects. Aromatherapy with peppermint oil also may tame nausea: Carry a small bottle of peppermint oil with you throughout the day and sniff it occasionally.

• **Urinary symptoms.** Drink cranberry juice (blended with other natural juices instead of sugar to improve taste) or take concentrated cranberry tablets to prevent urinary tract infections.

The Antioxidant Controversy

Using antioxidant supplements such as coenzyme Q10 or vitamin E during chemo has been controversial because of concerns that they might interfere with the oxidizing free radicals generated by chemotherapy drugs to kill cancer cells. But two major studies show that this controversy has no basis in science.

Dr. Block and his colleagues conducted an exhaustive review of every randomized controlled trial in which antioxidants were administered during chemotherapy. Not a single study showed evidence of a decrease in efficacy from antioxidant supplementation during chemotherapy. In fact, many of the studies showed that antioxidant supplements increased tumor responses to chemo, reduced toxicity, and increased survival times. They published their findings in *Cancer Treatment Reviews*.

Bottom line: When implemented under the supervision of an experienced integrative cancer specialist, you can take carefully selected antioxidants during chemotherapy without concern that they are interfering with your treatment.

•**Joint or muscle pain (myalgia).** Tart cherry juice concentrate may relieve muscle pain and improve sleep. Glutamine (10 to 20 g per day) may help with muscle pain due to treatment with paclitaxel.

•**Upper respiratory tract infections.** Chemotherapy patients may find that they are prone to colds because of a compromised immune system. Herbs that are commonly taken at the first sign of a cold include kan jang (*Andrographis paniculata*); echinacea or a combination of echinacea, wild indigo, and baptisia; *Pelargonium graveolens* (a South African herb called umcka); and *Sambucus nigra* (elderberry).

•**Congestion.** Soups containing garlic and hot pepper can help relieve congestion, and gargling with salt water helps relieve a sore throat.

SUPPORTIVE DIET

To prepare your body for chemotherapy, base your diet on unrefined and minimally processed foods with plenty of plants (which are anti-inflammatory) and minimal amounts of meat and dairy products (which are pro-inflammatory).

•**Eat a rainbow of vegetables,** emphasizing brightly colored ones (pigments contain cancer-fighting phytochemicals), leafy greens, cruciferous vegetables (like broccoli, cauliflower, and kale), onions, and garlic.

•**Consume plenty of whole grains,** the richest source of complex carbohydrates and fiber, which provide a slow, sustained supply of fuel for your daily activities while reducing fuel for cancer.

•**Avoid cancer-promoting foods,** including excess dietary fat (particularly saturated fats in meat and dairy, and trans fats found in many processed foods), and refined carbohydrates.

•**Consume plenty of legumes** (lentils, chickpeas, beans), soy foods, fish, and occasional omega-3 eggs. These choices have cancer-fighting properties, contain many of the nutrients found in meat, and are an excellent source of complex carbohydrates and digestion-regulating soluble fiber.

•**To satisfy meat cravings,** try grilling, barbecuing, or baking salmon, halibut, tuna, or haddock steaks. Try tofu hot dogs, veggie burgers, vegetarian bacon, and vegetarian cold cuts.

•**To satisfy cravings for sweets,** eat fruit (no more than two to three servings per day, because the high amount of natural sugar can make you gain weight and cause your blood sugar to fluctuate). You can also use small amounts of unrefined, healthful sweeteners, such as monk fruit, rice syrup, barley malt, agave, kiwi sweetener, stevia, or maple syrup.

•**Every day, drink eight cups of water,** three to five cups of green tea, plus other fluids such as vegetable juices and herbal teas. Green tea is even better for rehydrating than water. It contains many antioxidants and anticancer phytochemicals.

REDUCE STRESS

When dealing with cancer, you need a way to calm yourself to curb and counteract the stress hormones coursing through your body, which contribute to cancer's ability to multiply and spread and are linked to poor outcomes. One excellent way to relax is to use relaxed abdominal breathing.

3

Cures for Common Conditions

Don't Treat a Sprain with Ice...and Other Medical Counter-Wisdom for Everyday Life

Many things we do to heal ourselves and stay healthy are based not on modern science but on outdated theories and unproven practices. *We asked Dr. Paul Offit to tell us the truth about four supposedly "healthy" remedies...*

Belief: Treat a sprain with R.I.C.E. (Rest, Ice, Compression, Elevation).

Truth: Treating a sprain with R.I.C.E. can delay healing.

When an ankle is sprained, the damaged ligaments surrounding it release substances that promote inflammation, which triggers the body to boost blood flow to the injured area. Increased blood flow steers clotting fac-

tors and immune cells to the injury, where they help stop internal bleeding and remove damaged cells. Inflammation also promotes production of the protein collagen, which is needed for recovery. In other words, inflammation fuels healing.

But inflammation also causes pain. That's why the R.I.C.E. protocol, created by sports medicine physician Gabe Mirkin in 1978, gained traction, and many medical groups, including the American Academy of Orthopaedic Surgeons and National Athletic Trainers' Association, have endorsed it for treating sprains and other minor injuries. Rest, ice, compression (wrapping) and elevation all feel good in the moment, but ice and compression decrease blood flow to the injured area—the opposite of what is needed for healing.

Paul A. Offit, MD, attending physician in the division of infectious diseases at Children's Hospital of Philadelphia and the Maurice R. Hilleman Professor of Vaccinology at Perelman School of Medicine at University of Pennsylvania. He is author of *Overkill: When Modern Medicine Goes Too Far.* PaulOffit.com

Result: A prolonged period of healing and, possibly, improperly healed ligaments.

Important finding: There is "limited evidence supporting the efficacy" of the R.I.C.E approach, concluded a 2020 study in *World Journal of Orthopedics*. And in 2015, Dr. Mirkin himself renounced his own popular advice.

What to do instead: Try to tough out the pain without ice and compression. After the initial swelling has decreased, applying warmth to the area—a heating pad or a warm, damp cloth—for an hour may provide some relief. Elevation also may help.

Also: After a few days of rest and once the swelling has gone down, try gentle ankle movements to increase blood flow to the area.

Example: Draw an imaginary alphabet with your foot.

Belief: **Reducing your fever helps you get better faster.**

Truth: Treating a fever can prolong or even worsen an infection.

Say you've caught a bug and feel awful—fever, shivering, head and body aches. Your first goal may be to relieve your symptoms by popping aspirin, *acetaminophen* (Tylenol) or *ibuprofen* (Motrin, Advil). These medicines may reduce your fever and help you feel better in the short term, but they don't fight the pathogen that is making you sick. In fact, they may prolong the infection.

Here's why: When viruses, bacteria, parasites or other pathogens enter the bloodstream, the immune system releases proteins called *cytokines* that travel to the brain, where they enter the hypothalamus, the area that regulates body temperature. There, the cytokines set off a chain of events to reset the body's thermostat to a higher temperature, usually over 100°F, because the immune system is enhanced at higher temperatures. At this elevated temperature, the search-and-destroy immune cells *neutrophils* seek out and kill the foreign invaders.

Fever reducers, on the other hand, tell the brain to reduce your temperature. As your temperature drops, the neutrophils take a break, allowing viruses and bacteria to flourish.

Result: Mild infections may last longer, and severe infections can worsen or even become fatal.

Surprising: There are 5% more cases of influenza (and 5% more influenza-related deaths) per year in societies where fever reducers are frequently used.

What to do instead: The truth is, we're not supposed to feel good when we are sick. If possible, stick it out…stay in bed…hydrate…and let your body fight the infection the best way it knows how—by raising your temperature.

Caution: A high fever induced by infection is rarely dangerous—but in an older person, a high fever that lasts longer than two or three days can put stress on the heart, and fevers induced environmentally, such as those that occur in football players or outdoor laborers wearing heavy clothing, can cause heat stroke.

Belief: **Sunblock protects skin.**

Truth: "Sunblock" is a misnomer.

The FDA no longer allows products to be called "sunblock" because it implies that they "block" the sun. Besides staying indoors and wearing sun-protective clothing such as broad-brimmed hats and long-sleeved shirts when outside, there's no way to entirely block the sun from damaging your skin.

The appropriate term is "sunscreen"—these products help reduce the amount of damaging UV rays absorbed by skin. To convey the degree to which they prevent sunburn, sunscreens are labeled with numbers—products with a sun protection factor (SPF) of 15 screen out 93% of UVB rays…an SPF of 30 screens out 97%…and an SPF of 50, 98%. No sunscreens, not even ones with an SPF of 100, screen out 100% of UV rays.

These numbers are reliable measures of sun protection only if the sunscreen is used as it's designed to be used—at least one full ounce (enough to fill a shot glass) to cover all exposed skin on the face and body, applied 15 minutes before heading outside and reapplied every two hours and again immediately after swimming or perspiring, per the American Academy of Dermatology.

Reality: Most people apply less than half the recommended amount.

Added problem: Sunscreen gives people a false sense of protection, prompting them to stay out in the sun longer.

What to do: Cover as much of your skin as possible with sun-protective clothing. Regular clothing works, too, but it must be opaque—a sheer linen top won't block much, but a tightly woven long-sleeved denim shirt will. For any exposed skin, including often-overlooked places such as eyelids, tops of ears and the scalp, use ample sunscreen and reapply religiously.

Hand-Washing Mistake

About half of adults don't wash their fingertips…and nearly one-third neglect the backs of their hands.

Best: Cover your whole hands with soap and water—fingertips, thumbs, fronts and backs, and between each finger. Singing "Happy Birthday" or "Yankee Doodle" ensures that you scrub long enough.

Study of 190 adults by researchers at the School of Nursing, Tung Wah College, Hong Kong, published in *Journal of Environmental and Public Health.*

Tennis Elbow: Anyone Can Get It

Steve K. Lee, MD, Chief of the Hand and Upper Extremity Service at Hospital for Special Surgery in New York City.

You don't have to play tennis to get tennis elbow. In fact, most people who develop this painful condition are not racket-sports enthusiasts. Instead, they are hairdressers, gardeners, knitters, or anyone who puts repetitive strain on the muscles and tendons of the forearms. Some people develop tennis elbow after an injury. Others develop it without any apparent cause.

The condition, formally known as lateral epicondylitis, can be so painful that people abandon favorite sports or hobbies or can no longer do their jobs.

The good news: It's treatable, usually without surgery.

To understand what causes the pain in the first place, it helps to know a little anatomy. The muscles in your forearm are responsible for the extension of your wrists and fingers. Your forearm tendons, or extensors, attach these muscles to your upper arm bone at a bony point in your elbow called the lateral epicondyle. Over time, heavy use of your wrists and forearms can cause the tendon to pull away from the bone and develop small tears.

GETTING A DIAGNOSIS

The main symptom of tennis elbow is a distinctly painful spot on the outer elbow. The pain usually starts gradually and gets worse over time. It tends to be most noticeable when you use your wrists and forearms, especially with twisting motions. For some people, even shaking hands is painful.

If you go to your doctor with elbow pain in the spot typically associated with tennis elbow, he or she likely will press on the spot to confirm the location of the discomfort and ask how long you have had the pain and when you tend to notice it most. In many cases, you also will get an MRI scan to confirm the diagnosis.

If you have a clear-cut case of tennis elbow, you might not need any other tests. But if the diagnosis is not clear, you might get a more extensive workup. For example, you might get an X-ray to rule out arthritis in your elbow.

WHAT TO TRY FIRST

Once you know you have tennis elbow, the first thing to try is resting the affected arm for about a month. Stop or cut back on activities that aggravate your condition. That's not too hard if your pain is caused by recreational tennis or backyard gardening, but if the aggravating activities are part of your job, taking a break can be tougher. If needed, a doctor may write to your employer saying that you temporarily need different duties or a few weeks off.

During this time, try wearing a brace on your wrist. While wearing a wrist brace when your elbow hurts might seem counterintuitive, the idea is to support and rest the affected tendon at the point where it originates. Look for a brace that gently holds the wrist in a "cocked up" position. These are widely sold in drug stores and online.

You can take ibuprofen, naproxen, or other other-the-counter analgesics to control pain for a few days. But, because taking those medications for a long time can have side effects, such as ulcers and stomach bleeding, you might want to try an anti-inflammatory gel that you can apply directly to the painful area. Effective products containing the active ingredient *diclofenac* are available over the counter. Studies suggest they produce fewer side effects than pills do.

Some doctors also advise applying ice when your elbows hurt, especially when you first notice the pain. Apply ice or cold packs for 10 to 15 minutes several times a day. Put a cloth under the ice to protect your skin.

WHAT TO TRY NEXT

If you still have symptoms after a month of rest, bracing, and pain management, your next stop should be a physical therapy clinic. A therapist can work with you on gentle exercises to stretch and strengthen the muscles in your forearm.

If your pain persists, you may want to try a shot of cortisone, a potent anti-inflammatory agent that is injected directly into the painful area. Tennis elbow is not caused by inflammation, but the shots seem to help some people. If one shot does not provide adequate relief, your doctor may recommend a second shot after six to eight weeks.

Some doctors offer an additional therapy known as platelet-rich plasma (PRP). Platelets, which are blood cells that aid clotting and contain substances that might aid healing, are obtained from your own blood and injected into the affected area. Studies of the therapy have produced mixed results. Another experimental approach is using ultrasound or shock waves to promote healing.

Whatever approach you take, you should know that most patients get better within several months.

When Tennis IS the Cause

Sometimes tennis elbow is caused by playing tennis or other racket sports, but an aching elbow doesn't mean it's game over. Instead, you should work with a coach or trainer to see where you might make improvements in your equipment or technique that could ease the strain on your elbows. Common modifications include restringing your racket to reduce string tension, adjusting the grip size on your racket, or using a different backhand technique.

—Dr. Steve Lee

TURNING TO SURGERY

If you don't get better after six to nine months, you may be among the 10% to 20% of patients who are candidates for surgery. In the most common procedure, your surgeon will make one cut over your injured tendon and remove the damaged tissue. The tendon is then repaired. Less commonly, surgery is done with an arthroscope, a thin tube with a tiny camera and light that is inserted through a few small cuts. The surgeon uses a video monitor to see and remove the unhealthy part of the tendon. Neither kind of surgery requires an overnight hospital stay.

After surgery, you may need to wear a splint on your arm for a couple of weeks and then a wrist brace for a couple more. After that healing period, you will start gentle exercises to restore motion, followed by several weeks of strengthening exercises.

Hand Therapy for Arthritis and Carpal Tunnel

Timothy G. Havenhill, MD, a hand specialist and orthopedic surgeon at Northwestern Medicine McHenry Hospital, Crystal Lake, Illinois.

Physical therapy can be beneficial for both arthritis and carpal tunnel syndrome. For arthritis, physical therapy emphasizes range of motion, joint functionality, strength, flexibility, and dexterity.

ARTHRITIS EXERCISES

Try these simple exercises at home. For each one, do 10 repetitions on each hand.

• **Fist formation.** Fully extend your fingers, and then draw them in to form a fist with your thumb outside of your fingers. Don't squeeze. Hold the fist for three breaths; then slowly extend your fingers again.

• **Finger bends.** Fully extend your fingers, and then curl one finger at a time as far as you can into your palm. Hold each finger stretch three breaths and repeat 10 times.

• **Form an O.** Fully extend your fingers, and then slowly curve your fingers and thumb into an "O" shape. Release.

• **Hitchhiker bend.** Place your hand on a table with your thumb pointing up as if you are about to shake someone's hand. Curl your fingers into your palm to make a hitchhiker's sign. Release.

• **Finger lift.** Place your hand on a table, palm up. Raise each finger, one at a time, as high as it will go.

• **Wrist flex.** Extend your right arm and hand with your palm facing down. Use your left hand to press down on the back of the right hand until your palm is facing you. Hold for three breaths; then return to your original position. Repeat with your left arm.

• **Grip strengthener.** Squeeze a soft ball or rolled-up sock as hard as you can for three breaths. Release.

CARPAL TUNNEL EXERCISES

For carpal tunnel syndrome, physical therapists use what are called nerve-glide exercises. The carpal tunnel is a narrow passageway in the wrist. Carpal tunnel syndrome occurs when that passageway compresses the median nerve that runs through it. The nerve-glide exercise can help reduce pressure on the nerve to reduce symptoms, while tendon-glide exercises may improve range of motion.

• **Nerve-glide exercise.** Apply heat to your wrist and hand for 15 minutes. Make a fist with your thumb outside your fingers. Hold this and each subsequent position for three seconds.

Don't Delay

Exercises like these, as well as nighttime splinting, can effectively stop the progression of carpal tunnel syndrome symptoms, but only if they are caught soon enough. In most cases, once strength and sensation are lost, they can't be brought back, even with surgery. The most important thing you can do is seek an evaluation with a hand specialist or orthopedic surgeon. An occupational therapist can help develop strategies to work around hand impairments.

—Dr. Timothy Havenhill

• Extend your fingers while keeping your thumb close to the side of your hand.

• Keep your fingers straight and bend your hand back toward your forearm.

• Keep your fingers and wrist in position and extend your thumb.

• Keep your fingers, wrist, and thumb extended and turn your palm up.

• Keep your fingers, wrist, and thumb extended and use your other hand to stretch the thumb.

• Ice your hand and arm for 20 minutes.

• **Tendon-glide exercise 1.** Apply heat to your wrist and hand for 15 minutes. Hold your hand in front of you with your wrist straight. Your fingertips should be pointed to the ceiling. Straighten all of your fingers. Hold this and each subsequent position for three seconds.

• Bend the tips of your fingers into a "hook" position, with your knuckles up, and hold for three seconds.

• Make a fist with your thumb over your fingers and hold for three seconds.

• **Tendon-glide exercise 2.** Apply heat to your wrist and hand for 15 minutes. Hold your hand in front of you with your wrist straight. Your fingertips should be pointed to the ceiling. Straighten all of your fingers. Hold this and each subsequent position for three seconds.

• Bend your fingers at the bottom knuckle. On your right hand, the shape looks like the number seven. Hold for three seconds. Bend your fingers at the middle joint and touch your palm.

• When you've done the series, ice your hand and arm for 20 minutes.

MORE EXERCISES

•**Wrist extension.** Hold your hand as if you're telling someone to stop, and straighten your arm. Use the opposite hand to gently pull your palm toward you until you feel a stretch in your forearm. Hold for 15 seconds, release, and repeat five times.

•**Wrist flexion.** Keep your arm straightened, and bend your wrist so your palm and fingers are pointing down. Use your opposite hand to pull your hand toward your body until you feel a gentle stretch on the top of your forearm. Hold for 15 seconds, release, and repeat five times.

Better Showering with a Cast

Bad enough you broke a bone, but weeks of taping a garbage bag around your plastered limb adds insult to injury.

To the rescue: Reusable, waterproof cast covers will last until the cast comes off—and are watertight enough to let you swim. Mighty-X makes arm- and leg-cast covers that easily slip over a cast and stay up without the use of tape ($13 to $16). For kids, Bloccs waterproof cast cover has a watertight seal and is comfortable and less restrictive than many similar products ($30). Bloccs also makes a similar model for adults ($40).

LifeSavvy.com

Help for Chronic Concussion Symptoms

Chronic concussion symptoms are eased by yoga, meditation and mindfulness. These practices reduce fatigue and depression while boosting quality of life for patients dealing with long-term symptoms from brain injury, such as headaches, disturbed sleep and impaired academic/job performance. They are low-risk modalities that promote healing and can be used as part of a recovery plan.

Rebecca Acabchuk, PhD, a senior scientist at RoundGlass, a global holistic wellness company, and an associate research professor affiliate at University of Connecticut in Storrs. She is lead author of a meta-analysis of 22 studies published in *Applied Psychology: Health and Well-Being*.

Can Vitamin B-12 Reverse Poor Cognitive Function?

Mira Ilic, MS, RDN, LD, registered dietitian nutritionist in the department of gastroenterology, hepatology and nutrition at Cleveland Clinic. ClevelandClinic.org

Replacing B-12 in people who are deficient may improve their cognitive function, according to a recent study in *Cureus Journal of Medical Science*. Of the 202 participants, 84% reported that having their B-12 deficiency treated first with infusions and then with daily oral supplements for three months led to a significant improvement in their energy, concentration, memory loss and disorientation…and 78% had improved scores on the Mini-Mental State Exam (MMSE), which evaluates memory, attention and language. Even among those who said their symptoms didn't improve, more than half did better on the MMSE.

Causes of B-12 deficiency: Some medical conditions put you at risk for B-12 deficiency—the autoimmune disease pernicious anemia…diseases that affect the small intestine (where B-12 is absorbed), such as Crohn's and celiac disease…long-term use of PPIs for acid reflux…taking *metformin* for diabetes and *colchicine* for gout…resectioning of the stomach or terminal part of the small intestine… and weight-loss surgery. Because foods highest in B-12 are animal-based, being vegan or vegetarian can cause a deficiency.

Simply getting older also can increase incidence of the naturally occurring condition atrophic gastritis, when the stomach fails to produce enough of the acids needed to extract B-12 from food before it reaches the intestines. This condition may affect about 30%

of people over age 50, and the likelihood increases with age.

To prevent a B-12 deficiency: Adults generally need 2.4 micrograms of B-12 daily. Top sources include beef liver, clams, bluefin tuna, Atlantic salmon, milk, yogurt and eggs, fortified cereals and other enriched foods. Synthetic supplements are effective for people who can't absorb the B-12 in food.

Work with your doctor to determine what's best for you based on your bloodwork, health and medications you're taking. You also may need the B vitamin folate, which works in tandem with B-12.

Fatty Fish Helps Reduce Headache Frequency

A diet high in fatty fish and low in vegetable seed oils reduces headache frequency by up to 40%. Fatty fish such as tuna and salmon triggers production of molecules that seem to reduce pain in headache-relevant tissues… while the linoleic acid in vegetable oils has the opposite effect.

For cooking: Choose low linoleic acid oils such as olive, coconut and macadamia—or butter.

Daisy Zamora, PhD, assistant professor at University of North Carolina at Chapel Hill and co-lead author of a National Institutes of Health–funded study of 182 migraineurs published in *The BMJ.*

New Treatments for Migraine

Brian M. Grosberg, MD, director of the Hartford HealthCare Headache Center and professor of neurology at University of Connecticut School of Medicine, Farmington. HartfordHealthCare.org

I f you've ever had a migraine—almost 40 million people in the US suffer from them regularly—you know that it is far more than a typical headache.

Thankfully, new treatments are available now and more are in development.

New medications: Doctors used to believe that migraine was simply caused by overdilation and constriction of blood vessels in the head. But new research shows that migraine involves a cascade of events in the brain, including activation of the trigeminal nerve—a large nerve in the skull that is responsible for sensation in the face and motor functions such as biting and chewing—and the release of *calcitonin gene-related peptide* (CGRP). It appears that CGRP irritates nerve endings in the brain and inflames and dilates blood vessels. *This discovery has led to the development of new types of migraine-preventive medications…*

• **CGRP monoclonal antibodies.** One of the drugs in this class, *erenumab* (Aimovig), mimics the shape of CGRP and binds to the CGRP nerve receptors so that the peptide has no place to attach when it arrives at a nerve cell—this prevents pain. The other three drugs in this class—*galcanezumab* (Emgality) …*fremanezumab* (Ajovy)…and *eptinezumab* (Vyepti)—attach to CGRP itself, changing its shape so that it can't fit into the receptor. Aimovig, Ajovy and Emgality can be self-administered monthly or quarterly via an autoinjector. Vyepti is administered intravenously every three months by a health-care provider.

• **Gepants.** Also known as CGRP inhibitors, gepants work similarly to CGRP monoclonal antibodies, but they contain smaller molecules and so can be taken orally. *Ubrogepant* (Ubrelvy) and *rimegepant* (Nurtec) are taken as needed to stop migraine attacks. Recently, Nurtec received approval for use as a preventive treatment, too, meaning that it can be taken regularly during the month to help prevent migraine. *Atogepant* (Qulipta) also has received FDA approval for migraine prevention. Zavegepant is currently in clinical trials.

• **Ditans.** *Lasmitidan* (Reyvow) is the first approved drug in the "ditan" family, another new class of medication for migraine treatment. Ditans are close relatives of triptans (see next page) but are more selective in their effects on the brain—meaning that they work on different types of serotonin receptors than triptans. This allows them to have no effects on the cardiovascular system.

Warning: Ditans are potentially sedating, so lasmitidan has been labeled a controlled substance with a restriction against driving for eight hours after you take it. This side effect limits the drug's widespread use, but it may be helpful for people whose migraine attacks usually occur at night or awaken them from sleep.

Standard medications: Before CGRP inhibitors became available a few years ago, the class of drugs known as triptans was used to treat migraine. The first triptan—*sumatriptan* (Imitrex)—was approved by the Food and Drug Administration (FDA) in 1991. Others have since been released, including *almotriptan*, *eletriptan* (Relpax), *frovatriptan* (Frova), *naratriptan* (Amerge), *rizatriptan* (Maxalt) and *zolmitriptan* (Zomig). Depending on the triptan, these drugs are available as pills, injectables and nasal sprays. For some people, a single dose of a triptan can bring migraine relief within a few hours. But for 20% to 30% of people impacted by migraine, a second dose is needed.

Gepants vs. triptans: There are pros and cons for gepants and triptans…

Heart problems: Triptans may constrict blood vessels, which could cause heart attack or chest pain in people who have ischemic heart disease and/or poorly controlled high blood pressure. Gepants appear to be safer because they don't narrow blood vessels.

Rebound headaches: Gepants aren't as likely as triptans to cause rebound headaches from overuse of the medication.

Efficacy: Gepants often aren't as effective as triptans—only about 20% of people impacted by migraine find complete relief within two hours after taking a gepant (versus 64% for injectable sumatriptan).

But: Gepants are more likely to be effective when a migraine is already underway. Triptans, on the other hand, work best when taken at the very start of a migraine.

•**Nondrug treatments.** There are a number of brain-modulating devices that have recently received FDA clearance for migraine treatment. They can be used safely by all people impacted by migraine and are particularly helpful for people who don't find relief with medications or don't want to take medications. These devices effectively eliminate head pain in 30% to 40% of sufferers within two hours of using them. *Examples…*

•Cefaly Dual is a small device that is placed on the center of the forehead to prevent migraine as well as to stop an attack in progress. It delivers electric stimulation to small branches of the trigeminal nerve. It may take daily use for a few months to see a preventive benefit.

•Nerivio is an armband device that you control via a smartphone app to stimulate nerves in the arm and indirectly address migraine pain. It also is being studied for migraine prevention.

•Relivion is a headband that goes around the forehead to electrically stimulate nerve branches in the front and back of the head to treat headache pain.

Surprising Allergy Triggers

Jeffrey G. Demain, MD, a clinical professor at the University of Washington, Seattle and founder of the Allergy, Asthma and Immunology Center of Alaska.

For many people, allergy symptoms are getting worse with each passing year. Here are some surprising triggers for this spring misery—and what to do about it.

FRESH FRUITS AND VEGETABLES

Many people suffer from what is known as pollen food allergy syndrome (PFAS). Also known as oral allergy syndrome, PFAS is caused by allergens found in both pollen and raw fruits, vegetables, and some tree nuts. Your immune system can mistake the food for pollen and cause an itchy or tingling mouth, a scratchy throat, and swelling of the lips, mouth, and tongue. In some cases, you may develop hives where the food touched your skin. It is rare, but PFAS can trigger anaphylaxis, a severe and potentially fatal allergic reaction.

If you typically suffer spring allergies, you are likely allergic to birch-tree pollen. Up to

Allergy-Busting Steps

●**Treat before the symptoms begin.** To get ahead of the sneezing, congestion, watery eyes, and other troubling symptoms, start your allergy medications two weeks before allergy season typically begins.

Using a nasal steroid, such as *fluticasone* (Flovent), once a day starting at the beginning of pollen season can reduce your symptoms by about 35%. Taking an antihistamine, such as *loratadine* (Claritin) or *cetirizine* (Zyrtec), can lessen symptoms by 25%. Using both remedies provides a 45% to 50% relief in symptoms.

●**Eye drops that can help prevent itchy, watery eyes** before they start include *olopatadine hydrochloride* (Pataday). Once these symptoms appear, antihistamine eyedrops, including *ketotifen fumarate* (Zaditor), may be effective at alleviating them.

●**Keep your home allergy-free.** Close windows and doors and use an air purifier with a high-efficiency particulate air (HEPA) filter to remove pollens from indoor air. Take your shoes off at the front door to prevent tracking pollen into your house. Take a shower before bed to remove pollens from your skin and hair.

And don't forget pets: Animals can bring pollen in homes on their fur. Try to bathe them once or twice a month.

●**Perform outdoor exercise in the afternoon.** Tree pollen, primarily from birch trees, is the largest spring allergy trigger. Tree pollen cycles begin in the morning, so the best time of day to be outside for a walk, bike ride or some fresh air is the afternoon.

—Dr. Jeffrey Demain

70% of people with a birch-pollen allergy also experience an allergic reaction to apples, cherries, kiwi, peaches, pears, plums, carrots, celery, almonds, peanuts, and hazelnuts. You may have a reaction to these foods only during the spring, when pollen is the highest.

Other fruits, vegetables, and nuts may cross react with different tree and plant pollens that peak at other times of the year. For more information, visit AAAAI.org and search "oral allergy syndrome."

You may be able to eat fruits and vegetables that cause PFAS if you cook them. Heating affects the allergy-causing proteins. Unfortunately, cooking will not alter the proteins in tree nuts.

Most symptoms of PFAS resolve quickly on their own once you stop eating the offending food. However, if you have a reaction to a food, it is a good idea to consult your doctor to determine the cause. PFAS can be confused with a food allergy, so it is important to know what the allergy is and how to treat it. If you have a reaction when eating nuts, in particular, see a doctor as soon as possible. Nuts are more likely to cause anaphylaxis and require medical attention.

THUNDERSTORMS

While a spring rain may help alleviate allergy symptoms by washing pollen away, thunderstorms can exacerbate symptoms and lead to what is known as "thunderstorm asthma." When a heavy storm hits on a day with a high pollen count, grains of pollen get sucked into the storm clouds, where they absorb water and then pop, releasing even smaller grains. These particles are spread from the downdrafts of the thunderstorm and are easily inhaled.

Researchers in Georgia found that visits to the hospital for asthma were 3% higher after thunderstorms.

If you suffer from an allergy to pollen, and particularly if you also have asthma, stay indoors and keep windows closed when pollen counts are high and thunderstorms are predicted.

CLIMATE CHANGE

If you're allergic to pollen, which is an allergy trigger for one in five Americans, you may have noticed your symptoms are starting earlier than usual, getting more intense, and lasting longer. That's because allergy season lasts up to 27 days longer than it did only 10 years ago as it gets warm earlier in spring and cold later in winter. Increasing carbon dioxide levels, which are at an all-time high, make the already higher levels of pollen in the air more potent.

Because spring allergies are starting earlier and are more severe, you need to start your typical allergy-fighting regimen sooner and take extra precautions to successfully treat the symptoms (see sidebar). To determine when allergy season will begin in your area, consult the National Allergy Bureau, which tracks pollen and mold counts nationwide. Go to AAAAI.org and click on "check pollen counts" at the top of the home page.

Exercises to Increase Your Oxygen Intake

Meera Patricia Kerr, a yoga expert, singer, and songwriter. She is coauthor, with Sandra A. McLanahan, MD, of *Take a Deep Breath: A Simple Exercise Guide to Increasing Your Oxygen Intake* and author of *Big Yoga: A Simple Guide for Bigger Bodies.*

Most of us take the act of breathing for granted. It's an automatic bodily function that we barely notice, although we do it up to 30,000 times per day.

While breathing may appear to be simply the act of inhaling and exhaling, it's actually a complex physiological process involving various muscles, blood vessels and organs such as the lungs, heart, and brain. And in truth, many of us never learned how to breathe correctly when we were younger.

Common mistake: If you fill up your lungs and then your stomach with each breath, that's actually known as "reverse breathing" or "shallow breathing." Proper breathing starts deep in the abdomen and then moves up to the lungs.

When breathing is normal, there is little to think about. But when we are not able to get enough oxygen into our bodies, it can hinder our ability to function and it can be frightening.

Examples: Conditions such as asthma, chronic obstructive pulmonary disease (COPD), being overweight (especially if you carry a lot of weight in your middle section) and COVID-19 infection can impair breathing, causing shortness of breath, a recurring cough and constant pain in the chest.

Important: Even if your lungs are damaged by disease, proper breathing can reawaken portions of the lungs that haven't been used and may improve COPD, asthma and possibly COVID-19 symptoms.

HOW TO BREATHE CORRECTLY

Practicing this simple exercise, known as the diaphragmatic breath, for 20 to 30 minutes each day can strengthen your ability to breathe deeply and fully, deliver more oxygen to cells throughout your body and improve alertness and exercise endurance throughout the day. Improved breathing also helps keep stress and anxiety at bay. If you prefer, break it into two 15-minute sessions rather than all at once.

Sit in a comfortable chair that enables proper posture, with feet flat on the floor or on a pillow and your back supported.

1. Inhale for a count of four through the nose. It's better to breathe in through the nose than the mouth because the nostrils moisturize and warm air, purifying the breath as it goes into the body. Inhale from the bottom up as if filling a balloon with air—first expand the lower belly (below the belly button), then the rib cage, then the upper chest, which will fully expand your lungs.

Important: When your lungs are fully expanded, your collarbone may rise up, but keep your shoulders relaxed and below your ears to prevent tension in your neck.

2. Exhale through pursed lips for a count of four from the top down. Initially, the length of your exhalation should be equal to the length of your inhalation. Gradually increase the exhales to last up to twice as long as the inhales. Start by expelling air while pulling in the upper chest, then the rib cage and lastly the belly. At the end of the exhalation, your belly should be pulled in toward the spine. Breathing out in this order is a more effective way to expel all of the stale air and carbon dioxide from your body.

Keeping your lips pursed slows down the breath, giving you more control over the exhalation so you can breathe out more deeply. A secondary benefit is that it relaxes you, particularly beneficial for people with COPD and other lung diseases who become anxious and fearful when short of breath, making it even more difficult to breathe deeply.

Advanced: Work up to inhaling and exhaling for longer counts.

Goal: Inhale for a count of five, hold for a count of 20, and exhale for a count of 10.

RELAXATION AND DEEP BREATHING

If you prefer, you can perform diaphragmatic breathing while lying on your back. This "torso opener" exercise opens up the chest, which allows you to breathe even more deeply than when you are sitting in a chair. It even can improve digestion—when seated, having a big belly or hunching over with rounded shoulders can impede digestion.

1. Lie on a yoga mat or towel with your head on a pillow and your arms to your sides. Put a blanket or bolster under your knees or let your legs lie flat.

2. Place an eye mask over your eyes.

3. Practice diaphragmatic breathing and relax in this position for 10 to 15 minutes.

4. Come out of the position slowly to regain your bearings as you stand up.

STRENGTHENING EXERCISES

It is important to strengthen muscles that support breathing and improve circulation. When muscles are strong and breathing is deep, more oxygen is pushed out to the body's cells. *Perform three to five repetitions of each of the following seated exercises daily…*

● **Thoracic Toner.**

1. Inhale as you touch your fingertips to the tops of your shoulders with your elbows close together in front of your chest.

2. Exhale with pursed lips as you move the elbows out to the side of your body. Feel your

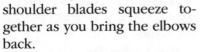

shoulder blades squeeze together as you bring the elbows back.

3. Move your elbows back to the first position, and repeat.

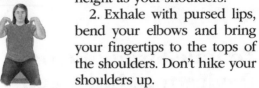

● **Elbow Bends.**

1. Inhale and extend your arms out to the front with your palms facing up. Keep your arms at about the same height as your shoulders.

2. Exhale with pursed lips, bend your elbows and bring your fingertips to the tops of the shoulders. Don't hike your shoulders up.

3. Return to the starting position, and repeat.

● **Shoulder Squeeze.**

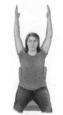

1. Inhale and bring your arms straight up overhead. They should be aligned with your ears and your palms should face inward. Don't tense up the shoulders.

2. Exhale through pursed lips, and swing your arms down behind your body keeping

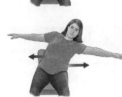

your palms facing inward. Squeeze the area between the shoulder blades.

3. Return to the starting position and repeat.

● **Side Stretch.**

1. Inhale and stretch your arms out to the side. Don't hike your shoulders up. Keep your arms relaxed and your palms facing down.

2. Exhale through pursed lips as you stretch to the left.

3. Inhale and return to the upright position.

4. Exhale through pursed lips, and lean to the right.

5. Return to the starting position, and repeat.

● **Side Twist.**

1. Inhale and extend your arms to the sides with palms facing in and down.

2. Exhale with pursed lips, and twist your upper body to the right slowly, progressively rotating from the waist up, bringing your head around last. Turn as far as is comfortable.

3. Inhale and return to the neutral position.

4. Exhale with pursed lips as you twist to the left.

5. Return to the starting position, and repeat.

Tongue-Strengthening Device for Mild Sleep Apnea Approved

People with chronic sleep apnea experience interrupted sleep because their tongues fail to keep their airways open. Now the FDA has approved a neuromuscular stimulation mouthpiece, called the eXciteOSA, that strengthens the tongue during waking hours to keep it from collapsing at night. In trials, snoring was cut by an average of 48% for 41 of 48 patients. The device is not for people with severe apnea.

U.S. Food and Drug Administration, Silver Spring, Maryland.

EASY TO DO...

Remember Hydrogen Peroxide?

This old home remedy is still good to have on hand. Keep a small bottle in your first-aid kit to clean wounds when soap and water isn't available. Put a few drops of peroxide in your ear to clear clogged earwax—wait a few minutes, then gently swish your ear canal with warm water. Treat swollen gums by rinsing daily for 30 seconds with one part 3% peroxide mixed with two parts water.

Also: Hydrogen peroxide effectively disinfects sinks, counters, cutting boards, toilets, toys and more. Just don't get it on your clothes or furniture, as it can bleach them.

MedicineNet.com and ClevelandClinic.com

Don't Brush Your Teeth Right After Eating

Acids in food temporarily weaken the protective enamel that covers and protects your teeth. Brushing while the enamel is still soft can permanently damage the enamel, leading to staining, sensitivity and decay.

Better: Rinse your mouth with water after a meal...and wait at least 30 minutes before brushing.

Richard Marques, BDS, dentist and founder, Dr Richard Clinics, London, UK, quoted in *New York Post.*

Time to Play Catch-Up with Your Dentist

Leila Jahangiri, DMD, Ira E. Klein Professor and Chair, department of prosthodontics at New York University College of Dentistry in New York City.

Many people try to get by with annual dental cleanings and checkups, but you're less likely to get a troubling diagnosis or a big bill if you make regular six- or nine-month appointments. These routine visits are great for identifying the most common dental problems—dental decay and/or gum (periodontal) disease. Most dental insurance plans cover such routine care on this schedule.

Frightening statistic: One in every four American adults has untreated cavities, and nearly half of people age 30 or older have signs of gum disease, according to the Centers for Disease Control and Prevention. If left untreated, these conditions can lead to tooth loss and more.

What you don't realize about teeth...

•**Dental problems don't always cause pain.** Even if your teeth feel fine, that doesn't mean they are healthy.

Here's why: The nerves that would alert you to pain are buried deep within the tooth beneath the enamel and other protective layers.

Once tooth pain occurs, the problem often is so far along that extensive dental treatments, such as root canal, bone grafting or an extraction, may be needed. These all are expensive. So don't be surprised if your dentist recommends treatment for a tooth that feels perfectly fine to you.

Also important: Your nerves shrink inside your teeth as you get older, which means that even more damage can occur before your teeth finally become painful.

•**Your medications may cause "silent" damage.** Antidepressants, antihistamines and some blood pressure drugs are among the medications that can cause dry mouth, which increases your risk for tooth decay. That's because saliva helps neutralize acids created by bacteria in your mouth and even can help repair tooth enamel.

Helpful: If you take a medication that makes your mouth feel dry, ask your dentist about getting a prescription for high-fluoride toothpaste. This may help strengthen teeth and reduce the risk for significant dental decay.

DO YOU REALLY NEED THAT TREATMENT?

If you're behind on your routine visits, be prepared for your dentist to recommend unexpected tests and treatments. This is especially true if you're seeing a new dentist for the first time.

Here's how to ensure that recommended tests and treatments are necessary…

•**Keep track of your X-rays.** Most adults with no ongoing dental issues may need X-rays only every two to three years, while those who have gum disease may require them more often. What's important is knowing that you have access to your X-rays if you switch clinicians.

If you're seeing a dentist for the first time for any reason, it's wise to get your dental records and past X-rays so that he/she will have a baseline to help identify any developing problems and won't have to do a new set of X-rays.

Note: You may have to pay a small fee to your former dentist to digitize or copy your printed records.

•**Ask the right questions.** If your dentist doesn't tell you why your teeth need the treatments he is recommending, don't be shy about asking. To prompt the conversation, you can say something like, "Can you please explain to me what the problem is you're seeing in the imaging? And why are you recommending that course of treatment?"

Similarly, if your dentist recommends that a filling needs to be replaced, it's perfectly reasonable to ask why. Generally speaking, you don't need to replace an older filling that's still intact simply for a newer and "safer" material. Dental fillings should be replaced only if they are chipped, broken or there is leakage underneath the filling that's causing decay and deterioration.

Important: As with other dental problems, a filling doesn't have to cause pain for damage to occur.

•**Don't downplay "aesthetic" work.** Many people assume that treatments designed to fix crowded or misaligned teeth are done to simply improve one's smile. But that's not always the case. Some orthodontics work is recommended to help prevent future problems, such as increased dental decay, jaw pain, gum disease or tooth damage, all of which can occur if your bite is not aligned properly or if teeth are crowded.

•**Get a second opinion.** If you think your dentist's diagnosis is extreme—or he can't adequately explain why you need the work he is recommending—you should feel comfortable seeing another dentist to confirm that the diagnosis and treatment are appropriate. This recommendation applies mostly to very complex situations that often require multiple extractions, numerous restorations or many implants. In these situations, the treatment may be costly and time-consuming, giving a greater justification for a second opinion.

You can ask the staff for a copy of your records and the X-rays to take to the second-opinion provider.

Kidney-Stone Prevention Plan

David S. Goldfarb, MD, a professor of medicine at New York University Grossman School of Medicine. He is chief of nephrology at New York Harbor VA Medical Center and the co-founder of Moonstone Nutrition.

A round the world, the incidence of kidney stones is rising. In the United States, the lifetime risk of having at least one kidney stone is now about 10%, up from 3.8% in the 1970s, according to the National Kidney Foundation.

Among possible reasons: the warming climate and the migration of people to warmer urban areas. But heat isn't the whole story. The way we eat and drink and the rise of obesity and diabetes likely play roles, too.

FROM UNNOTICED TO UNBEARABLE

Typical stones may be as small as a grain of sand or as large as a chickpea. More rarely, they can be as large as golf balls. A small stone may sit in your kidney unnoticed for months or years before it gets big enough or starts moving enough to cause trouble. Often, that happens when a stone moves from a kidney to a ureter, one of the tubes leading to the bladder. The stone may get stuck there, blocking urine flow or causing irritation as it makes its way through the ureter and bladder and out through the urethra. *Once a stone becomes problematic, symptoms can start suddenly…*

• **Intermittent mild to severe pain in the side, back, or groin for five to 15 minutes**

• **Stomach pain, nausea, and vomiting**

• **Blood in the urine**

• **Fever, chills, and bad-smelling or cloudy urine**

• **Kidney damage that may linger.**

DIAGNOSIS AND TREATMENT

If you show up in an emergency room or doctor's office with a possible kidney stone, expect to get a CT scan, an ultrasound, or an X-ray to confirm the stone as well as its size and location. You also will get blood and

Four Kinds of Kidney Stones

Not all kidney stones have the same causes. Knowing which type you're prone too can help you tailor your prevention plan.

• **Calcium oxalate.** Most kidney stones form when calcium in urine combines with oxalate, a salt. Calcium oxalate stones make up as many as 85% of cases. They are linked to inadequate fluid intake and diets that are high in oxalates and salt but, paradoxically, low in calcium.

• **Uric acid.** These stones are linked with conditions including type 2 diabetes, obesity, and gout and with diets high in animal protein.

• **Struvite.** These stones occur mostly in women with chronic urinary tract infections. That's because some bacteria secrete enzymes that make urine less acidic, allowing stones to form.

• **Cystine.** These rare stones are found only in people with a genetic disorder called cystinuria that causes the kidneys to excrete excessive amino acids. They tend to recur.

—Dr. David Goldfarb

urine tests to check for kidney function, levels of stone-forming substances, and infection.

Unless the stone is quite large or causing unmanageable pain or other complications, your doctor is likely to send you home to see if the stone will pass, which will happen within a few weeks in 80% of cases in which stones are no larger than 4 millimeters. Larger stones are less likely to pass. While some people will need prescription painkillers to get through the process, others will do fine.

ADVANCED INTERVENTIONS

When stones appear unlikely to pass unaided or are causing complications, the next step is a procedure to remove or destroy them. *There are several options…*

• **Ureteroscopy.** A small instrument, called a ureteroscope, is inserted through your urethra and bladder to reach the stone. Then, in most cases, a laser is used to break up the stone so it can be easily expelled.

8 Steps to Prevent Stones

1. Drink up. Staying hydrated is important for everyone, but especially for people prone to kidney stones. Aim for 12 cups of fluid (96 ounces) every day. Water is better than sodas or tea. If you are sweating a lot, drink more.

2. Get enough calcium. Even though the most common stones contain calcium, a calcium-rich diet helps prevent them. That's because calcium in food binds with oxalates in your digestive tract, preventing these minerals from reaching high concentrations in your kidneys. Good sources include low-fat milk, cheese, yogurt, sardines, and fortified cereals and juices. Calcium supplements may increase stone risk, but you can blunt that risk by choosing calcium citrate rather than calcium carbonate products. Taking them with food helps, too.

3. Limit sodium to 2,000 milligrams per day. Excessive sodium leaches calcium from the bones and concentrates it in the urine. Watch out for the salt hidden in restaurant meals and processed foods, such as soups, bread, and sandwich meats.

4. Limit foods that are high in oxalates. If you are prone to stones containing oxalate (see sidebar on previous page), your doctor may suggest that you limit foods such as strawberries, spinach, beets, nuts, organ meats, chocolate, tea, coffee, and cola.

5. Limit animal protein to about 80 grams per day. Diets heavy in meat and seafood are linked with both calcium and uric acid stones (see sidebar on previous page).

6. Watch out for sweeteners. High-fructose corn syrup, found in many foods and drinks, is linked with uric acid stones.

7. Talk to your doctors about medications and supplements that might help prevent your type of stone. These can include pills or drinks containing citrate and medication to reduce uric acid levels. Some medications can increase your risk of kidney stones. Talk to your doctor or pharmacist to review all of the medications that you take.

8. You can also try a home remedy to reduce your risk. Mix one-half cup of lemon juice with two quarts of water and drink throughout the day.

—Dr. David Goldfarb

• **Shockwave lithotripsy.** For this procedure, you lie on a surgical table or in a tub of water while shockwaves are aimed at the stone to break it apart.

• **Percutaneous nephrolithotomy.** This less-common procedure is used for large or irregularly shaped stones or in other special circumstances. A surgeon makes a small incision on the back, uses instruments to see and break up stones, then suctions out the fragments.

WHAT CAN YOU DO?

Anyone who's ever suffered through a kidney stone shares one fervent wish: They never want to do it again. Yet, half will develop another stone within a few years. Those who've had two or more stones are at even higher risk.

One reassuring fact: Most kidney stones can be prevented, no matter the season. See the sidebar to the left to learn how.

Exercising with Back Pain

Carol B. Espel, MS, program and wellness director at the Pritikin Center for Longevity in Miami. In 2012, she was named "Fitness Director of the Year" by the World IDEA Health & Fitness Association.

Back pain: It's become a reality for many people as poor posture, excessive sitting, and slouching have had deleterious effects on the back, core, and hips. While exercise is undoubtedly healthy, it's important to take special care of your back.

Don't make the mistake of thinking you can work through the pain, believing it's due to muscle inactivity. Working through pain leads to poor form and exercise execution and, in the end, leads to serious and chronic injury and more pain. It's important to ease into exercise slowly, and to heal, strengthen, and stretch the back and core muscles first. You can then start to add exercise and activities that are appropriate, effective, and safe.

BRACE YOURSELF

Bracing the core muscles (primarily the abdominal and oblique muscles) is critical to alleviating back pain when standing. An easy way to activate the "brace" is to take a deep breath in and then exhale fully. At the end of the exhalation, to expel any remaining air, forcefully exhale, making a "huh" sound. This will tighten and tone the abdominal wall. Supporting your body posture this way sets you up for pain-free movement, activity, and exercise. The following exercises are gentle and safe for people with back pain.

CAT COW

Start and end each session with this exercise. Start on all fours. Inhale as you round your back up like a cat, fully contracting your abdominals. Drop your chin into your chest and look at your belly button. Try to stay there for two to four counts. Exhale as you slowly lengthen your spine, lifting your head up and out, gazing slightly upward, and arch your back. Stay for two to four counts. Slowly repeat as many times as you enjoy.

BIRD DOG

Start on all fours. Look slightly forward and down. Brace your abdominal muscles and then slowly and fully extend your right leg straight back. Return to the starting position. Next, slowly extend your left arm in front of you, then return to the starting position. Repeat on the other side. Complete one to three sets of six to 12 repetitions on each side.

MODIFIED CURL-UP

Lie on your back. Place both hands behind your head, lightly supporting it. Let your elbows drop and open out, as close to the floor as possible. Bend both of your knees and place your feet flat on the floor. Contract your abdominals in and down as you slowly lift your entire torso off the floor. Return to the floor completely. This should be a small movement. Your focus must be up toward the ceiling throughout the exercise. Complete one to three sets of six to 12 repetitions.

HIP EXTENSIONS

Lie on your back, with both knees bent and your feet flat on the floor. Place both hands on top of your pelvis. Better yet, place a foam block on top of your lower belly and pelvis. The purpose of the foam block is to make sure both hips are pressing upward equally, avoiding one side dropping lower than the other. Lift both hips off the floor, squeezing the gluteal muscles, but not arching the rib cage. Return to the starting position. Complete one to three sets of six to 12 repetitions.

The key to long-term success for better back health involves a daily commitment to performing regular back and core strength, flexibility, and mobility exercises. These moves will help you to enjoy doing the things you like to do with greater ease, freedom of movement, and joy.

Credit Card Debt Causes Pain—Literally

People with consistently high unsecured debt, such as credit cards and payday loans, were 76% more likely to have pain and stiffness later in life, according to a recent study. Even if they managed to mostly pay off such debt, risk for pain and stiffness was 50%. Taking on new unsecured debt during middle age was particularly damaging.

Adrianne Frech, PhD, associate professor of health sciences at University of Missouri in Columbia and leader of a study of 8,000 adults published in *Social Science & Medicine—Population Health*.

How to Stop Achilles Heel Pain

Mitchell Yass, DPT, creator of The Yass Method, which uniquely diagnoses and treats the cause of chronic pain through the interpretation of the body's presentation of symptoms. Dr. Yass is author of The Yass Method for Pain-Free Movement: A Guide to Easing through Your Day without Aches and Pains. MitchellYass.com

In most cases, Achilles' heel pain is caused by weakness in the muscles that support the hips or in the leg muscles. Because the Achilles tendon connects the calf to the heel, strain in the calf often leads to pain in and above the heel.

If you have Achilles heel pain on both sides, there's likely a strength imbalance between the hip flexor/quad muscles and the gluteus maximus/hamstrings. Such an imbalance can develop from running, stair-climbing and exercises that tend to overdevelop muscles in the front of the legs while neglecting those in the back. This imbalance causes a forward center of mass that must be picked up by a muscle in the back of the body or you would fall forward. In this case, the excess load ends up being supported by the calves, resulting in pain in both Achilles tendons.

THREE EXERCISES FOR RELIEF

The exercises below and on the next page will strengthen your gluteus medius muscles, gluteus maximus muscles and hamstrings—all the muscles involved in creating optimal posture. The descriptions below are for single-sided weakness, but if your pain is bilateral, perform the exercises on both sides.

Complete three sets of 10 repetitions for each exercise (resting 45 to 60 seconds between sets). Repeat the workout three times a week with one day between workouts. The level of resistance should feel like you are working reasonably hard to complete the set. Stay with this resistance level until it feels fairly easy to complete the set, then increase the resistance. This process can continue until you are strong enough to perform your daily activities without pain.

Important: For single-sided pain, work the leg that is opposite the side where the heel pain occurs. If you work the same side, you'll inadvertently increase the imbalance between the two sides and the pain will continue.

For pain on only one side, the most important exercise is the hip abduction exercise. For pain in both Achilles tendons, perform the three exercises with both legs.

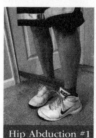
Hip Abduction #1

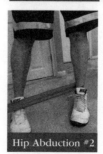
Hip Abduction #2

HIP ABDUCTION (GLUTEUS MEDIUS)

Knot both ends of a resistance band together and put the knot behind a closed door at ankle height. Standing perpendicular to the door, place the loop of the band around the ankle farthest from the door (the working gluteus medius). Start with your feet together. Turn the toes of the working leg in so that the foot is pointing about 10 degrees in front. Keeping your nose aligned over the standing leg, lift the moving leg slightly and move it until the outside of the ankle is aligned with the outside of the hip. Put the foot down. Now shift your weight until your nose is over the moved foot. Immediately move the foot and your body to the start position with your nose over the standing leg again.

HIP EXTENSION
(GLUTEUS MAXIMUS)

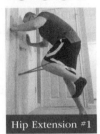

Hip Extension #1

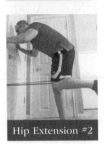

Hip Extension #2

Close the knot of the resistance band in the door at about knee height. In a standing position facing the door, place the loop of the resistance band behind your knee. Start with the hip flexed to about 60 degrees. Bring the knee about 10 degrees behind the hip. Then return to the start position. Make sure your back is rounded and the knee of the leg you are standing on is not locked.

HAMSTRING CURL
(HAMSTRINGS)

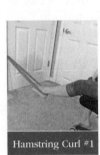

Hamstring Curl #1

Close the knot of the resistance band in the door at about knee height. In a seated position facing the door, place the resistance band around the back of the ankle. Begin with the exercising leg pointing straight out with the knee unlocked. Be-

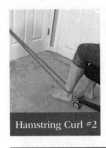

Hamstring Curl #2

gin to bend the knee until it reaches 90 degrees, then return to the start position. To isolate the hamstrings better, the toes of the exercising leg should point upward toward the face as the exercise is being performed.

How to Beat Bunion Pain...

A bunion is a deformity of the metatarso-phalangeal joint that causes a large bump on the outside of the big toe. *The first step to treating pain is always conservative management...*

• **Wear well-fitting, comfortable shoes** with ample space for your toes and the widest part of your foot.

• **Use over-the-counter arch supports or prescription orthotic devices to help position the foot correctly.**

• **Avoid walking barefoot.**

• **Use warm soaks and ice packs for pain relief.**

• **Take nonsteroidal anti-inflammatory drugs if needed.**

• **Maintain a healthy weight.**

Samuel K. K. Ling, assistant professor, department of orthopaedics and traumatology, faculty of medicine, The Chinese University of Hong Kong. Dr. Ling developed a type of minimally invasive bunion surgery that has provided pain relief for up to 10 years in his patients.

4

Diet and Fitness

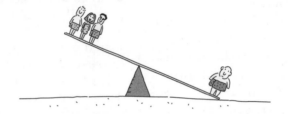

Sneaky Vegetable Secrets

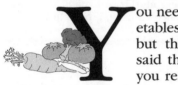 Y ou need to eat your vegetables for good health, but that can be easier said than done. Even if you really like the taste of veggies—which many people don't—it can be hard to get the recommended amounts into your day. That's where the concept of hiding them in other foods comes in. You can sneak veggies into just about anything you're making, boosting the health value of meals for you and your family—and the pickiest of eaters won't even taste them.

BREAKFASTS

Add zucchini or carrots to breakfast baked goods such as muffins. Try scrambling your eggs with minced broccoli or grated cauliflower. These additions don't change the texture of your eggs, and they give you your daily dose of anti-cancer cruciferous veggies. Try adding canned pumpkin puree to pancakes.

SMOOTHIES

Add extra greens to a fruit smoothie. A large bunch of raw spinach will wilt down to nothing and the taste is easily hidden if you add other naturally sweet ingredients, especially pineapple and banana.

SANDWICHES

Bulk up ground meat with carrot puree or chopped mushrooms. Or replace burgers with grilled portobello mushrooms. Choose Mexican-style tacos or quesadillas: Cut the cheese in half, and add lots of corn, onions, peppers, spinach, beans, and salsa.

SOUPS, STEWS, AND CASSEROLES

Thicken soup and add vegetables with pureed tomatoes, carrots, sweet potato, butternut

Janet Bond Brill, PhD, RDN, FAND registered dietitian nutritionist and nationally recognized nutrition, health and fitness expert who specializes in cardiovascular disease prevention. Dr. Brill is the author of *Intermittent Fasting for Dummies, Blood Pressure DOWN, Cholesterol DOWN*, and *Prevent a Second Heart Attack*. DrJanet.com

squash, beans, and greens. Add corn, extra tomatoes, onions, garlic, and peppers to chili. Cauliflower, pumpkin, butternut squash, and carrots are all excellent additions to macaroni and cheese. The colors blend with the traditional dish and provide a nice nutrition boost.

BAKED GOODS AND DESSERTS

Greens can be pureed and added into cake and brownie batter. Beets make a great addition to chocolate cake—the cocoa flavor disguises the beet's earthy flavor; plus the beets add sweetness. Sweet breads can be made using zucchini. Cookie batter does well with pureed pumpkin. Dark chocolate brownies taste great with added pureed beans.

SNACKS

Instead of potato chips, try making kale chips. You get all the crunch and a huge nutrition boost. Zucchini is an incredibly versatile, mild-tasting vegetable that can be transformed into a variety of snacks. Zucchini chips are super simple to make. Slice and season with salt,

pepper, and parmesan cheese; then bake in a hot oven until deeply golden and crisp.

PASTA SAUCE

Add canned pumpkin to pasta sauce for large amounts of vitamin A to sustain sharp eyesight, the antioxidant beta-carotene to fight cancer, and vitamin C to maintain a healthy immune system.

How to Eat Your Fruits and Veggies

Five produce servings a day are not enough to promote good health. The balance of fruits and vegetables also matters—and so do the specific items eaten. Two servings a day should include fruits with high levels of beta-carotene and vitamin C, such as berries and citrus fruits. The other three servings of produce should be vegetables—such as spinach, other leafy greens and carrots. Other starchy vegetables—including peas, corn and potatoes—are not associated with reduced risk for death or chronic diseases.

Study by researchers at Harvard Medical School and Brigham and Women's Hospital, both in Boston, published in Circulation.

Creamy Pumpkin Pasta Sauce

Ingredients...

- 1 tsp. of extra virgin olive oil
- 2 shallots, minced
- 3 cloves of garlic, minced
- 15 oz. can pumpkin purée
- 8 oz. cannellini beans
- 1 Tbsp. oregano
- 1 tsp. cracked black pepper
- 15 oz. low-sodium vegetable broth

Directions...

In a small saucepan, heat the olive oil over medium-low heat. Cook the shallots until soft and translucent (about 10 minutes). In a blender, add the cooked shallots and the rest of the ingredients in the recipe. Blend sauce until it is a smooth purée.

Yield: 8 servings (½ cup per serving).

Nutrition information per serving (pasta sauce only): *Calories:* 63 kcal, *Fat:* 1 g, *Cholesterol:* 0 mg, *Carbohydrate:* 12 g, *Dietary Fiber:* 3 g, *Protein:* 3 g, *Sodium:* 158 mg

---

When the Only Food Is Fast Food...

Joel Fuhrman, MD, board-certified family physician and expert on nutrition and natural healing. A seven-time New York Times *best-selling author, his books include* Fast Food Genocide: How Processed Food Is Killing Us and What We Can Do About It...Eat for Life...*and* Super Immunity. *He also runs the Eat To Live Retreat in San Diego. DrFuhrman.com*

Fast food is never good for you, but sometimes you just don't have a choice. When that happens, knowing the best options at the better restaurant chains means having a meal with the least negative impact on your health...and the least remorse about having to refuel this way.

Many fast-food restaurants still specialize in the equivalent of a heart attack on a bun (think double cheeseburger with bacon), but more progressive chains such as Panera and Starbucks have made improvements to their menus for both their customers' health and the environment. All fast-food chains post nutrition information on every menu choice on their websites, and many, such as Chipotle, allow you to customize their offerings—eliminating cheese, for instance, and doubling up on veggies. It's easy when you order on the restaurant's website or app, and making your selections in advance rules out any last-minute temptation—but also keep these guidelines in mind when you visit in person.

MAKE-IT-HEALTHIER GUIDELINES

When you can, the best choice is to head for a salad bar, freestanding or perhaps within a supermarket, where you can create your own meal. Search the Internet for salad bar locations when you're close to home or traveling. *But if you must go to a chain restaurant…*

•**Look up nutritional information before making your selections.**

Example: At Chick-fil-A, a packet of Light Italian Dressing has 25 calories while Zesty Apple Cider Vinaigrette has 230 and Avocado Lime Ranch has 310.

•**Choose healthful beans and bean-based menu items instead of meat options whenever possible.**

Example: A bean burrito with avocado and salsa (skip the sour cream) is tasty and filling.

•**Avoid special sauces and salad dressings,** particularly those made with mayonnaise or soybean/canola vegetable oils. Look for olive oil and vinegar or dressings with a base of tahini, avocado, nuts or tomato. Or opt for a plant-based salsa—a nutritional powerhouse naturally low in fat and cholesterol-free…it makes a great topping for almost anything.

•**Avoid foods prepared with toxic cooking methods**—char-broiling, flame-broiling, barbecuing and deep-frying all use high heat, which contributes to the formation of harmful compounds called advanced glycation end products (AGEs). The best choice is

baked, and lightly grilled is better than flame-broiled. Soups, stews and vegan or beef chilis are good choices because they're made with water-based cooking methods, which limits AGEs. Avoid deep-fried fillets. Instead, opt for sashimi or sushi (order rolls with crab stick and cooked fish or veggie rolls with lots of avocado if you're concerned about the freshness of raw fish).

•**Order platters instead of white-bread/ roll sandwiches.** Unless specifically whole-wheat flour, eating foods made with white flour is like eating sugar because they're absorbed so rapidly.

•**Have fresh fruit for dessert,** instead of pies and tarts laden with artificial ingredients and unhealthy fats and sugars.

Caution: Frozen yogurt can have a surprising amount of sugar.

ON THE MENU

Go with these healthier options at the following popular fast-food restaurants…

•**Panera.**

Breakfast: Fresh fruit, steel-cut oatmeal and Greek yogurt parfaits…or an egg-based baked Spinach and Artichoke Soufflé with red peppers and artichoke hearts.

Lunch and dinner: A wide array of salads with healthy ingredients, including the Mediterranean Bowl with Chicken…and the Baja Bowl with brown rice, quinoa, black bean and corn salsa, and assorted vegetables.

Another option: Slow-cooked All-Natural Turkey Chili with chickpeas and kidney beans, tomatillos and tomatoes. Panera also is known for its soups, such as the hearty Ten Vegetable Soup and the Autumn Squash Soup.

•**Starbucks.**

Breakfast: Variations on oatmeal such as Hearty Blueberry Oatmeal and Strawberry Overnight Grains with oatmeal, quinoa and chia seeds…or a Spinach, Feta and Egg White Wrap made with cage-free egg whites in a whole-wheat wrap. Avoid the baked goods.

Lunch: Chicken & Quinoa Protein Bowl with Black Beans and Greens…the plant-based Chickpea Bites & Avocado Protein Box with snap peas, mini carrots, dried cranberry and nut mix.

For the ease of a sandwich: Antibiotic-free Turkey & Pesto Panini on a ciabatta roll.

•Chipotle.

Chipotle's menu is built on bean-based offerings that can be customized.

Examples: With the Burrito Bowls, you can request extra beans (black and pinto), fajita vegetables (peppers and onions) and guacamole. The Lifestyle Bowls build on greens and guacamole and offer a Keto option, too. Add steak, chicken or pork if you're a meat eater and want the protein, or check out the vegan or vegetarian options. There's both white and brown rice.

•Chick-fil-A.

Breakfast: Healthier morning fare is limited to the fruit cup or Greek yogurt parfait.

Lunch or dinner: Grilled chicken comes as no-utensils-needed nuggets, a fillet and slices in salads such as the Spicy Southwest Salad with roasted corn, black beans, poblano chiles and red bell peppers…and the Market Salad with blue cheese, red and green apples, and berries. (Avoid the breaded versions of chicken.)

Also: Traditional Cobb salad…and the Cool Wrap—a flaxseed-flour flatbread filled with grilled chicken breast, green leaf lettuce and Jack and Cheddar cheeses.

•Subway.

Stories of no tuna in Subway's tuna sandwiches sparked a lot of news, but the company maintains that its tuna is real and even wild-caught. And it is a better choice than Subway's processed deli meat sandwiches.

Even better: Recently added items such as slow-roasted turkey and rotisserie-style chicken. You can order them in a protein bowl loaded with vegetables or on the multigrain bread made with whole grains, rye, cracked wheat, oats and seeds.

For vegetarians: Veggie Delite wrap. A great add-in is "smashed avocado"—just avocado and sea salt.

•Taco Bell.

Not necessarily known for healthy fare, Taco Bell has bean-based offerings that can be customized—order the bean burrito loaded with tomatoes, lettuce, black beans and jalapeño peppers, for instance…or put together your own combo of guacamole and a side serving of black beans with rice and onions.

•Wendy's.

The chain offers mostly burgers, but two of its fresh-made salads—the Southwest Avocado Salad and the Apple Pecan Salad—are built around grilled chicken.

•McDonald's.

Breakfast: Fruit and Maple Oatmeal with whole-grain oats, diced apples and a cranberry-raisin blend (there's no actual maple in it, but light cream and brown sugar).

Lunch or dinner: A plain hamburger (skip the bun)—far better than the various crispy chicken sandwiches.

Note: That chicken patty is not pure chicken—it contains flour, oil and more than a dozen other ingredients.

Fast-food places to avoid: KFC…Burger King for anything other than a plain hamburger …Popeyes…and In-N-Out Burger.

Intermittent Fasting: Eat Less, Get Healthier, Live Longer

Janet Bond Brill, PhD, RDN, FAND registered dietitian nutritionist and nationally recognized nutrition, health and fitness expert who specializes in cardiovascular disease prevention. Dr. Brill is the author of *Intermittent Fasting for Dummies, Blood Pressure DOWN, Cholesterol DOWN,* and *Prevent a Second Heart Attack.* DrJanet.com

---

What's all the buzz about intermittent fasting providing health and longevity benefits? Is there scientific proof that a program of intermittent fasting can help prevent disease and even help us live longer? The answer is a resounding yes. A review article recently published in the prestigious *New England Journal of Medicine* revealed that intermittent fasting has many health benefits.

WHAT EXACTLY IS INTERMITTENT FASTING?

Years ago, scientists discovered that mice put on a low-calorie diet or caloric restriction (CR) lived longer and were healthier than mice on a regular diet. Intermittent fasting is a remake and much more palatable form of fasting that consists of repetitive, short-term fasts. Methods of intermittent fasting dictate when you eat rather than what you eat. There are a variety of recommended strategies, but one of the most popular is the 16:8 method, which stands for 16 hours of fasting and eight hours of eating each day. You may eat breakfast at 8 a.m. and finish your final meal of the day by 4 p.m. and abstain from any foods or drinks with calories until 8 a.m. the next morning. Or you may eat your first meal at noon and finish by 8 p.m., not eating again until noon.

EFFECTS ON THE BODY

Once you're done eating for the day, the body transitions into a fasted state and the liver converts fat into ketones for use as fuel. The phenomenon is called the metabolic switch, which affects two important hormones: insulin and norepinephrine. Insulin levels increase when you eat and decrease dramatically when you fast. Lower levels of insulin increase fat burning. (Long-lived people tend to have unusually low insulin levels.)

Numerous additional health benefits that have been associated with intermittent fasting include improved cellular stress response to free-radical damage; reduced inflammation and oxidative stress; improved markers of cardiovascular disease such as blood pressure, resting heart rate, and levels of high-density and low-density lipoprotein (HDL and LDL) cholesterol, triglycerides, glucose, and insulin; and prevention and treatment of autoimmune diseases such as arthritis, asthma, and multiple sclerosis. Intermittent fasting can also promote brain health by enhancing production of a protein called brain-derived neurotrophic factor, a substance that prevents stressed neurons from dying.

GET STARTED

If you'd like to try intermittent fasting, first get your doctor's go-ahead and stock up on plenty of fruits and vegetables, lean meats, nuts, and seeds to follow a healthful plant-based Mediterranean dietary plan during your eating hours. Set your eating window for the time that works best for you. If you wake up hungry, set an early window. If nighttime hunger is a problem, move your eating window later so you can eat when you are most hungry. To stave off hunger in your fasting periods, drink plenty of calorie-free liquids and keep busy with hobbies and exercise. Also, remember that it takes about a month for your body to adjust to fasting.

5:2 Diet Plan Is an Easier "Sell"

Individuals with obesity who participated in a weight-loss program were given instructions for either a traditional weight-management diet and exercise...or the 5:2 diet, which involves two nonconsecutive days a week of calorie restriction and five days of sensible eating. Both groups lost about the same amount of weight—15% of participants in the standard group and 18% in the 5:2 group lost at least 5% of body weight in a year. But those on the 5:2 diet said they were more likely to recommend that approach to others and were more willing to continue the diet after the study ended. Researchers suggest that at least some of the appeal of the 5:2 plan is that it can be explained briefly, which makes it seem less complicated.

Study of 300 adults with obesity by researchers at Queen Mary University, London, England, published in PLOS ONE.

Why You Still Feel Hungry After Eating

If you frequently have the munchies soon after a meal, here are likely reasons. *Not enough protein*—a high-protein meal helps you feel fuller than a high-carb or high-fat meal. *Not enough fiber*—fiber takes longer to digest than other carbs and slows your stomach's emptying rate. *Not enough volume*—"stretch receptors" in your stomach sense how much you've eaten. Vegetables, chicken breast and turkey are good high-volume/low-calorie choices. *Eating too quickly or while distracted*—not chewing thoroughly and not focusing on your eating make you feel less full. *Leptin resistance*—your brain may have trouble recognizing the hormone that signals fullness. Plentiful sleep and exercise helps, but see a doctor if you suspect this is the problem.

HealthLine.com

Selenium Protects Against Weight Gain

Mice fed high-fat diets lived longer and were less obese if their diet included selenium. The selenium group also showed physiological benefits similar to consuming a vegan diet. Selenium is known to decrease gut inflammation, which contributes to weight gain.

Food sources of selenium: Nuts, fish, beef and poultry. Selenium supplements also are available. The safe upper daily limit for selenium is 400 micrograms.

Andrew Rubman, ND, medical director of Southbury Clinic for Traditional Medicines, Southbury, Connecticut, commenting on a study by researchers at Orentreich Foundation for the Advancement of Science.

Turmeric: The Anti-Inflammatory Spice

Janet Bond Brill, PhD, RDN, FAND registered dietitian nutritionist and nationally recognized nutrition, health and fitness expert who specializes in cardiovascular disease prevention. Dr. Brill is the author of *Intermittent Fasting for Dummies, Blood Pressure DOWN, Cholesterol DOWN,* and *Prevent a Second Heart Attack.* DrJanet.com

Turmeric has been used in India for thousands of years as both a spice and medicinal herb. It lends both flavor and rich color to dishes like curries, and, thanks to a compound called curcumin, provides a sol-

id dose of anti-inflammatory and antioxidant effects, too. *Here are some of its promising health benefits…*

•**Alzheimer's disease and brain cancer.** Curcumin can cross the blood-brain barrier and has been shown to help battle the disease process of both Alzheimer's disease and brain cancer. Curcumin can disrupt the brain plaques that are the hallmark of Alzheimer's disease, and it can inhibit the growth of malignant brain tumor cells.

•**Arthritis.** Because of its anti-inflammatory properties, turmeric has shown promise for easing the joint pain and stiffness associated with both osteoarthritis and rheumatoid arthritis.

•**Irritable bowel syndrome (IBS).** Some research has demonstrated that turmeric can help improve symptoms of IBS, such as abdominal pain. It is also being studied as a treatment for other inflammatory bowel diseases like Crohn's and ulcerative colitis.

•**Type 2 diabetes.** Turmeric has been shown to help fight inflammation and keep blood sugar levels steady.

Studies have shown that just 50 mg of curcumin, consumed over a three-month period, provides significant health benefits. But while curcumin makes up just 3% of turmeric, it is best not to consume curcumin by itself, as it is very poorly absorbed. Instead, use the whole spice and add black pepper, which contains a compound called piperine. This natural substance has been shown to increase the absorption of curcumin by 2,000%.

One caveat, turmeric contains oxalates, which can increase the risk of kidneys stones. Turmeric may also interfere with the action of drugs that decrease stomach acid. Consult your physician if you have these conditions.

Tofu Scramble with Turmeric

2 Tbsp. extra virgin olive oil

7 oz. soft tofu

½ tsp. ground turmeric

½ cup egg substitute

½ tsp. salt-free seasoning blend

⅛ tsp. black pepper

½ avocado, cubed

½ cup grape tomatoes, quartered

In a large non-stick skillet, heat oil over medium-high heat. Pat the tofu dry with a paper towel, and then crumble into the skillet. Sprinkle with turmeric. Cook, stirring gently, until most of the moisture is cooked out of the tofu, about four minutes.

Meanwhile, in a bowl whisk together the egg substitute, salt-free seasoning blend, and pepper. Set aside.

When the tofu appears dry, reduce the heat to medium. Pour the reserved eggs over the tofu. Cook, stirring occasionally for about two minutes until set. Divide between two plates and serve with avocado and tomatoes.

Makes 2 servings.

Nutrition per Serving: *Calories:* 208, S*odium:* 95 mg, *Potassium:* 523 mg, *Magnesium:* 45 mg, *Calcium:* 120 mg, *Fat:* 15 g, *Saturated fat:* 2 g, *Cholesterol:* 0 mg, *Carbohydrate:* 9 g, *Dietary fiber:* 4 g, *Sugars:* 1 g, *Protein:* 13 g.

Do You Really Need That Supplement?

Renee Miranda, MD, DABMA, ETSU Health provider, assistant professor of family medicine, integrative medicine and medical acupuncture at East Tennessee State University, Johnson City, Tennessee. She also is an emergency medicine physician with SCP Health in Smyth County and Russell County, Virginia.

According to the Centers for Disease Control and Prevention (CDC), 58% of US adults report taking a dietary supplement in the past 30 days…and one-quarter of people age 60 and older take four or more daily. In fact, Americans spent nearly $60 billion on dietary supplements in 2020 alone.

There was a time when swallowing handfuls of supplements was seen among older adults as evidence of their dedication to a healthy lifestyle. But we now know that people who consume a balanced diet and are in good health are likely getting all the nutrients they need.

Still, some supplements can fill in nutritional gaps for people who have food allergies…eat lots of junk food and eschew healthy produce…or avoid entire categories of food—picky eaters, vegans or people who skip, say, soy or dairy products because they fear they're unhealthy (they're not).

We asked integrative medicine specialist Renee Miranda, MD, who should be taking supplements…and which ones.

DO YOU NEED A SUPPLEMENT?

When a patient asks me about supplementation, my first two questions are, "What does your diet look like?" and "What is your goal?"

What does your diet look like?

A varied diet rich in whole foods such as fruits, vegetables, beans and legumes, grains, dairy and protein provides all the required nutrients, so theoretically the only people who need supplementation are those with gaps in their diets.

To evaluate your diet: Keep a food log for three consecutive days, including at least one weekend day. Note portion sizes and preparation methods. This log can give you and your doctor an idea of any nutrient gaps.

To improve your diet, a good place to start is the American Heart Association recommendations (Heart.org). I recommend six to nine servings of fruits and vegetables daily… two to three servings of quality protein mainly from plant sources such as legumes (if you prefer animal products, lean toward unprocessed meats)…one to three servings of whole grains…and an occasional serving of nuts and seeds.

What is your goal?

Some people want to improve their heart health, and they have read that a supplement might help…or they have been told that multivitamins boost overall wellness. New research is constantly emerging about whether certain supplements live up to the hype. Oftentimes, they don't.

A 2018 meta-analysis in *Journal of the American College of Cardiology* determined that supplementing with a multivitamin, vitamin D, calcium or vitamin C does not significantly reduce risk for heart attack or stroke or of dying from any cause. Also, supplementing with large amounts of certain antioxidants—found naturally in fruits and vegetables—may work *against* your goals by increasing risk for certain types of cancer or chronic diseases. This may be because some fat-soluble vitamins—such as A, D, E and K—are stored in the body for long periods and can accumulate to toxic levels when taken in large doses. And new research suggests that high doses of supplemental antioxidants may even protect cancer cells from the body's natural cancer-fighting process.

There are, however, instances when supplements make sense.

Example: Many older adults are deficient in vitamin B-12, especially those who regularly take acid-suppressing medication, such as *esomeprazole* (Nexium), *omprasole* (Prilosec) and *lansoprazole* (Prevacid). Vitamin B-12 is critical for healthy functioning of the brain and nervous system.

WHICH SUPPLEMENTS SHOULD YOU TAKE?

Here are the supplements that I recommend for certain patients and why...and how to get the most out of them...

•**Vitamin D** does everything from boost calcium absorption from foods (crucial for bone strength) to strengthen the immune system. Yet nearly one-half of Americans are deficient.

Reasons: Vitamin D isn't found in many foods besides oily fish such as salmon, fortified milk and juice, and UV-B-light–boosted mushrooms...we spend so much time indoors (depriving our skin of sunlight, which the body needs to produce vitamin D)...and when we are outside, we use sunscreen.

Also: Older adults, people with obesity, darker-skinned individuals and people living in colder, grayer climates are at increased risk for deficiency.

What to do: Ask your health-care provider for a blood test to assess your vitamin D level. If it is low, the doctor may recommend 400 international units (IU) to 600 IU daily...or a 50,000-IU pill weekly for four weeks. If your level is around 40 ng/mL—the lower end of normal—and you feel tired, that also suggests supplementation may be useful.

Encouraging: New research shows that older people in China who maintain healthy

vitamin D levels had less cognitive impairment and healthier lipid levels than their deficient counterparts.

Note: Vitamin D is fat-soluble—it needs to be combined with a little fat to be absorbed. Swallow the supplement with a plant-based source of fat such as avocado or some almonds, walnuts or other nuts and seeds. Vitamin D also needs magnesium to be activated, so get enough of this mineral.

•**Vitamin B-12.** As you age, the stomach produces less and less *hydrochloric acid*, a compound needed to absorb B-12 from food. For the same reason, people taking acid-reducing medications may have lower levels of B-12.

Vegans (people who eat no animal products) and some vegetarians (people who don't eat meat) may need supplemental B-12 because B-12 is available only in animal products or fortified foods such as breakfast cereal and nutritional yeast. Individuals with celiac disease or Crohn's disease also may be deficient because their gut doesn't absorb the nutrient efficiently from food.

The average adult needs 2.4 micrograms (mcg) of vitamin B-12 a day. Supplements contain about 1,000 mcg to 2,000 mcg—so you'll need to supplement only a few times a week. Any excess will be excreted in your urine. Ask your doctor for guidance.

•**Magnesium.** About half the US population is magnesium-deficient, yet this mineral has a hand in dozens of bodily systems. It promotes regular bowel movements, calms anxiety, promotes sleep and more. Magnesium also converts food into energy, so low levels can cause fatigue.

Foods high in magnesium: Nuts, seeds, beans, whole grains, leafy green veggies and some fortified foods.

Adults absorb less magnesium as they grow older. People with type 2 diabetes lose magnesium in their urine, and certain medications can reduce magnesium levels. These include bisphosphonates such as *alendronate* (Fosamax) for osteoporosis...loop diuretics such as *furosemide* (Lasix) for high blood pressure...

and prescription proton pump inhibitors such as *esomeprazole* (Nexium).

A blood test can check for magnesium deficiency, but there's little risk from supplementing. These supplements come in different forms, including *magnesium citrate* (recommended for constipation) and *magnesium chloride* (better suited for sleep and anxiety). Start with 200 mg a day, and see if symptoms improve. You can slowly move up to 400 mg/day. Toxicity symptoms at higher doses or due to inability to eliminate excess magnesium (common among people with kidney disease) include gastrointestinal upset, flushing, weakness and palpitations.

Warning: Start low, and go slow—magnesium citrate supplements can have a laxative effect. If you take any of the previously mentioned medications, space them several hours apart from your supplement.

Avocados Reduce Dangerous Belly Fat in Women

It is difficult to lose visceral fat, the deep belly fat that surrounds inner organs and raises risk for diabetes.

Recent finding: Overweight and obese women who consumed a daily meal that included one fresh avocado showed a reduction in abdominal fat and improvement in the ratio of visceral fat to subcutaneous fat, indicating that fat was redistributed away from the inner organs. A similar group of women who ate a similar daily meal equal in nutrition and calories that did not include avocado had no change in abdominal or visceral fat...nor did men in the study, regardless of whether they ate avocados.

Study by researchers at University of Illinois at Urbana-Champaign, published in *Journal of Nutrition*.

Skin Nutrition: What to Eat to Keep the Glow

Janet Bond Brill, PhD, RDN, FAND registered dietitian nutritionist and nationally recognized nutrition, health and fitness expert who specializes in cardiovascular disease prevention. Dr. Brill is the author of *Intermittent Fasting for Dummies, Blood Pressure DOWN, Cholesterol DOWN*, and *Prevent a Second Heart Attack*. DrJanet.com

Scientists are increasingly learning more about the relationship between diet, skin health and aging. *Let's look at the top foods known to contribute to better skin from the inside out...*

1. Avocado. Avocados are chock full of healthy monounsaturated fat, which the skin needs to stay supple and moisturized. Avocados also are a good source of vitamins E and C, two of the most important antioxidants for your body. Both vitamins are involved in creating new, healthy skin. Some research links antioxidant compounds in avocado with preventing UV sun damage, thereby warding off wrinkles and premature aging.

2. Fatty fish. Salmon, tuna, halibut and herring are full of omega-3. A deficiency of this "good" fat has been shown to cause extremely dry skin, illustrating the necessity of getting this type of fat to keep skin flexible and moisturized. The high-quality protein content in fish contributes to the strength and creation of new, healthy cells. The exceptional amount of omega-3 fat, zinc, and vitamin E in fatty fish tame inflammation—a key cause of skin disorders and wrinkles.

3. Walnuts. Walnuts are packed with the plant version of omega-3 fat called ALA. Walnuts contain a nice cache of vitamins and minerals such as vitamin E, selenium, and zinc. These nutrients help the skin heal, and they fight off bacteria and inflammation, creating a natural defense system that contributes to clearer, smoother skin. Try the walnut encrusted salmon recipe on the next page to get a double dose of skin-healthy nutrients.

4. Soy. Soy contains a plant chemical called isoflavones, which can either block or mimic estrogen in the body. Research has shown that consuming soy daily improves wrinkles and skin elasticity. In postmenopausal women, regular soy consumption has been shown to improve skin dryness and increase the collagen content, leading to smoother, stronger skin.

Take care of the largest organ in the body from the inside with a nutritious diet and from the outside by routinely using a good sunblock to prevent UV damage.

Walnut Encrusted Salmon

Ingredients…

3 cloves of garlic
¾ cup walnuts
½ cup fresh cilantro
2 Tbsp. extra virgin olive oil
4 wild salmon fillets (about 6 oz. each)
1 tsp. kosher salt
¼ tsp. freshly ground pepper
Fresh lemon slices for garnish

Directions…

Preheat oven to 450°F. Mince the garlic in a food processor. Add in the walnuts and process to a fine consistency. Add cilantro until mixture is thick and pasty. Add olive oil and process until blended. Place salmon on a foil-lined baking tray and season both sides with salt and pepper. Spread the walnut mixture evenly over the fish. Bake for 20 minutes or until fish flakes easily with a fork. Garnish with lemon slices.

Yield: 4 servings (*serving size:* 1 salmon filet)

Nutritional Information Per Serving (1 salmon filet): *Calories:* 456, *Fat:* 32 g, *Cholesterol:* 94 mg, *Sodium:* 658 mg, *Carbohydrate:* 4 g, *Dietary Fiber:* 2 g, *Sugars:* 0 g, *Protein:* 37 g

---

Coffee Makes Sweets Taste Sweeter

Researchers tested the taste sensitivity of 156 subjects before and after they drank coffee.

Result: Participants reported increased sensitivity to sweetness and blunted sensitivity to bitterness after consuming either regular or decaf, thanks to the bitter substances found in coffee.

Wise: If you've been trying to switch to dark chocolate to reap its health benefits but can't handle its bitterness, eating it as you sip coffee might get you over the hump.

Alexander Wieck Fjældstad, MD, associate professor of clinical medicine, Aarhus University, Holstebro, Denmark, and leader of a study published in *Foods.*

Effective Ways to Halt Sugar Cravings

Eat *well-balanced meals*—the desire for sugar often is because some important food component, such as protein or fiber, is deficient in your diet. *Do not skip meals*—that causes the body to need fuel quickly and so it may crave sugar. *Stay well-hydrated*—the body sometimes misinterprets thirst as a sugar craving. *Avoid high-salt foods*—they can trigger a desire for sweetness to balance the salt. *Figure out the reason for the craving*—it often is emotional or habitual. Try to determine if you tend to want sweets when you are unhappy or bored or upset, and then find ways to deal with the underlying feeling. *Give in to the craving, and then move on*—if you really want some chocolate or ice cream, have a modest amount and go on with your day. Trying to deflect the craving or restrict what you eat only makes the desire stronger.

Roundup of nutritionists and dietitians reported at EatThis.com.

Drink Without Derailing Your Diet

Rachel Beller, MS, RDN, founder of Beller Nutrition, based in Culver City, California. She is a spokesperson for the American Cancer Society, and creator of the *Beller Method 8-week Transformation Masterclass.* BellerNutrition.com

---

A glass of wine with dinner or a cocktail when out with friends doesn't have to undermine otherwise healthy eating habits.

Summer Ginger Zinger

This summer cocktail is low calorie, sneaks in nutritional value, and is delicious.

    1½ oz. vodka
    3 oz. soda water
    2 Tbsp. pomegranate juice
    1 tsp. 100% pure ginger juice
    Squeeze of lime
    Mix and pour over ice.
Serves one.

Per serving: 115 calories, 0 g total fat, 0 g saturated fat, 0 g protein, 4 g carbs, 4 g sugar, 0 g fiber, 0 g cholesterol, 14 mg sodium

Source: Recipe courtesy of Rachel Beller, RDN

Virgin Mojito

Try this mocktail recipe when you want a festive drink, but not the alcohol or extra calories.

    6 cups soda water
    2 Tbsp. lime juice
    15 ice cubes
    1 cup fresh mint leaves
    1 Tbsp. pure maple syrup
    Mix in a large pitcher.
Serves four.

Per serving: 14 calories, 0 g total fat, 0 g sat fat, 0 g protein, 4 g carbs, 3 g sugar, 0 g fiber, 0 g cholesterol, 47 mg sodium

Source: Recipe courtesy of Rachel Beller, RDN

If you're watching your calories, it can be confusing to choose the best option: Should you stick to a glass of wine? Have a light beer? Or try a spiked seltzer or seemingly healthy fancy cocktail?

WINE

Whether you choose white, red, or rose, a 5-ounce glass of wine contains about 100 to 130 calories. Watch out for port wines or sweet dessert wines, which can contain up to 300 calories in the same serving.

Best choice: Go red. Because many of the healthful compounds are found in the grape skin, red wine contains more of the beneficial plant compounds found in those skins, such as resveratrol. Resveratrol contains antioxidant and anti-inflammatory properties, which help reduce heart disease risk, increase HDL "good" cholesterol levels, and slow age-related mental decline.

BEER

Whether it is a pale ale, a lager, a stout, or other type, beer generally contains about 150 calories in a 12-ounce can or bottle. In a bar or restaurant, a pour may be a larger 16-ounce pint.

Best choice: If what really quenches your thirst on a hot day is a nice cold beer, consider choosing a light beer. The calories in a 12-ounce serving typically range from about 50 to 100 calories. Squeeze in a little lime, lemon, or orange for a small shot of vitamin C.

HARD SELTZER

These popular canned drinks, such as Truly and White Claw, are made with brewed cane sugar and/or malted rice, with added soda water and flavorings. A typical 12-ounce can contains about 100 calories. Some hard seltzers contain real fruit juice, but it is not enough for any nutritional benefit.

Best choice: If you want to enjoy this fruity option, feel free to choose your favorite flavored hard seltzer, but don't overdo it. They are easy to overdrink.

LIQUOR

A 1.5-ounce (shot glass) serving of gin, rum, vodka, tequila, or whiskey is 100 calories. The mixers you choose, however, can quickly add up. For instance, 4 ounces of orange juice will add nearly 60 calories, and many sodas, such as Coke or Sprite, have about 45 to 50 calories in the same amount. A mojito or margarita on the rocks can be as low as 150 calories, but a pina colada, daiquiri, or other frozen drink can pack as many as 500 calories into one drink.

Best choice: If you crave a cocktail, pick no-calorie mixers such as fruit-flavored sparkling water, club soda, or plain sparkling water.

To add some flavor, squeeze in a little lime or lemon. To pack a nutritional punch, try a splash of pomegranate juice, which adds flavor plus the cancer-fighting compound ellagic acid, with few calories. Or consider a teaspoon of 100% ginger juice, which contains anti-nausea and anti-inflammatory properties.

Switch to a Vegetarian Diet the Easy Way

Start slow—swap one meat serving for vegetables this week, two next week, etc. *Beans are your friends*—they're filling, packed with fiber and protein, and great substitutes for ground beef or chicken. *Eat whole, unrefined grains*—don't overload on empty carbs just because they're meatless...instead choose farro, buckwheat and oats, which have high amounts of vitamins, protein and fiber. *Don't worry about protein*—a varied vegetarian diet will deliver all the proteins and amino acids you need because nuts, grains, beans and everyday vegetables all have protein. *Use supplements as needed*—most vegetarians are low on iron and vitamin B-12, which are easily supplied by supplements.

Roundup of dietitians reported on Shape.com.

Copious Protein Doesn't Build Extra Muscle

The Recommended Dietary Allowance for protein is about 0.36 grams of protein per pound of body weight per day (about 56 grams for the average man, 46 grams for the average woman). In a study of 50 weight-lifting novices ages 40 to 64, those on a high-protein diet saw no benefit in strength or body composition after 10 weeks of training versus those on a moderate-protein diet.

Nicholas Burd, PhD, associate professor of kinesiology at University of Illinois at Urbana-Champaign and leader of a study published in *American Journal of Physiology: Endocrinology and Metabolism*.

Limitations of BMI

William Yancy, MD, associate professor of medicine, Duke University School of Medicine, and medical director of the Duke Lifestyle & Weight Management Center.

Body mass index (BMI) has become the most commonly used measurement to assess the relative healthiness of one's weight.

It delineates where normal weight crosses into overweight, and where obesity—and its associated health risks—begins. But taken as a single measure, its accuracy and validity can vary widely.

BMI BASICS

BMI is calculated as (weight in kilograms [kg]) / (height in meters [m] squared). Ideal BMI is between 18.5 kg/m^2 and 25 kg/m^2 (BMI is usually written without the unit of measure). A person with a BMI between 25 and 30 is considered overweight, and a person with a BMI 30 or over is considered obese. Generally, people with higher BMIs have a higher risk of diabetes, arthritis, fatty liver disease, hypertension, some cancers, high cholesterol, and sleep apnea.

Studies show that BMI can accurately reflect the health risks of obesity at high levels (over 30), but is less reliable in the overweight (25 to 30) category. That's because BMI only represents weight by height. It doesn't differentiate between lean and fat mass. A weightlifter or athlete, for example, could be very lean and muscular but show a high BMI because of overall weight.

Further, BMI doesn't take into account the location of fat. Visceral (or belly) fat is associated with more health risks than higher fat in other parts of the body. The value of BMI has also been questioned in older adults because height and body composition change as we age.

Even one's ethnicity can affect the validity of BMI. Asians have higher health risks at substantially lower BMI levels, so different risk cutoffs are used. In addition, studies have shown that at the same BMI, people who are

Body-Fat Scales

Scales that use bioelectric impedance are widely available and inexpensive. They send a small electric current through the body and measure the resistance. (The current faces more resistance passing through body fat than it does passing through lean body mass and water.) These measurements can be affected by hydration, so be careful hanging your hat on one measurement. Following a trend may be more useful.

African American have lower levels of body fat than those who are Caucasian.

OTHER MEASURES TO CONSIDER

• **Waist size.** The National Institutes of Health concluded that a waist larger than 40 inches for men and 35 inches for women increases the chances of developing heart disease, cancer, or other chronic diseases. Waist measurement is fairly easy to use, but there is less information available about race/ethnic variations.

• **Waist to hip ratio.** You can also take your waist measurement and divide it by your hip measurement to get a waist-to-hip ratio. According to the World Health Organization, a healthy result is 0.9 or less in men and 0.85 or less for women. Waist-to-hip ratio is not substantially more accurate at determining risk than waist size alone but is more difficult to interpret.

• **Relative fat mass index (RFM).** Researchers at Cedars Mount Sinai developed a formula to compare height and waist circumference…

Men: 64 - (20 x height/waist circumference) = RFM

Women: 76 - (20 x height/waist circumference) = RFM

Men who score over 30 and women who score over 40 would be considered obese and at elevated risk for health problems and even death.

Core Curriculum: 5 Pilates Exercises to Maintain Strength and Vitality Forever

Erica Christ, founder/owner of EC Wellness in Port Chester, New York. Erica is a fully certified, advanced Pilates instructor, exercise physiologist, health and fitness instructor certified through the American College of Sports Medicine, certified diabetes educator (CDE) and registered dietitian (RD). EricaChrist.com

If you want to be able to turn around in your car and grab something in the back seat without throwing out your back…if you want to be able to pick up a heavy, over-sized box without getting hurt…if you want to keep doing all the things you were able to do when you were 20 years old when you reach 90, consider taking up a Pilates routine at home.

The Pilates method is an excellent form of low-impact exercise to strengthen the multitude of muscles that surround the spine, from the top of your neck to the tip of your tailbone. In addition, Pilates can improve posture and balance to help protect your body from falling and other injuries.

CORE PRINCIPLES OF PILATES

Pilates, developed by Joseph Pilates, a German physical trainer, in the 1920s, often is associated with the use of large pieces of studio equipment with bars, straps and springs that create resistance. But you can also do Pilates exercises at home using just a thick padded mat.

The Pilates philosophy has evolved substantially beyond Joseph Pilates' original concept of using movement to help people heal their bodies from injury. Today, there is a distinct intellectual component to the practice of Pilates, in which participants are encouraged to continuously think about their body alignment as they do each exercise to ensure proper movement and avoid further injury. *The core Pilates principles…*

• **Centering.** All Pilates movements start from and are sustained through the Center, known as the core or Powerhouse. This is true even if you are working other muscle groups such as the arms or legs. Your Powerhouse includes all of your musculature from shoulder to shoulder and hip to hip, from the front to the back of the body.

•**Concentration.** With Pilates, the mind guides the body. Razorlike focus on what you are doing is essential to executing the exercises to their fullest benefit.

•**Precision.** To gain the most benefit from each exercise, you have to do them precisely. Pay attention to the form, structure and quality of your movements. If you are doing an exercise in the optimal manner, you don't need a lot of repetitions to tire the muscle.

•**Control.** Gravity must never be allowed to control the exercises. You can control gravity by moving slowly through the motion.

•**Breath.** Pilates breathing is about increasing your lung capacity, inhaling to increase oxygenation of muscles and exhaling to rid the body of stale air. By supplying fresh oxygen during an exercise, the muscles of the Powerhouse become stronger and more flexible.

•**Flow.** As you progress with your Pilates practice, your goal is to move continuously and gracefully from one exercise to the next.

ESSENTIAL EXERCISES

This powerful five-exercise workout takes a mere 15 minutes. It stretches and strengthens nearly every muscle in your body—all the muscles of the Powerhouse in your core as well as neck, legs and arms, glutes (buttocks) and inner thighs, hamstrings (back of the thighs) and hip flexors. It even massages the spine. Do the exercises at least once a week formally, but try to bring the principles of the practice into your everyday movement as often as possible. As explained above, do them slowly and thoughtfully with an emphasis on maintaining good form—keep your abdominal muscles pulled in and your spine lengthening rather than compressing. You don't want to increase repetitions…you want to enhance the effort by engaging the muscles with more depth and control. You may not feel like you're moving very much at first,

and that's OK. Your goal with each exercise is to fatigue your muscles without feeling pain—which could mean as few as five repetitions. If your muscles shake, that's also OK—it is a sign of painless fatiguing.

Helpful: Look online for a beginner Pilates mat class, or book a virtual session with an instructor to learn proper form so you do the exercises safely.

My favorite online resource: PilatesAnytime.com, $22 per month after a 15-day free trial.

If a move hurts, stop doing it—never try to work through pain. Part of the progression with Pilates is learning how to self-correct if something hurts. Meeting with an instructor also can help you learn how.

Warning: Yoga mats are too thin to cushion pressure points and protect the back.

Preferred mat: EcoWise ⅝-inch thick ($92.35 Aeromats.com).

1. HUNDRED

Lie on your mat, and center your body. Bring your knees into tabletop position (knees over your hips, shins parallel to the

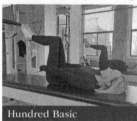
Hundred Basic

floor), and raise your head and neck up toward your knees. Be sure to raise your head and neck from your core and not by simply tucking your chin, which can put undo strain on your neck. Vigorously pump your arms up and down to above the level of your hips and then down to the floor while you inhale deeply for five counts and then exhale deeply for five counts up. Start with one to five repetitions, and work up to a max of 10 repetitions, which is 100 pumps.

Important: Inhale through your nose, exhale through your mouth as if you're breathing through a straw to support your upper body. If you feel neck strain, lower your head and neck a bit and continue the exercise. Count breaths, not hand pumps.

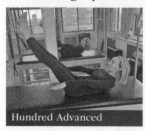
Hundred Advanced

To advance the movement: Perform the exercise with your legs straight, toes relaxed. The higher your legs, the more you support your back.

2. SINGLE LEG CIRCLES

Lie on your back on your mat, arms at your sides, palms down. Extend one leg up to the ceiling as high as you can. The bottom leg can

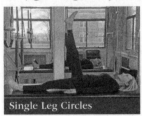
Single Leg Circles

be straight, or bend it to support the back and help straighten the lifted leg. Keep the knee soft, and push the heel of the lower leg gently into the mat to stabilize the hips. Start making a circle with your extended leg, staying within the frame of the body. Your goal is to keep the hips stable on the mat. Repeat five times, and then reverse the circle for five repetitions. Switch legs, and repeat on the other side.

To advance the movement: Straightening the bottom leg and/or increasing the diameter of the circle can both increase the challenge of this exercise, but you never want to go wider than your shoulders, and your hips always should stay on the mat.

3. ROLLING LIKE A BALL

Sit on your mat, knees bent, feet on the mat. Place your hands behind your knees, and lift your feet off the mat a few inches. With a

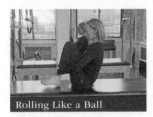
Rolling Like a Ball

small rhythmic rocking motion, gently roll back as far as feels comfortable and then come back up in a continuous flow. The motion drives from the abdominals. Keep your abdominal muscles pulled in and up. Inhale as you rock back, and exhale as you rock forward. Progress to rolling farther back toward the floor and back up again, keeping arms behind your knees.

To advance the movement: Hug your shins so your body is in a tighter ball. Repeat five to 10 times.

4. SINGLE LEG STRETCH

Lie on your mat, and bring your knees into your chest. Lift your head and shoulders off of the mat using your abdominal muscles rather

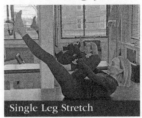
Single Leg Stretch

than your neck muscles to avoid straining your neck. Place both hands on one knee with your elbows out wide. Extend the other leg out at no more than a 45-degree angle while you continue to hug the knee toward your chest. Exhale and pull the extended leg toward your shoulder. Inhale and shift your hands, and extend the other leg. Exhale and pull the extended leg toward your shoulder. If your neck is compromised with lifting, keep your head on the mat. Repeat eight to 10 times for each leg.

To advance the movement: You can hold your position during your breath work and increase the movement flow.

5. SPINE STRETCH FORWARD

Sit up tall on your mat. Open your legs a bit wider than your mat, keeping your knees slightly bent and your feet flexed, so that the

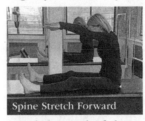
Spine Stretch Forward

heels are digging into the mat. Reach both of your arms forward at shoulder height and shoulder-width apart with your fingers stretching toward the end of the mat. The arms should be at shoulder height and parallel to the mat at all times during this exercise. Shoulders should remain neutral. Inhale and lift your spine. Exhale and curl your nose toward your naval and the top of your head toward the mat. Let the shoulders move naturally, and keep your lower back straight as you stretch forward—curl from your upper back and shoulder blades. Inhale as you roll back up to sitting tall. Exhale and repeat three to five times.

To advance the movement: Deepen your exhalation so it reaches further into the abdominals to deepen the stretch of the spine.

Afternoon Workouts Are Better for You

If you struggle to drag yourself out of bed for an early-morning workout, you can stop beating yourself up.

Recent finding: Of 32 men at risk for or who had type 2 diabetes, those who worked out between between 3:00 pm and 6:00 pm did better on tests of insulin sensitivity, body composition, weight loss and exercise performance than those who worked out between 8:00 am and 10:00 am.

Study by researchers at Maastricht University Medical Center, the Netherlands, published in *Physiological Reports*.

Try Tai Chi

Rudolph Tanzi, MD, Joseph P. and Rose F. Kennedy Professor of Neurology, Harvard Medical School, and Tara Stiles, founder of Strala Yoga, and author of *Clean Mind, Clean Body: A 28 Day Plan for Physical, Mental and Spiritual Self-Care*.

Tai chi is a gentle, low-impact exercise that involves a series of graceful movements accompanied by deep breathing. It is gentle enough for anyone, and research suggests that it offers substantial benefits.

• **Cognitive functioning.** A study led by Peter Wayne, PhD, a professor of medicine at Harvard Medical School, reported that tai chi shows potential to enhance cognitive function in older adults by improving attention and processing speed.

• **Osteoarthritis.** Tai chi can reduce pain and stiffness while increasing physical function. The American College of Rheumatology recommends it for osteoarthritis of the hip and knee.

• **Lung disease.** Several review articles reported that tai chi can improve asthma and chronic obstructive pulmonary disease, according to a report in *Canadian Family Physician*.

• **Stress relief.** The exercise can also promote the relaxation response, which can help lower blood pressure, heart rate, breathing rate, oxygen consumption, adrenaline levels, and levels of the stress hormone cortisol.

GIVE IT A TRY

All of these benefits are pretty impressive for an exercise that won't cause you to break a sweat. *Here are a few simple exercises you can try at home…*

• **Breathing exercise for relaxation.** Sit or stand comfortably. Close your eyes and relax your knees, elbows, and shoulders. Remain soft and moveable. Imagine that if someone nudged you gently, you would sway like a tree in the wind. Stay in this state for a moment before taking a single, deep breath through your nose. Notice your body lifting up and expanding with your inhalation. Exhale through your mouth and notice your body relaxing downward. Repeat this breathing twice more. Notice how your body moves after your breath. The movement follows the breath. Keep your eyes closed. How does your body feel? Softer? Do you feel tension anywhere? Take note. When you're ready, gently open your eyes.

• **Movement exercise.** Stand comfortably, with your knees, elbows, and shoulders soft. Let your arms hang by your sides. Move your hips from side to side, letting your arms sway gently like windshield wipers. Let your breath guide your motions.

• **Touch the sky.** Sit up straight in a comfortable chair. Place your hands in your lap, palms up. Take a slow, deep breath and raise your hands in front of you to chest level. Then turn your palms outward and lift your hands above your head. Keep your elbows soft. As you exhale slowly and deeply, lower your arms to your sides.

TAI CHI SEQUENCES

Tai chi instructors create routines that combine a variety of gentle movements with fanciful names, such as Grasp the Bird's Tail, White Crane Flashes Its Wings, and Step Back to Repulse the Monkey. These more advanced programs, which you've likely seen in movies or television shows, offer additional benefits

Quick Bouts of Exercise Are All You Need

Four Seconds of Exercise Is Good...

Bouts of intense exercise lasting as little as four seconds can have surprising benefits—especially for people who spend hours at a time sitting at a desk, which can make it harder to burn fat even during exercise. A small study found that such micro-sessions conducted five times per hour over an eight-hour period improved fat metabolism and lowered triglycerides. Study participants used a specialized exercise bike that allowed them to hit maximal energy exertion quickly.

Study by researchers at University of Texas at Austin published in Medicine & Science in Sports & Exercise.

12 Minutes of Strenuous Exercise Is Better...

Twelve minutes a day of strenuous exercise can be enough to boost life expectancy and lower the risk for heart disease and diabetes. After a twelve-minute burst of intense physical activity, levels of the biomarker *DMGV*—which is linked to risk for diabetes and fatty liver disease—dropped 18%. And levels of *glutamate*—associated with heart disease, diabetes and shorter life expectancy—decreased 29%. The exercise needs to be intense and done on a regular basis—but does not need to continue for a long time.

Study of 411 men and women by researchers at Massachusetts General Hospital, Boston, published in Circulation.

as you shift your weight from side to side, stretch, and gently strengthen muscles. There are different styles and sequences, and a class is an excellent place to learn them. Look for programs at the local hospital, fitness center, or community center, or find instructional videos online.

Avoid These Workout Mistakes

Stretching same-hand to same-foot. When doing a seated one-leg stretch, always reach for your toes with the opposite-side hand. *Leaning forward when you squat.* If you tend to bend forward at the waist while doing squats, try crossing your arms in front of your chest to correct your form. *Working your neck during ab exercises.* You should never feel strain in your neck while you're doing crunches. If you do, you're probably pulling upward on the back of your head with your hands. Instead, make an X in front of you by crossing your forearms at the wrists, palms inward, and move this X behind you to the base of your neck to use as a cradle during the exercise. It'll keep you from tugging up on your head.

Celebrity trainer Joel Harper. JoelHarperFitness.com

For Better Health, Walk with a Purpose

People who walk from home to work or for other specific purposes, such as to the grocery store, report better health than those who walk for leisure. Those who walk for targeted purposes walk faster—an average of 2.7 miles per hour, versus 2.55 miles per hour for people who walk for recreational reasons. Trips from home also are longer—64% last at least 10 minutes, compared with 50% of walks that begin elsewhere.

Study of the walking habits of more than 125,885 people, ages 18 to 64, by researchers at The Ohio State University, Columbus, published in Journal of Transport & Health.

Foot Muscles Need Exercise, Too

Strengthening moves: Stand barefoot with feet flat on the floor, and pull your arch upward to shorten your footprint and raise your instep.

Toe scrunch: Place a dish towel on the floor, and stand barefoot on it, then scrunch your toes to bunch up the towel.

Run on uneven terrain: Running on trails, sand or grass gives your feet a workout because they need to support your body at a variety of angles on varied terrain.

Lifehacker.com

Can't Manage 10,000 Steps a Day? That's OK!

Recent study: Walking at least 7,000 steps a day reduced risk for premature death by 50% to 70%. Walking between 7,000 and 10,000 steps daily improved health even more...but walking more than 10,000 steps a day did not add any additional benefit.

What you might not know: The often-cited guideline to walk 10,000 steps a day is not based on scientific research. That number of steps originated from an ad campaign for a Japanese pedometer.

Eleven-year study of 2,100 participants by researchers at University of Massachusetts Amherst, published in *JAMA Network Open.*

5

Natural Health News

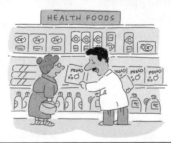

Eat for Your Brain

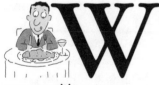**W**hat we eat affects our weight, our energy levels, our susceptibility to diseases and, we now know, our cognition, too.

But while a poor diet can set off a chain reaction that leads to memory loss, all evidence suggests that we may be able to improve and protect cognition by swapping foods that compromise our gut bacteria—which directly affects the neurochemicals involved in memory—with foods that enhance it. Diet may even prevent or slow down cognitive decline and conditions like Alzheimer's disease (AD).

FIRST, DO NO HARM

Both high-fat and high-glycemic-index foods (those that cause a rapid rise in blood glucose) can alter brain pathways that are necessary for learning and memory. Neurons in the hippocampus—the part of the brain most involved in remembering things such as a new acquaintance's name or facts about the world—are particularly sensitive to diet. High-fat and high-sugar consumption can hamper the expression of critical growth factors and other hormones that promote healthy function in the hippocampus and can affect insulin signaling and insulin sensitivity in the body's tissues. The traditional fatty, sugary, and processed Western diet can even cause the hippocampus to shrink.

Research is showing that neuro (brain) inflammation has been linked to both age-related cognitive decline and the risk of developing AD.

Uma Naidoo, MD, instructor in psychiatry at Harvard Medical School, director of nutritional and lifestyle psychiatry at Massachusetts General Hospital, and author of *This Is Your Brain on Food: An Indispensable Guide to the Surprising Foods That Fight Depression, Anxiety, PTSD, OCD, ADHD, and More.*

75

THE MIND DIET

Thankfully, it appears that dietary changes can halt these processes and even reverse them, protecting against cognitive decline. For five years, a team of researchers from Rush University Medical Center and the Harvard School of Public Health studied the link between diet and cognition. They concluded that a combination of two established dietary plans, the Mediterranean diet and the Dietary Approaches to Stop Hypertension (DASH), provided clear and significant cognitive benefits. They named the combination of the two the MIND diet (short for the Mediterranean-DASH Intervention for Neurodegenerative Delay).

The investigators discovered that people who followed the MIND diet the most closely were 7.5 cognitive years younger than those who followed more of a standard American diet. They showed better episodic memory (long-term recall of personal facts), working memory (short-term recall of information that is still being acted upon), semantic memory (memory of facts and knowledge about the world), visuospatial ability (the ability to see and understand the size and space of their surroundings), and perceptual speed (how quickly things are seen). The effects were most pronounced with episodic memory, semantic memory, and perceptual speed.

The MIND diet was also associated with a reduced incidence of AD. The higher the adherence to the MIND diet, the slower the rate of cognitive decline. In 2019, another research team reported that the diet was also associated with a reduced incidence and delayed progression of Parkinson's disease.

BRAIN-BOOSTING FOODS

The basic tenets of the diet are simple. *Strive to base your diet on 11 foundational foods…*

1. Green leafy vegetables (kale, collards, greens, spinach, lettuce, tossed salad, microgreens). Six or more servings per week

2. Other vegetables (peppers, squash, carrots, broccoli, celery, potatoes, tomatoes, tomato sauce, string beans, beets, corn, zucchini, summer squash, eggplant). One or more servings per day

3. Berries (strawberries, blueberries, raspberries, blackberries). Two or more servings per week

4. Nuts. Five or more servings per week

5. Whole grains. Three or more servings per day

6. Fish (not fried, particularly high-omega-3 fish such as salmon). One or more meals per week

7. Beans, lentils, soybeans. More than three meals per week

8. Poultry. Two or more meals per week

9. Wine. One glass per day

10. Fruit. At least one or two servings per day

11. Use olive oil as your primary oil

At the same time, there are some foods you should limit or eliminate…

- **Margarine or butter-like spreads.** Less than 1 tablespoon per day

- **Cheese.** Less than once per week

- **Fried food.** Less than once per week

- **Red meat and pork.** A few times per week

- **Limit sweets such as ice cream, cookies, brownies, snack cakes, donuts, and candy.**

ADDITIONAL FOOD RESEARCH

Outside of the MIND diet, researchers have identified some specific foods that may add even more protective benefits…

- **Coffee.** Caffeine, which increases the neurotransmitters serotonin and acetylcholine, may stimulate the brain and help stabilize the blood-brain barrier. The polyphenols in coffee may prevent tissue damage by free radicals. Trigonelline, a substance found in high concentration in coffee beans, may activate antioxidants that protect blood vessels in the brain.

Research suggests that three cups of coffee per day may lower the risk of cognitive decline, dementia, and AD. Keep your overall caffeine consumption (which includes chocolate, cola, tea, and guarana) under 400 milligrams per day.

•**Turmeric.** The active ingredient of this spice is curcumin, which has antioxidant, anti-inflammatory, and neuron growth-promoting properties. A 2019 review of curcumin studies showed that consumption of curcumin improved attention, learning, overall cognition, and memory. It improves cognitive function in people with AD and may help prevent it.

When you consume plain turmeric or curcumin, however, very little of it is absorbed into the blood. Boost absorption by combining it with black pepper or a fat such as olive oil. Cooking with it also makes it easier for your body to use.

•**Black pepper and cinnamon.** Black pepper and cinnamon suppress inflammatory pathways and may act as antioxidants. They increase the availability of acetylcholine, which improves memory, and help clear amyloid deposits. (A build-up of these deposits is a hallmark of AD.)

•**Saffron.** Several studies suggest that saffron has cognitive benefits, from enhancing memory to increasing cognition in people with AD. It has antioxidant and anti-inflammatory properties. Saffron can be used in cooking or taken as a supplement.

•**Ginger.** Ginger has been shown to enhance working memory in middle-aged healthy women. In animals, it has increased the levels of adrenaline, noradrenaline, dopamine, and serotonin contents in the cerebral cortex and hippocampus, so it may work through these brain chemicals to enhance memory.

These first four spices work well together in a variety of savory dishes, including Indian curries. (This stew-like dish with meat or vegetables in a spiced gravy is not the same thing as the spice called curry.) That may be part of the reason why the incidence of AD for people ages 70 to 79 is four times lower in India than in the United States.

•**Rosemary.** One study found that the aroma of rosemary changes brain waves so that people become less anxious, more alert, and better able to compute math problems. Rosemary can also boost acetylcholine, which is instrumental in memory. You can use it in

cooking (try it on roasted potatoes or chicken) or aromatherapy.

•**Sage** decreases inflammation in the brain, reduces amyloid deposits, decreases oxidative cell damage, increases acetylcholine, and helps neuronal growth. It can enhance memory, attention, word recall, and speed of memory in healthy adults. It can make people feel more alert, content, and calm. You can use it in cooking or aromatherapy.

Beat Brain Fog

Brain fog occurs when you struggle to concentrate, think clearly, or multitask. It can also affect both short- and long-term memory. Experts believe it comes from excessive brain inflammation and suggest that it can be alleviated by following a whole-foods diet, such as the MIND diet, and avoiding processed, fatty, and sugary foods. *Some additional nutrients may help too…*

•**Luteolin** is an antioxidant and anti-inflammatory agent that prevents toxic destruction of nerve cells in the brain. You can find it in Mexican oregano, juniper berries, fresh peppermint, sage, thyme, hot and sweet peppers, radicchio, celery seeds, parsley, and artichokes.

•**Citicoline.** If your brain fog is due to acetylcholine and dopamine depletion, foods such as beef liver and egg yolks may help.

•**Phosphatidylserine** is required for healthy nerve cell membranes and coverings, and its protective effects can prevent brain fog. You can find it in soybeans or supplements.

•**Probiotics** are often beneficial, but sometimes they can cause slower digestion that leads to brain fog. If you're taking a probiotic and finding your thoughts sluggish, consider switching supplements. Better yet, get your probiotics from dietary sources like plain yogurt with active cultures.

•**Gluten.** After consuming gluten, some people find themselves thinking less clearly and wanting to sleep all day. If you are suffering from brain fog, cut out gluten to see if you improve. It may turn out that you have celiac disease or non-celiac gluten sensitivity.

Drinking Tea Boosts Brain Health

Brain regions of people age 60 and older who had been drinking tea at least four times a week for 25 years were more efficiently interconnected than the brain areas of people who did not drink tea. The type of tea did not matter—the effect was found with green, oolong and black tea. This means that long-term tea drinking may help protect against age-related declines in cognitive function.

Study by researchers at National University of Singapore, published in *Aging*.

Pollution Protection

David Carpenter, MD, the director of the Institute for Health and the Environment at University at Albany (State University of New York), a Collaborating Centre of the World Health Organization in Environmental Health.

No matter where you live, you're likely exposed to pollutants such as heavy metals, pesticides, phthalates, and flame retardants. Scientists have found that exposure to these substances can cause oxidation, a kind of internal rust, and put your immune system into overdrive, causing chronic, low-grade inflammation. The end result is cellular damage and a higher risk of disease.

Illnesses linked to pollution include all the big killers, such as high blood pressure, heart disease, and stroke. Exposure to some air pollutants for even one day can quadruple the risk of dying from a heart attack. That's just the start. Pollution is linked to cancer, diabetes, obesity, Alzheimer's disease, respiratory illness, attention deficit and hyperactivity disorder, age-related macular degeneration, infertility, acne, psoriasis, and Parkinson's disease.

Foods that are high in fiber—such as fruits, vegetables, whole grains, beans, bran cereal, popcorn, and nuts—reduce the absorption of pollutants and help you excrete those that have been absorbed.

LET FOOD BE THY PROTECTION

While you can't entirely avoid pollution, you can take steps to protect yourself. Scientists at major universities around the world are rapidly accumulating evidence that some foods can help prevent, slow, or reverse the cellular damage caused by pollutants.

• **Fruits and vegetables.** Polychlorinated biphenyls (PCBs) have been used in hundreds of industrial applications and products, and they permeate the soil, water, and air. Once they're ingested, they're stored in fat. Research links high blood levels of PCBs with a higher risk of type 2 diabetes, but the risk is much lower in people with a high intake of fruits and vegetables, which deliver a wide range of antioxidant and anti-inflammatory compounds, including vitamins, minerals, and phytochemicals (plant compounds). PCBs are also linked to heart disease and cancer, and researchers from the College of Medicine at the University of Kentucky say that eating more fruits and vegetables may lower the risk of pollutants triggering those diseases.

Aim for at least five servings of fruit and vegetables each day. If you're not a fan, try hiding them in other foods. A handful of spinach disappears in chili, while minced cauliflower blends seamlessly into just about any recipe. Also, since PCBs are stored in fat, minimize your consumption of fatty meats, such as strip steak and ribeye.

• **Vitamin C.** One reason fruits and vegetables are protective is that they are rich in vitamin C, which is particularly protective for some of the people most vulnerable to air pollution—those with chronic obstructive pulmonary disease (COPD) and asthma. In one study, researchers from the United Kingdom noted that exposure to air pollution increased hospital admissions in people with COPD and asthma, but people with the highest blood levels of vitamin C had a 35% lower risk of being hospitalized. Boost your vitamin C by eating citrus, strawberries, broccoli, and tomatoes.

- **High-fiber foods.** Foods that are high in fiber, such as fruits, vegetables, whole grains, beans, bran cereal, popcorn, and nuts, reduce the absorption of pollutants and help you excrete those that have been absorbed. Aim for 21 to 25 grams a day for women and 30 to 38 grams a day for men.

- **Green tea.** In a scientific paper published in the *Journal of Nutritional Biochemistry*, researchers from the University of Tennessee and several other institutions cited more than 70 studies that detailed how green tea—rich in the phytochemical epigallocatechin gallate (EGCG)—may help protect against environmental toxins of all kinds, including pesticides, smoke, mold, PCBs, and arsenic. (More than 2 million Americans have well water with a high level of arsenic, a carcinogen.) Try to drink two cups per day.

- **Beer contains hops,** which are rich in xanthohumol, an antioxidant and anti-inflammatory phytochemical that can protect cells from pollution-induced damage to DNA, which can trigger cancer. Xanthohumol is also found yogurt, chocolate, and muesli.

- **Sesame-based foods.** According to a scientific paper recently published in *Reviews on Environmental Health*, sesame is uniquely protective against disease processes triggered by pollutants. The "bioactive" components in sesame seed and oil include lignans, sasamin, sasamol, and sesamolin. These components reduce oxidation, boost the antioxidant power of vitamin E, kill cancer cells and stop them from multiplying, lower high cholesterol and blood pressure, strengthen the liver, a detoxifying organ, protect brain cells against damage, and downregulate inflammatory immune factors.

You can use sesame oil like any vegetable oil. Sesame-based foods include tahini (a nut butter), hummus, baba ghanoush (a dip with mashed cooked eggplant, olive oil, lemon juice, and seasonings), and halva (a dessert).

- **Cranberry.** Several types of air pollutants—including sulfur dioxide, nitrogen dioxide, ozone, carbon dioxide, and particu-

The Power of Fish and Fish Oil

A study published in the Aug. 25, 2020, issue of *Neurology* showed the protective power of fish and fish oil against the cell-damaging, disease-causing particulates in air pollution. A team of researchers from eight leading medical schools tracked 1,315 women, ages 65 to 80, for 10 years and assessed their exposure to particulate pollution, the amount of omega-3 fatty acids in their red blood cells (both docosahexaenoic acid [DHA] and eicosapentaenoic acid [DHA]), and the size of the hippocampus and the white matter of the brain. Brain shrinkage in those areas is a sign of aging and increases the risk of cognitive decline.

They found that the women with the most exposure to air pollution had the greatest degree of brain shrinkage—unless they had high blood levels of omega-3s. The researchers also found that the women with the greatest dietary intake of omega-3s—from non-fried fish and fish oil supplements—had greater brain volume.

In a new study published in the *American Journal of Cardiology*, Chinese scientists found that people who took a fish oil supplement maintained normal biomarkers after exposure to air pollution—but people who didn't take the supplement had several signs of circulatory dysfunction, including blood inflammation, thicker blood, and tighter arteries.

The best food sources of omega-3s are fatty fish such as wild-caught salmon, sardines, and anchovies. The American Heart Association, which has issued a formal scientific statement linking air pollution to cardiovascular illness and death, recommends that all adults eat fatty fish at least twice a week. Omega-3 supplements containing DHA and EPA are also widely available, and research shows they are effective. Look for a supplement that delivers a daily minimum of 250 to 500 milligrams of combined EPA and DHA.

—Dr. David Carpenter

lates—have been linked to a wide range of respiratory problems, including lung and esophageal cancers. According to Bernard Hennig, PhD, at the University of Kentucky, cellular studies have shown that cranberry can protect against those and other cancers, including cancers of the colon, prostate, and brain (glioblastoma). You can ingest cranberry as a food, in juice (choose a low-sugar variety), or in supplemental form.

•**Selenium.** Research shows that this trace mineral binds to toxic metals such as lead, cadmium, and methylmercury, forming a so-called "insoluble precipitant" that is easily excreted. Seniors are more likely to be deficient in the mineral.

•**Brazil nuts and seafood** are the richest sources of selenium. Other good sources include red meat, grains, and dairy products. Seniors may want to include a selenium supplement. Look for a product with at least 55 micrograms (mcg) and take it once a week. (Too much selenium can be toxic.)

•**Quercetin.** Cellular studies show that quercetin can protect the arteries from PCBs. This phytochemical is found in apples, onions, cherries, citrus fruits, red grapes, and green leafy vegetables.

•**Curcumin.** This anti-inflammatory compound is the active ingredient in turmeric. Several cellular and animal studies show that curcumin—also available in supplement form —can help prevent lung and heart damage from air pollution, including diesel exhaust. Curcumin can also prevent inflammation from cadmium, a heavy metal.

Curcumin is very difficult for your body to absorb, so when using it in cooking, combine it with a fat and/or black pepper to boost its bioavailability. If taking a supplement, look for one that is formulated for enhanced bioavailability, such as products with added oil, piperine (a pepper extract), or a smaller particle size.

Diet Changes Can Lower Your Risk for Gout

Chris Iliades, MD, retired ear, nose, throat, head, and neck surgeon who now dedicates his time to educating patients through his medical writing.

When gout strikes your toes, feet, ankles, or knees, the pain can be so intense that a bedsheet on your skin can be unbearable. Redness, swelling, and pain intensify for the first 24 hours and then linger for a week or more. Over time, untreated gout can destroy joint tissue, causing long-term pain, disability, and deformity.

UNDER THE SURFACE

Gout starts with a basic molecule called a purine. Humans need purines to build DNA. You make some purines naturally and get more from your diet. After your body uses purines, they are broken down into uric acid. Normally, this acid is removed by your kidneys and causes no problems. But in some people, such as those with kidney disease or overconsumption of high-purine foods, the uric acid level can get too high and forms crystals that resemble microscopic needles. Those crystals can get trapped inside a joint, where they cause a sudden and severe attack of inflammation and pain.

PEOPLE AT RISK

Not everyone with high levels of uric acid forms these crystals. In fact, researchers have discovered that several inherited genes may be to blame for those who do. If you have a family history of gout, you'll want to be extra careful to reduce other modifiable risk factors. You can't do anything about your age (the risk of gout increases as you grow older) or your sex (it's more common in men than women up to the age of menopause), but you can control your diet. *There are three diet changes to help reduce gout...*

•**Limit your calories and get adequate exercise to prevent obesity.**

•**Avoid purines in your diet.**

• **Follow the Dietary Approaches to Stop Hypertension (DASH) diet** to lower your risk of gout, even if you have gout genes.

AVOIDING PURINES

• **Avoiding purine-rich foods** can lower your risk of developing gout and, if you already have it, help manage the condition.

• **Avoid alcohol, especially beer.** Having two or more beers per day more than doubles your gout risk. If you want to drink, the safest choice is a glass of wine.

• **Avoid sugar-sweetened beverages** and anything sweetened with fructose to decrease your gout risk by about 80%.

• **Avoid eating shellfish and ocean fish,** which increase gout risk by about 50%.

• **Avoid red meat,** especially wild and organ meat to reduce risk by about 40%.

You may be able to lower gout risk by about 50% by eating more low-fat dairy products and foods high in vitamin C and drinking six or more cups of black coffee every day.

THE DASH DIET

At the 2021 meeting of the European Congress of Rheumatology, researchers presented a study that showed that the typical American diet, which is rich in red meat, saturated fat, processed foods, refined grains, and sugar-sweetened beverages, was associated with a higher risk of gout than the DASH plan, even in people who had a genetic risk for gout. The DASH diet was originally developed to reduce high blood pressure and the risk of heart disease, but studies published in 2016 and 2017 found that it also lowers uric acid levels.

This diet limits calories to an average of 2,000 per day and outlines a target number of servings by food group...

• **Six to eight servings of whole grains**

• **Four to five servings of fruits and vegetables**

• **Two to three servings of low- or fat-free dairy foods**

• **Six or fewer servings of lean meat, poultry, and fish**

• **Two to three servings of fats and oils, but no trans fats**

• **No more than 2,300 milligrams of sodium**

The diet also limits nuts, seeds, dry beans, peas, and sweets to five or fewer servings per week. (See the sidebar for examples of serving sizes.)

Not only can the DASH diet help prevent and control gout, but it can help you maintain a healthy blood pressure and body weight, too.

WHAT'S IN A SERVING?	
Whole grains	One slice of bread, 1 oz. of dry cereal, ½ cup of cooked rice or pasta
Vegetables	1 cup of raw leafy greens, ½ cup of raw vegetables
Fruits	One medium piece of fruit, ¼ cup of dried fruit
Low- or fat-free dairy foods	1 cup of milk or yogurt, 1½ oz. of cheese
Lean meat, poultry, or fish	1 oz. of meat, poultry, or fish, 1 egg
Fats and oils	1 tsp. of soft margarine or vegetable oil, 1 Tbsp. of mayonnaise
Nuts and seeds	⅓ cup of nuts, 2 Tbsp. peanut butter or seeds
Beans and peas	½ cup cooked legumes
Sweets	1 Tbsp. sugar, 1 Tbsp. jelly or jam, or 1 cup of lemonade

Home Remedy for Knee Pain: Pectin and Grape Juice

Although there is no scientific research to back up the claims, many people swear that this folk remedy eases arthritis knee pain.

To try it: Liquid pectin, such as Certo brand used for making jams and jellies, is easiest to use. Mix one tablespoon of liquid pectin in eight ounces of purple grape juice, and drink daily.

Alternative: Some people get more relief taking the mixture two or three times a day. To do that, mix two teaspoons of liquid pectin in three ounces of purple grape juice per dose.

Terry Graedon, PhD, medical anthropologist and leading authority on the science behind folk remedies, and cohost of *The People's Pharmacy* radio show and website, writing at PeoplesPharmacy.com.

The Science Behind Acupuncture

Ania Grimone, MS, a licensed acupuncturist and Chinese herbalist with the Northwestern Medicine Osher Center for Integrative Medicine in Chicago.

For 3,000 years, acupuncture has been a staple of Chinese health care, where it is regularly used to treat conditions as diverse as insomnia, pain, and the symptoms of menopause.

In the United States, the history of the practice is shorter—the first legal acupuncture center opened in 1972—but acupuncture is now the most widely used alternative medical practice in the nation.

It's supported by an impressive body of research, offered by some of the most respected academic medical institutions, including the Mayo Clinic and Harvard Medical School, and covered by several major insurers. Even the U.S. Army endorses it as a treatment for chronic pain.

THEORY OF ACUPUNCTURE

In acupuncture, thin, sterile needles are gently inserted through the skin at different points in the torso, limbs, and head. These points are positioned along a network of pathways called *meridians* that are dotted with acupuncture points, also called acupoints.

Traditional Chinese medicine practitioners believe that organs, tissues, muscles, and ligaments are all connected, and that meridians run the length of the body, so the needle placement is often unexpected. For example, chronic headaches may be treated with needles on the hands and ankles as well as the head. Upper back and shoulder pain, for instance, is associated with a blockage in the bladder meridian, which has 67 acupoints starting at the eye, crossing the forehead, running down the back of the head, past the buttocks, and ending at the pinky toes.

When an acupuncturist stimulates acupoints with needles, it signals the brain and body to produce endogenous opioids, powerful pain-relieving chemicals, anti-inflammatory compounds, immune-boosting compounds, hormones, and vasodilators that increase blood circulation. Traditional acupuncturists also believe that stimulating acupoints releases blockages in the body's flow of energy, called *qi* (pronounced chee). For many people, that stimulation translates to pain relief.

PROVEN PAIN RELIEF

In a report published in the *National Institute for Health Research Journals Library*, researchers reviewed 29 clinical trials and concluded that adding acupuncture to standard medical care (anti-inflammatory medications and physical therapy) reduced the severity of neck and lower back pain, significantly reduced the number of headaches and migraines, and eased the pain and disability of osteoarthritis. The American College of Physicians recommends acupuncture and other non-pharmacologic therapies as first-line treatments for patients experiencing chronic low-back pain.

It's even used for pain relief in veterinary medicine. Studies show it can ease chronic spinal and osteoarthritic pain, as well as acute pain from neuromusculoskeletal injuries and surgery. Since animals don't have expectations for a treatment to work, veterinary applications offer exciting evidence that acupuncture offers more than a placebo effect.

ALZHEIMER'S DISEASE

In a 2019 review article published in *Frontiers in Psychiatry*, researchers reported that acupuncture may be beneficial for people with Alzheimer's disease. They cite multiple small studies that have found that acupuncture can improve mood and cognition and increase verbal and motor skills. A clinical trial with

87 patients found that acupuncture improved cognitive function better than the medication *donepezil* (Aricept), with benefits that lasted for 12 weeks.

HOT FLASHES

Acupuncture also appears to ease hot flashes from breast cancer treatment and menopause. In a *Journal of Clinical Oncology* study of breast cancer patients experiencing treatment-related hot flashes, those who received weekly acupuncture as part of a three-month self-care regimen including exercise, nutrition, and psychological support had hot flash scores (calculated as the frequency of hot flashes multiplied by the average severity) that were 50% lower than those in the acupuncture-free self-care protocol. Importantly, the benefits continued for six months after the acupuncture ended.

In another study, women who underwent five weeks of acupuncture had fewer hot flashes, less frequent and less severe night sweats, and fewer sleep, skin, and hair problems than women in the control group.

Acupuncture may provide these benefits by dilating blood vessels, similar to what hormone replacement therapy does, and triggering the release of endorphins (stress- and pain-relieving chemicals) and hormones related to mood regulation.

FIGHT INSOMNIA AND DEPRESSION

After reviewing 46 clinical trials, researchers reported in the peer-reviewed *Journal of Alternative and Complementary Medicine* that acupuncture independently improves sleep quality and duration and amplifies the benefits of other insomnia interventions. Last year, a different team reported that eight weeks of electroacupuncture (acupuncture with mild electrical stimulation) improved the quality and quantity of people's sleep, and significantly improved depression symptoms.

DEPRESSION AND ANXIETY

Many studies have reported that acupuncture can ease depression. At least one has found that it may be more effective than medication. Similarly, studies show that it can treat both general and preoperative anxiety. The quality of these studies, however, tends to be low—but so are the risks as long as you visit a certified acupuncture practitioner who uses sterile or single-use needles. (To find an acupuncturist, visit NCCAOM.org.)

WHAT TO EXPECT

For many people, the largest barrier to trying acupuncture is a fear of needles, but the most you should feel is a small pinch, if anything at all. Once the needle is in, you may have a mild awareness that something is there, but you won't experience pain.

On average, sessions last about 25 minutes. Many acupuncturists will treat acute issues twice a week and chronic conditions once a week, continuing until the problem is resolved or you've hit a plateau in improvement. In general, newer health problems resolve more quickly than chronic issues.

Acupuncture tends to have very few side effects, although some people may experience minor bleeding or soreness at the insertion sites. It can lower blood pressure and blood sugar levels, depending on which acupoints are stimulated, so be sure to hydrate and eat before your session.

Acupuncture for COVID Relief

Joseph Audette, MD, chief of pain management at Atrius Health, assistant professor of medicine at Harvard Medical School, board member of the American Academy of Medical Acupuncture and a physical medicine and rehabilitation specialist.

E merging research indicates that acupuncture can be a powerful tool for helping patients suffering the lingering effects of COVID.

How it works: In traditional Chinese medicine (TCM), when a person contracts a virus, an energy system within the body called *qi* (pronounced "chee") works to ward off the pathogen. This energy flows throughout the body along channels called meridians. If a patient has only mild COVID symptoms, it indicates that his/her qi was strong enough to keep the virus on the surface level of the body, manifesting as a sore throat, congestion, perhaps fever.

But if a person's qi is weaker—due to a comorbidity such as heart disease or obesity, for instance—it may not be able to prevent the virus from descending into the lungs and causing labored breathing, pneumonia, even blood clots. Weakened qi can leave a patient vulnerable to the post-COVID illness "long-haul COVID." Symptoms include shortness of breath, headaches, joint pains, brain fog, changes in smell and taste, and more.

How acupuncture helps: Acupuncture needles unblock and strengthen qi. The points where needles are introduced are chosen based on the organs involved.

Example: In TCM, excess phlegm is the result of imbalanced energy between the lungs and spleen. A combination of points such as SP 6 in the lower leg and PC 6 at the wrist can help relieve this symptom.

Acupuncture is an adjunct COVID treatment, not a replacement for medication or hospitalization. Some practitioners treat patients in the midst of an active COVID-19 infection, but in the US and Europe, it's more commonly used for long-haul COVID. Expect weekly treatments for long COVID…twice a week for lingering symptoms.

Findings from a 2021 Chinese study suggest acupuncture may have benefits for COVID-19 patients who also have cancer or heart disease or are obese. Trials are underway to see if it can improve loss of smell. Some clinics offer acupuncture before/after COVID vaccination to prepare the body to respond strongly to the vaccine.

Grow a Home-Remedy Garden

Elizabeth Millard, co-owner of Bossy Acres, an organic farm in Minnesota, and author of *Backyard Pharmacy*, which details how to grow and use dozens of herbs.

Even if you've never put a tulip bulb in the ground, it's easy to create your very own home-remedy garden with herbs, flowers and more. In fact, it's much easier to grow herbs than vegetables, regardless of your current green thumb status.

HERBS TO START WITH

People tend to think "exotic" when it comes to healing herbs, but many of the culinary ones that you already reach for have medicinal properties, so they're a great place to start. You can find out about other medicinal herbs at the National Library of Medicine's website, NLM.nih.gov/about/herbgarden/index.html, or consult my book, *Backyard Pharmacy. Here are some of the most popular and easiest-to-grow medicinal plants…*

• **Basil.** Chewing on basil leaves can freshen breath and even ease cold symptoms. There are dozens of varieties of basil, but holy basil is the variety most often used for medicinal purposes including reducing inflammation and fighting aging caused by free radicals. It is widely available in garden centers and supermarkets in small starter plants that grow very well when planted in your garden. Pluck larger leaves at the bottom, and leave tiny ones at the top to help the plant regenerate. Snip off flowers as they appear in order to prolong growth.

Ideal conditions: Six to eight hours of sun daily and well-drained, loosened soil.

• **Cayenne peppers** are rich in capsaicin and have antibacterial and anti-inflammatory properties. They are easy to dry and grind for year-round use. They're a great anti-cold remedy all winter long, particularly when mixed with warm water, honey and crushed garlic. Buy small plants at garden centers in mid-spring.

Ideal conditions: Eight to 10 hours of full sun daily and well-drained, loosened soil.

• **Chamomile's dried flowers** make a great infusion for easing anxiety and helping you get to sleep. I recommend German chamomile over the more common Roman. It tends to have more flowers, and that's what you will be using for remedies.

Ideal conditions: Eight to 10 hours of sun daily and well-drained soil.

• **Echinacea's dried flowers** support the immune system and can ease cold symptoms. The flowers of both echinacea and its cousin chamomile will add beauty and attract birds and butterflies to your garden.

Ideal conditions: Six to eight hours of sun daily and loamy soil.

•**Garlic,** important for boosting heart health and relief from colds and flu, is surprisingly easy to grow. In a shallow trench and spacing them about eight inches apart, plant the largest individual cloves from one or more heads (buy those grown specifically for propagation)—root-side down, pointy end up. If you love garlic, set aside an eight-foot-by-three-foot patch for your trenches to be able to harvest at least a three-month supply.

Garlic should be planted in fall, left to develop root structure over the winter, and harvested in summer. Stored in a cool dark cabinet, the heads will last for months.

Ideal conditions: Six to eight hours of sun daily and well-drained, loosened soil.

•**Lemon balm** has been used for centuries as a calming agent, including to ease a queasy tummy, and it also can help manage seasonal allergies. It thrives in cool weather so you can get a head start on it in early spring. It also makes a great addition to hot and iced teas or other beverages and even can be used as a flavoring for desserts.

Ideal conditions: Six to eight hours of sun daily and well-drained, loosened soil.

•**Mint** provides an energy boost and can soothe stomach issues. Chew on the leaves or brew them into a tea. Mints of all varieties are hardy and easy to grow from seed. It can be invasive so you might want to keep it in pots or place it in the garden where it has plenty of room to grow.

Ideal conditions: Full sun or partial shade and well-drained, loosened soil.

•**Oregano's dried leaves** make a wonderful tea that is high in antioxidants and is used to treat digestive complaints. Fresh leaves can be turned into a poultice to soothe itchy skin. It is best to plant oregano at the margins of your garden because its low-lying branches spread easily between vegetables. It gets bushy, so you'll need to thin it every few years.

Ideal conditions: Full sun and well-drained, loosened soil.

SEED OR STARTER PLANT?

Plants that you start from seed may take hold better outdoors because they develop in the local environment, but there are no guarantees! Seeds usually are less expensive than starter plants, even when you buy organic, which I recommend. How many starter plants to buy depends on your needs and uses and the space you have. But two or three of each should be a good start. Avoid buying large transplants, such as those in six-inch or larger containers. Small ones are less likely to experience shock when you replant them. Look for two- or four-inch starters.

If you're buying seeds: Good seed sellers include Johnny's Selected Seeds…Seeds of Change…Strictly Medicinal Seeds…and Hudson Valley Seed Company.

Hint: Once you have started growing your seeds and transplanted them outside, make your own planting notes right on the packets and store the packets in a dedicated bin as you would recipe cards.

If you're buying starter plants: Small transplants from a local nursery, state fair or farmers' market are a great option if you're getting a late start…are less experienced…or you want to try an herb you've never grown before. Ask the seller for tips about what grows best in your local area and soil and how much space it will need.

ENJOYING YOUR HERBS

There's nothing quite like plucking fresh herbs for a relaxing afternoon tea or to enhance home cooking. But if you don't use them frequently, regularly trim the plants back to encourage new growth, and dry the cuttings for future use.

At the end of your growing season, harvest your herbs. You can cut fresh herbs, chop them and put them in ice cube trays with a little olive oil and water, then freeze and transfer to freezer bags for storage. You also can dry them on a mesh screen or in bundles by tying the stems together and hanging them, stem end up, to dry. Or freeze the fresh or dried herb in a plastic bag in the freezer.

Store dried herbs in airtight glass jars, and keep them out of the light. Enjoy them as teas…or as tinctures, made by putting the herb in a container of two-thirds alcohol such as vodka and one-third water for at least two weeks. Or make balms or salves by placing your herbs in a jar of olive oil for a period of weeks to create an essential oil, then heating the oil with beeswax or coconut oil (once cool, it solidifies). Always do your research before using herbs to be sure they're safe for you.

How to Make Fire Cider

The Old Farmers' Almanac. Almanac.com

Fire cider is a traditional mix of apple cider vinegar and herbs that has been used to boost health and ward off colds.

To prevent colds: Drink one tablespoon per day…add it to tea or juice.

For a scratchy throat: Use as a gargle. You also can sprinkle it on salads and add it to vegetables, soups, chilis and cocktails.

Recipe: In a one-quart jar, combine one-third cup of grated-together horseradish and ginger, one-quarter cup peeled and diced turmeric (or two tablespoons of dried turmeric powder), six cloves of minced garlic, one-half cup peeled and diced onion, one or two habanero chiles cut in half (or one-half teaspoon cayenne pepper), one large lemon sliced including the rind, two tablespoons each of fresh chopped rosemary and thyme (or one teaspoon each of dried), one-half cup parsley, one cinnamon stick, a few allspice berries, a few cloves and one teaspoon of black peppercorns. Then add enough raw unfiltered apple cider vinegar to cover the ingredients by an inch or so (about four cups). Shake well, and let it sit for a few weeks in a cool dark place, shaking the mixture daily. Next, strain and add honey to taste. Store it in the refrigerator and use within one year.

NATURAL HEALING

Natural Remedies for Warts

Aloe vera—remove a leaf from an aloe plant, apply the gel to the wart, and repeat daily. *Apple cider vinegar can help peel away infected skin*—mix two parts of the vinegar with one part water, soak a cotton ball in the solution, place it on the wart and leave it on for three to four hours. *Banana peel*—try rubbing the inside of the peel on the wart daily. *Dandelion weed*—break apart a dandelion, squeeze out the sticky white sap from the stem, and apply to the wart once or twice a day for two weeks. *Garlic*—crush a clove, mix with water, apply to the wart, cover with a bandage, and repeat daily for three to four weeks. *Pineapple*—rub fresh pineapple on the wart daily. *Potato*—cut a small one in half, rub the cut side on the wart, and repeat twice a day. There is little or no scientific evidence for most of these remedies, but they are easy to try and some people report success using them.

Healthline.com

Bananas for Poison Ivy

If you've been exposed to poison ivy, first wash the area with soap and water to remove the urushiol resin that causes the extremely uncomfortable blisters and itching. If you start to get itchy, you may get some relief by rubbing the rash with the inside of a banana peel—the riper, the better. Scientists have yet to study this, but there's plenty of anecdotal evidence that it helps.

Joe Graedon, pharmacologist and cofounder of The People's Pharmacy. PeoplesPharmacy.com

Natural Relief for Gas and Bloating

Jamison Starbuck, ND, is a naturopathic physician in family practice in Missoula, Montana, and producer of *Dr. Starbuck's Health Tips for Kids*, a weekly program on Montana Public Radio, MTPR.org. She is a past president of the American Association of Naturopathic Physicians and a contributing editor to *The Alternative Advisor: The Complete Guide to Natural Therapies and Alternative Treatments.*

"I feel like I'm six months pregnant! It's so embarrassing and my doctor says nothing is wrong!"

This is a frequent refrain at my office. I see many patients who are miserable with gas and bloating shortly after meals but have normal lab tests, scans, colonoscopies, and endoscopies. Suggestions from conventional medical providers are often limited to antacids, weight loss, and sometimes antidepressants. I have a different approach.

If you have gas and bloating after meals daily, something is wrong. It's entirely appropriate to get a physical exam and tests to rule out serious conditions such as Crohn's disease, ulcerative colitis, and even cancers of the digestive tract. But if all of those are normal, your solution may lie in naturopathic medicine. *Consider these possibilities…*

•**Digestive deficiency.** Gas and bloating happen when foods are not thoroughly broken down inside the digestive tract. The first step in digestion is chewing and mixing food with saliva. As it moves to the stomach, food is bathed in hydrochloric acid and dissolved from solid into liquid form. Partially digested food then moves to the small intestine, where it is coated with pancreatic enzymes and bile released from the gallbladder. As food moves through the intestines, nutrients are absorbed and the remaining waste is eliminated via stool.

When any step in this process is deficient—if you don't chew your food thoroughly, don't make adequate saliva, or don't secrete enough hydrochloric acid, bile, or pancreatic enzymes to digest your food—gas and abdominal distention occurs. A naturopathic physician can assess the specific nature of your digestive deficiency and help you choose the most effective natural medicine to correct your problem.

Over-the-counter gas remedies, such as charcoal capsules, chewable papaya tablets, peppermint, and chamomile tea are very safe and surprisingly effective. But readily available digestive enzymes and gut "cleansing" formulas can make things worse. It's best to consult with a physician before tinkering with your digestive health, especially if you have a history of an ulcer or gut inflammation.

•**Food allergy.** I have many patients whose digestion is just fine as long as they avoid their food allergens. If they eat even a little bit of whatever they are allergic to, they know it pretty quickly. The top three food allergens are dairy, wheat, and eggs. The next tier includes peanuts, almonds, citrus, coffee, and sugar. You can determine food allergens by a process of elimination and reintroduction or by undergoing food allergy blood testing.

•**Excessive dietary sulfur.** Sulfur is an essential nutrient that is abundant in our foods. It plays an important role in protein metabolism, DNA formation, and the repair and protection of our cells. But too much sulfur causes gas: the stinky kind. If that's your trouble, try eliminating high-sulfur foods, such as garlic, onions, meat, peanuts, legumes, horseradish, and mustard, for one week. If your gas subsides, reintroduce these foods slowly, and in small quantities. Most folks tolerate them, but only in reduced doses.

Prebiotics Could Help with Sleep Disruption

According to a recent study, rodents with disrupted sleep cycles slept better when fed prebiotics—starchy foods such as artichokes and onions that allow gut bacteria to flourish. While further research may uncover more about the effects of prebiotiotics on sleep, including them in your diet might help with jet lag or if you work a night shift.

Michael Breus, PhD, clinical psychologist and sleep expert in private practice, Manhattan Beach, California, commenting on a study published in *Brain, Behavior and Immunity*.

Beat Insomnia Naturally

Jamison Starbuck, ND, naturopathic physician in family practice in Missoula, Montana, and producer of *Dr. Starbuck's Health Tips for Kids*, a weekly program on Montana Public Radio, MTPR.org. She is a past president of the American Association of Naturopathic Physicians and a contributing editor to *The Alternative Advisor: The Complete Guide to Natural Therapies and Alternative Treatments*.

Insomnia is a torturous medical condition that is often the result of another condition, rather than its own illness. Common causes include pain, allergies, hormone changes, indigestion, excess caffeine, sugar, or alcohol, medication side effects, irregular work patterns, inadequate exercise, and, of course, stress. Successfully treating those issues might cure your insomnia.

If you think stress is the chief cause of your sleep concerns, try my natural medicine approach. It's designed to enhance bedtime relaxation while simultaneously buoying stress management.

•**Daytime stress support.** When using natural medicine to treat stress-induced insomnia, you must support your daytime stress demands without overly revving up your nervous system. Limit caffeine to two cups a day, and drink it at least 10 hours before bedtime. Help your adrenal glands, your major stress support system, to manage the day by taking 500 milligrams (mg) of vitamin C and a B complex containing at least 75 mg of B5 (pantothenic acid) with breakfast each morning. If you do not have high blood pressure, take licorice root throughout the day, either in tea (16 ounces in 24 hours) or a tincture (¼ teaspoon in 24 hours), away from food. Licorice is a non-stimulating botanical medicine that nourishes the adrenal glands, enabling them to efficiently use the stress hormone cortisol. (People with high blood pressure should avoid licorice root and may benefit instead from the herb astragalus.)

•**Dietary guidelines.** Have your largest meal at midday, with a light supper, and a small plant-protein snack (such as hummus and crackers or nut butter on celery) at bedtime. This allows your digestive system to work optimally, eliminating the disruption that middle-of-the-night indigestion can cause. Bedtime plant-protein snacks gently support your body in replenishing your stress hormones, reducing the 2 a.m. stress wake-up response that adrenal deficiency can cause.

•**Evening movement.** As your day winds down, engage in gentle physical movement. Walk home from work if you can. Take an evening yoga class, a bike ride, or walk with your family or the dog after dinner.

•**Botanical support.** Take rest-inducing botanicals and amino acids in the late afternoon or early evening.

Natural medicines are not like drugs: They rarely kick in with immediate effects, but instead, work gently over several hours. If you have insomnia, you must encourage your body to start relaxing as soon as the sun begins to set.

An effective and safe protocol for most people is to take 60 drops of the botanical medicine skullcap tincture in 3 ounces of water, along with 200 mg of L-theanine and 500 mg of L-tryptophan sometime between 4 and 6 p.m., at least 30 minutes away from food. Repeat this dosing 30 minutes before bed. If you wake in the middle of the night, you may repeat the skullcap tincture dose of 60 drops.

Melatonin: Sorting Fact from Fiction

Cinthya Pena-Orbea, MD, a sleep specialist at the Cleveland Clinic, Ohio.

For anyone who has ever suffered from insomnia, an over-the-counter supplement like melatonin is alluring. But before you stock up, it's helpful to have a realistic understanding of what this hormone can—and can't—do.

NATURAL MELATONIN

Your body already makes its own melatonin. Nestled in the center of the brain, the pineal gland communicates with receptors in the retina—the back of the eye—to know when it's light or dark. When it senses darkness, it releases high levels of melatonin to prepare you for sleep. When it senses light, it shuts melatonin production down.

Around age 40, your body begins to produce less melatonin, which can lead to age-related sleep problems. By age 90, melatonin levels are a mere 20% of what they were in your young adult years.

Whatever your age, you can help melatonin do its job by taking a few simple steps…

• **Keep the lights low before bed.** Even dim light can interfere with a person's circadian rhythm and melatonin secretion. Just eight lux—less than a table lamp—has an effect.

• **Avoid blue light from computers, smartphones, and tablets for two to three hours before bed.** If you can't avoid them, try using a blue-light filter or an app, like F. Lux or Night Shift to adjust your screens to nighttime mode. Compact fluorescent lightbulbs and LED lights produce more blue light than incandescent lightbulbs.

• **Dim red light is the best choice for nightlights.**

• **Get exposure to daylight during the morning.** Sunlight helps your body produce serotonin, which is the precursor to melatonin.

• **Melatonin can also be found in various foods,** including corn, cucumbers, asparagus, olives, pomegranate, nuts, seeds, barley, and rolled oats. Studies have reported that consumption of kiwis, tart cherry juice, and salmon may improve sleep, too.

SUPPLEMENTAL MELATONIN

Melatonin affects when you fall asleep, not how quickly, so taking a melatonin supplement is far from a cure-all for insomnia. In fact, studies show that it may shave a mere seven or eight minutes off your wait to fall asleep and lengthen sleep time by about the

---

Cognitive Behavioral Therapy for Insomnia

Cognitive behavioral therapy for insomnia (CBT-I) helps people with insomnia identify and replace thoughts and behaviors that cause or worsen sleep problems with habits that promote sound sleep. *The therapy has multiple components…*

• **Sleep hygiene.** These are practices that foster and maintain sleep, such as keeping the bedroom dark and quiet, participating in regular exercise, and limiting the consumption of caffeine, alcohol, and tobacco.

• **Stimulus control therapy** trains your brain to associate your bed with sleep or sex and nothing else. It means no working, watching television, or worrying while lying in bed.

• **Relaxation training** uses practices such as progressive muscle relaxation and diaphragmatic breathing to create a positive state for sleep.

• **Cognitive therapy** helps you identify and challenge incorrect and unhelpful thoughts about sleep, such as "I know this is going to be a bad night. I won't feel rested tomorrow. Why can't I sleep like everyone else?"

To find a CBT-I provider, visit https://cbti. directory/index.php/search-for-a-provider. The Cleveland Clinic offers a 6-week-long online program, Go to Sleep. Learn more at https:// clevelandclinicwellness.com/pages/GoTo Sleep.htm

---

same—hardly a cure for standard insomnia. The American College of Physicians guidelines strongly recommend the use of cognitive behavioral therapy for insomnia (CBT-I) instead. (See sidebar.)

But sleep disorders that aren't simple insomnia are different. Because melatonin affects your circadian rhythm, it can help with issues such as delayed sleep phase syndrome, which is when you consistently fall asleep very late and wake up late the next day.

It may help shift workers, who often struggle to work at night when melatonin levels naturally rise and to sleep during the day when they fall. Studies suggest, however, that light therapy is more effective than melatonin supplements.

The strongest case for supplemental melatonin comes from studies on jet lag. Multiple studies show that taking melatonin close to bedtime when you arrive in a different time zone can help reduce lag symptoms.

DOSAGE

There is no general consensus regarding dosage. Melatonin supplements often come in doses of 3 to 5 milligrams (mg), but studies suggest that as little as 0.3 to 0.5 mg per day might be more effective than higher doses in many people. Taking too much of the hormone can cause morning grogginess, headaches, reduced focus, and dizziness, so it's best to start small. (You might have to get a 1 mg tablet and cut it in half to do so.)

Take melatonin about an hour or two before bedtime to give it time to work. Don't take it in the morning, as it can reset your internal clock in an unintended way.

SAFETY

Short-term use of melatonin supplements appears to be safe, but there isn't enough data to assess long-term safety. Be careful of mixing it with other drugs. Melatonin can have interactions with other drugs such as blood thinners, anticonvulsants, some blood pressure medications, and diabetes medications. Melatonin may stay active for a longer time in older people, and it can cause dizziness and drowsiness that can increase the risk of falls.

In 2017, researchers tested 31 melatonin supplements and found that the amount of melatonin in the product didn't match what was listed on the product label in most cases. They found serotonin in more than a quarter of sampled products.

6

Aging Well

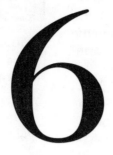

The Truth About Living to 100

Wouldn't it be nice if those headlines about living vibrantly to age 100 were true? And, even better, if it didn't require voodoo or new-age machinery to do it? Well, it is...and it doesn't. You just need to understand the root causes of deterioration as we age, most of which are because the body accumulates pro-aging toxins faster than it can eliminate them.

A PRIMER ON PREMATURE AGING

At the cellular level, aging is caused by free radicals, unstable molecules that break down our bodies' cells and damage DNA. By doing this, they create a sort of cellular chaos—called oxidative stress—that can hasten aging and fuel the development of disease.

Most approaches to fighting oxidative stress involve antioxidants—restorative vitamins and minerals in food and supplements—to counter the effects of free radicals. But all the kale in the world won't help you keep pace with the alarming rate with which free radicals infiltrate the body.

Best defense: Integrate smart, science-backed strategies into your daily life to reduce the amount of pro-aging toxins that enter your body and eliminate the ones that do get in.

STRATEGY #1: **Reduce consumption of advanced glycation end products (AGEs).** AGEs are inflammatory compounds formed when high-heat cooking methods (grilling, broiling, browning, roasting, frying) alter the fat and proteins in food. AGEs also are created when proteins and fats in certain foods—particularly animal-based fats (butter, meat, cheese) and processed foods—mix with fruc-

Ann Louise Gittleman, PhD, CNS, a holistic nutritionist based in Post Falls, Idaho, and *The New York Times* best-selling author who has written more than 35 books, including *Radical Longevity: The Powerful Plan to Sharpen Your Brain, Strengthen Your Body, and Reverse the Symptoms of Aging.* AnnLouise.com

tose and glucose in the bloodstream. The resulting "sticky" molecules promote oxidative stress and signs of aging in the body, from the skin (that sagging skin on your upper arm) to the heart (arteries stiffened by AGEs can nearly double the chance of dying from heart disease). *Self-defense...*

•**Choose the right fats**—olive oil and avocados...and avoid the wrong ones—bacon and fried foods. You can eat nuts and seeds raw or lightly toasted—roasting can double their AGE content.

•**Eat plant-based foods.** Fruits and veggies are low in AGEs and rich in detoxifying enzymes, fiber and antioxidant vitamins and minerals. Avoid high-fat animal products such as bacon and cheese.

•**Limit "high and dry" cooking methods,** such as grilling and roasting. Go for low-heat, wet cooking methods including simmering, braising, steaming, poaching and slow-cooking to maximize nutrients while limiting AGEs. If you grill, first marinate the fish or meat in an acidic medium such as citrus juice, organic grass-fed broth, apple cider vinegar—even olive oil will work. Per pound of meat or fish, use four to six tablespoons of liquid (plus enough water or other ingredients to cover the food), and add herbs and spices for flavor. This can slash AGE formation in half.

STRATEGY #2: **Minimize heavy metals and misbehaving minerals.** Metals and minerals such as aluminum, mercury and copper suppress the immune system, speeding aging and development of degenerative diseases.

•**Aluminum** increases osteoporosis risk and is linked to neurodegenerative diseases, such as Parkinson's and Alzheimer's. It enters the body in aluminum-containing medicines and foods cooked using aluminum products. *Self-defense...*

•Minimize use of aluminum-containing medications and products. Many antacids, antidiarrheals, OTC painkillers and deodorants contain aluminum.

•Use parchment paper instead of aluminum foil when cooking.

EASY TO DO...

Moves to Help You Live Longer

Exercise Barefoot

Exercising barefoot helps balance and mobility. The neural feedback to the brain provided by thousands of nerve endings in our feet encourages subtle muscle adjustments to optimize strength and balance. Wearing shoes smothers those communications.

To start: Walk barefoot in your house for 10 minutes a day...stand barefoot on both feet and turn your head from side to side...balance barefoot on one foot for five seconds and work up to a minute on each side.

Stacey Vachon is a certified personal trainer and owner of Core First Studio in Vail, Colorado. COREV3.com

Add In Just 10 Minutes of Exercise...

According to a recent study, more than 110,000 lives could be saved by adults over age 40 if they added just 10 minutes of moderate-to-vigorous activity to their daily routines. Even more lives would be saved if they increased that activity by 20 or 30 minutes daily. Research shows that even a very small amount of moderate-to-vigorous exercise can have a big impact on health.

Study of nearly 5,000 adults by researchers at National Cancer Institute, Rockville, Maryland, published in *JAMA Internal Medicine*.

•Replace aluminum pots, pans and cookie sheets with stainless steel, glass, Pyrex and ceramic nonstick cookware.

•**Mercury** exposure occurs through consumption of certain fish and seafood...medications and personal-care products...and dental amalgams (mercury fillings). Mercury damages nerves' protective covering, which impacts cognitive function and may lead to Alzheimer's. It also can cause tinnitus (ringing in the ears) and hearing loss. *Self-defense...*

•Avoid eating large fish (swordfish, ahi tuna, orange roughy, king mackerel and shark).

•Skip mercury-containing self-care products, including Preparation H and some contact lens solutions.

• Consider having mercury fillings removed. Mercury vapors may be released from fillings. Visit the website of the International Academy of Biological Dentistry and Medicine (IABDM. org/location) to find a dentist trained in mercury filling–removal protocols.

• **Copper comes in two forms**—monovalent, or food-based (found in avocado, asparagus, mushrooms, nuts, liver and chocolate)… and divalent, or synthetic (mostly in environmental sources such as drinking water from copper pipes, multivitamin/mineral supplements, copper-lined cookware and copper IUDs). Monovalent copper is essential for healthy bones, connective tissue, red blood cells and the immune system. But divalent copper accumulates over the years and is highly inflammatory, paving the way toward the destruction of brain cells and possibly leading to Alzheimer's disease. *Self-defense…*

• Test levels of copper in your drinking water. It should be a conservative 0.01 ppm (0.01 mg/L) or less. Home-testing kits are available at WaterCheck.com. If the copper level is over 0.01 ppm, install a copper filter (such as a reverse osmosis filter) on the tap used for drinking and cooking water.

• Avoid copper-containing supplements. Multivitamin/mineral supplements often are enriched with copper.

• Supplement with resveratrol, a plant compound that binds and removes copper. I like the Longevinex brand (one to two capsules per day).

***STRATEGY #3:* Reduce exposure to "smart" radiation.** Cell phones, smart devices (including smart thermostats and doorbells), Wi-Fi and cordless phones emit electromagnetic fields (EMFs), a form of radiation linked to fatigue, migraines, back pain, cognitive issues, problems with the heart, digestive system and sleep, cataracts—even brain tumors and cancer. They also raise levels of the stress hormone cortisol, which can accelerate aging, disrupt sleep and increase risk for cardiovascular disease. *Self-defense…*

• Hard-wire your home using Ethernet cables instead of Wi-Fi. If you have Wi-Fi, turn it off at night to slash exposure while you are sleeping. Keep cell phones away from your head—instead use a speaker phone or an air-

More from Ann Louise Gittleman…

Age-Proof Your Bones

Calcium gets all the attention, but your body requires other key minerals to properly deposit that calcium where it's needed. *Here are the key players**…

• **Magnesium,** found in leafy green vegetables, nuts, seeds, and legumes, helps create strong, more flexible bones.

Recommended: 400 mg to 800 mg of magnesium per day.

• **Boron** plays a key role in maintaining calcium and magnesium levels. Prunes are an excellent source.

Recommended: 3 mg/day—about 10 prunes.

• **Selenium.** Selenium is an antioxidant protector that helps support bone health. Found in Brazil nuts, fish and beans.

Recommended: 100 mcg/day to 200 mcg/day—about two or three Brazil nuts, depending on size.

• **Vitamin D,** found in eggs, fatty fish, beef liver and mushrooms, supports calcium absorption.

Recommended: 2,000 IU/day to 5,000 IU/day. You also can get the recommended amount by exposing your arms and legs to 15 to 20 minutes of midday sunshine.

• **Vitamin K** activates the critical protein osteocalcin, which integrates calcium into bones. Food sources include green leafy vegetables such as collards, kale, and spinach.

Recommended: 90 mcg per day—up to one cup.

*Be sure to ask your doctor before starting to take any new supplements. Vitamin K, in particular, can interfere with medications such as *warfarin*.

tube headset, rather than wireless ear buds. Keep your phone off or on airplane mode when not in use, and never leave it next to your bed when you're sleeping. If you need an alarm clock, get a battery- or electricity-powered one. Try to limit cell-phone or smart-device use to areas that have excellent reception—these devices use more power (and emit more radiation) in areas with poor reception. Avoid 5G-enabled devices. Until now, the wavelengths of all generations of wireless telecommunications technology, including 4G, have traveled along the surface of the skin, but 5G wavelengths are absorbed by the skin.

• Eat hemp seeds, rosemary and miso soup, all of which absorb radiation and mitigate its effects in the body.

• Supplement with magnesium, which helps offset the effects of EMFs. Take 5 mg of magnesium per pound of body weight per day.

• Decorate with plants that absorb electromagnetic radiation—snake plants, aloe vera, rubber plants and cacti.

Survival of the Fittest: It Doesn't Take Much

Barry A. Franklin, PhD, director of preventive cardiology/cardiac rehabilitation at Beaumont Health in Royal Oak, Mich. He is a long-standing member of the *Bottom Line Health* advisory board. DrBarryFranklin.com

Regular exercisers and endurance athletes live about three to six years longer than the general population.

But what is conferring this survival advantage: Simply being more active or working hard enough to experience improvements in aerobic fitness?

ACTIVITY VERSUS FITNESS

To find out, researchers compared the cardiovascular benefits of progressive levels of physical activity versus the body's ability to take in and use oxygen, or what we more commonly call aerobic fitness. They found that the most physically active people had a 30% lower risk of heart disease than the least active, showing that physical activity of any kind is beneficial.

But it's not nearly as effective as improving fitness. There was a 64% decline in the risk of heart disease from the least to the most fit participants. Put another way, a low level of fitness or aerobic capacity increases the risk of heart disease more than twice that of merely being physically inactive. Subsequent stud-

Keep Improving

Start where you can and work up to a total of 150 minutes of exercise per week. As your fitness increases, keep challenging yourself to continue to lower your risk by eating better and stopping smoking.

ies have shown that aerobic capacity is one of the strongest prognostic markers in people with and without heart disease. At any given risk-factor profile, low-fit individuals are two to three times more likely to die during the study follow-up than their more fit counterparts.

IMPLICATIONS FOR THE EXERCISER

In these studies, fitness level is measured by metabolic equivalents (METs). One metabolic equivalent (MET) equals the amount of oxygen your body uses at rest. A person with a fitness level that is less than 5 METs (or five times the energy expenditure at rest) generally has a higher risk of mortality. Examples of lower METs activities include billiards and bowling (2 to 3 METs) and bicycling at 5 to 6 miles per hour (mph; 2 to 4 METs).

In contrast, an aerobic capacity of 8 to 10 METs or higher signifies an excellent long-term prognosis. That's equivalent to participating in activities such as bicycling at 12 to 14 mph, jogging at 6 mph, or playing competitive handball or squash.

START SMALL

If you're not yet fit, don't worry: It doesn't take a lot of work to see big rewards. The biggest reductions in the risk of heart disease are seen in people who move from the "lowest" (bottom 20%) to the "low" (below average) aerobic capacity category. To do that, you just need to regularly exercise at 3 METs or higher. That is the equivalent of walking on a flat treadmill at 3 mph or on a 3.5% grade at 2 mph. Other comparable activities include bicycling at 6 mph, golf (pulling a golf bag), or pushing a light power mower.

Dance Away Old Age

Dancing improves health and self-esteem after menopause. A three-times-a-week dance program helped postmenopausal women better manage weight and other health risk factors, such as high cholesterol…improved their functional fitness (coordination, agility, aerobic capability)…and also boosted their self-image and self-esteem. Dance therapy is low-cost and has low injury risk, and many women are more likely to stick with dancing than with other forms of exercise.

Study of 36 postmenopausal women by researchers at São Paulo State University, Brazil, published in *Menopause*.

Improve Your Functional Fitness

Karl Knopf, EdD, former director of fitness therapy and senior fitness for the International Sports Sciences Association and retired director of adaptive fitness at Foothill College in Los Altos Hills, California. He is author of 16 books on functional fitness including *Resistance Band Workbook* and *Injury Rehab with Resistance Bands*.

Have you stopped riding a bike, bowling or playing golf or tennis because these activities are too hard to perform? Do your muscles sometimes struggle when you're going up the stairs? Or raising yourself up from a low chair, the toilet or the car? Do you find yourself losing your balance more often than you used to? These all are telltale signs that you need to improve your functional fitness—the ability to perform everyday tasks that use multiple muscle groups and require balance, strength and dexterity.

Although our physical capabilities naturally decline with age, our increasingly sedentary lifestyle also significantly impacts our strength and flexibility. If you have trouble carrying groceries into your home or feel winded after a short brisk walk, this decline in physical function can mean the loss of the ability to live independently as you age.

But it doesn't have to be this way. *Starting a functional fitness program can improve your ability to live a full life…**

CREATING YOUR ROUTINE

To design your routine, start by assessing which activities you do regularly that you find challenging. Then choose from the exercises described on these pages. Start with two or three repetitions of each exercise, rest and then repeat several times, eventually working up to two to three sets of 10 or 15 repetitions.

Important: Maintaining proper form and posture through each exercise is critical to its effectiveness.

These exercises require only exercise bands (buy at least two—one that is open and one that is a closed loop) and dumbbells (start with one- to three-pound weights depending on your current strength). Resistance bands normally come in sets of low-, medium- and high-resistance. Experiment to see what's right for you. When you get comfortable, challenge yourself with more resistance, more weight and/or more repetitions.

If you have trouble going up stairs or getting up from a chair or if your legs are weak, you need to strengthen the leg and core muscles. *Doing so can help to reduce the load on your knees and possibly reduce knee pain…*

LUNGES

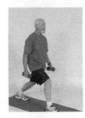

1. Stand up tall on a nonslip surface holding a dumbbell in each hand at your sides or while wearing a weighted vest. Inhale.

2. As you exhale, lunge forward with your right leg while keeping your left leg stationary. Only lunge forward as far as comfortable and be sure to keep your front knee aligned with your ankle.

3. Inhale and step back to your starting position. Repeat.

*Note: Get clearance from a doctor before starting any exercise program to determine if you have an underlying dysfunction that is contributing to your limitations.

Then switch sides. Be sure to maintain erect posture as you do each repetition.

LEG PRESSES

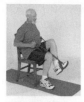

1. Sit in a chair and wrap an exercise band around your left foot. Hold on to both ends of the band with your elbows bent and shoulders relaxed.

2. Exhale and slowly extend the left leg forward. Do not lock your knee.

3. Inhale and return your leg to the starting position. Repeat, and then switch sides.

WALL SQUATS/SLIDES

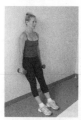

1. Lean your back against a wall with your feet about 12 to 18 inches away from the wall. Hold a dumbbell in each hand with your arms at your sides. Inhale.

2. Exhale as you slide yourself down along the wall, going no farther than feels comfortable or until your thighs are parallel with the floor. Do not let your knees extend beyond your toes.

3. Inhale and return to the upright position...or for greater challenge, hold for a count of five before inhaling and returning to the starting position. Keep your head straight and eyes looking forward.

Note: Skip this exercise if you have heart or blood pressure issues. Instead, try a Mini Chair Squat. Just stand in front of a chair or tall stool to hold onto for balance and only lower yourself slightly, rather than doing a full squat.

If you have trouble opening heavy doors or carrying groceries, you need to strengthen your arms and shoulders...

CHAIR PUSH-UPS

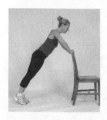

1. Stand behind a sturdy chair or countertop. Lean forward, and place your hands on the chair back/countertop shoulder-width apart. Extend your arms fully, without locking your elbows, as you walk your legs back until your body is at a 45-degree angle to the floor. Your heels will be raised slightly. Keep your legs straight but not locked. Inhale.

2. Exhale and slowly lower your chest to the chair. Keep your elbows close to your body and your torso in a straight line with your legs.

3. Inhale and press your body away from the chair, fully extending your arms without locking them, returning to the starting position.

PULL-DOWNS

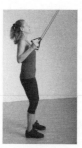

1. Tie a knot in the middle of an open exercise band, and anchor it at the top of a closed door, leaving both ends hanging down. Sit in a chair or stand and reach overhead, arms straight, to grasp each end of the band at a point that will provide resistance when stretched. Inhale.

2. Exhale as you pull your elbows back, bringing your hands to shoulder level. Be careful not to arch your back and to keep your shoulders down.

3. Inhale. Return to starting position.

SHOULDER RETRACTIONS

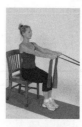

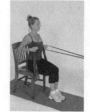

1. Position a chair near a closed door. Tie the middle of an open exercise band around the doorknob leaving two long ends. Grasp an end in each hand about halfway up so you feel a comfortable level of resistance. Inhale and suck in your stomach to stabilize your back.

2. Exhale and slowly pull your elbows back toward your sides. Keep your shoulder blades together throughout.

3. Inhale and return to the starting position.

BOW & ARROW

1. Stand with your feet about hip-width apart. With your left hand, grab one side of a closed-loop exercise band and extend that arm out to your side at shoulder height. Now grab

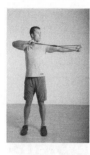

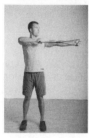

the opposite side of the band with your right hand, keeping your right hand near your left shoulder and your right elbow at shoulder height. You should be positioned as though holding an archery bow.

2. Inhale and stretch the band back across your chest with your right hand as if you were pulling a bow. Your right elbow will be bent, left arm extended. Keep shoulders relaxed/down.

3. Exhale. Return to the starting position. Repeat and switch to the other side.

If you have trouble reaching things on high shelves, you need to stretch and strengthen the arms and shoulders…

WALKING FINGERTIPS

1. Stand sideways to a wall about an arm's distance away…or stand facing it.

2. Reach out to the wall. Slowly walk your fingertips up the wall as high as you can.

3. Crawl your fingers down to the starting position, repeat and switch sides.

GOOD TO KNOW…

One-Stop Shop for Age-at-Home Products

Home-improvement chain Lowe's partnered with AARP to launch Livable Home in 2022—a program that offers products, services and DIY expertise to help seniors stay in their own homes instead of moving to assisted-care facilities. The program includes specially trained Lowe's employees wearing AARP-branded badges available to help customers as well as products and information for installing shower grab bars, non-slip floors, wheelchair ramps and walk-in bathtubs. The program is launching in 500 stores in 50 metro areas.

Information: Lowes.com (search "livable home").

CNBC.com

WALL CIRCLES

1. Stand facing a wall with one arm extended touching it at shoulder level.

2. Draw small circles clockwise, increasing to larger circles as feels comfortable. Repeat, and switch sides.

APPLE PICKER

1. Stand tall with your hands on your shoulders.

2. Reach your right hand up to the ceiling, stretching as high as is comfortable.

3. Return your right hand to your shoulder, and reach up with your left hand.

A Single Head Injury Increases Dementia Risk

Researchers recently discovered that a person with a single head injury had a 1.25 times higher risk of developing dementia than someone with no head injuries. A history of two or more injuries more than doubled the risk. Overall, 9.5% of all dementia cases in the study population could be attributed to a head injury.

Andrea L.C. Schneider, MD, PhD, assistant professor of neurology, University of Pennsylvania School of Medicine, Philadelphia, Pennsylvania.

Your Brain Works Best in the Morning

Older adults are mentally sharpest and less distracted in the morning. Researchers are not sure why this is so but believe it may be to do with circadian rhythms. If you need to do a cognitively challenging activity, tackle it first thing in the morning, when you're at your best.

Mind, Mood & Memory, reported in *Harvard Heart Letter.*

What About the New AD Drug?

Dharma Singh Khalsa, MD, president and medical director of the Alzheimer's Research and Prevention Foundation in Tucson, Arizona, and prevention editor of *Journal of Alzheimer's Disease*.

At first blush, the FDA's recent approval of the first treatment for early-stage Alzheimer's disease (AD) since 2003 offers a glimmer of hope for the six million Americans with AD. Marketed under the name Aduhelm, *aducanumab* removes amyloid, a sticky compound often found in the brains of people with AD. Amyloid can clump and form plaques that disrupt cell-to-cell communication.

Theory: By removing amyloid, you may be able to slow or reduce cognitive decline. Aducanumab is not a cure, and it cannot bring back lost cognitive function. One year of aducanumab, given intravenously every four weeks for 45 to 60 minutes at a time, costs $28,000 (lowered from the original cost of $56,000).

Concerns: The new drug was approved via an accelerated approval pathway, meaning that despite uncertainty about its efficacy, the FDA wanted to provide access to a treatment that it believes is "reasonably likely" to help. This approval came after trials of the drug were initially halted because it seemed aducanumab wasn't working as well as hoped. Subsequent reanalysis of the data suggested some potential, and, despite the FDA's own advisory committee being against it, the accelerated approval happened.

Aducanumab has some side effects, including headaches, brain swelling and increased risk of falling.

Note: The Cleveland Clinic and the Mount Sinai Health System do not plan to carry aducanumab due to safety and efficacy concerns.

Perhaps even more important is that more and more high-level AD researchers now suggest that amyloid deposits may not be the only cause of AD. Many patients live long, cognitively healthy lives despite having those plaques. Amyloid may be a marker of aging, but many holistic- and integrative-minded brain experts believe that AD results from lifestyle factors, including stress, poor diet, lack of exercise, lack of mental stimulation, lack of meditation and more.

Keep Your Driving Skills Sharp as You Age

William Van Tassel, PhD, manager of driver-training programs at the national office of the American Automobile Association (AAA) in Heathrow, Florida, where he is also three-time chair of The Association of National Stakeholders in Traffic Safety Education, funded by the National Highway Traffic Safety Administration (NHTSA). AAA.com

Americans are living longer these days, and we want to maintain our independence and mobility for as long as possible. By staying current with new car technology, keeping driving skills up to date and caring for our bodies and minds, we don't have to lose that independence.

Driving expert William Van Tassel's tips to extend our safe-driving years…

THE ELEMENTS OF DRIVING

Driving consists of three components—perception, decision and action. You perceive a car braking ahead of you…you decide to decelerate…and you act by tapping your brakes. *To maintain your skills in each of these three areas…*

•**Perception.** Our eyesight begins to diminish as early as our 40s. We start losing some of our peripheral vision…our ability to see well in low light declines…and cataracts, macular degeneration and other conditions can make things even worse. *Steps to keep your perception sharp…*

•Get screened. Every senior driver should have his/her vision tested at least once a year and, of course, stay on top of eyewear prescriptions and any new vision problems.

•Drive only when visibility is good. Many seniors are retired and therefore have flexible schedules. Take advantage of that by being selective about when you drive to avoid crowded roadways and poor weather conditions.

• Brighten your headlights. You might be surprised at the improved visibility after simply changing to a new set of factory bulbs. Xenon or high-intensity discharge (HID) bulbs are especially good for seniors because they can improve visibility at night. *Also:* Be sure to clean your headlights regularly.

• Modify your rig. If your peripheral vision has diminished, you can install special mirrors that help you see better out to the sides. If your neck hurts when you turn around to back up, have a rear-view camera installed. *Caution:* These cameras can take some getting used to—be sure to practice in a safe, off-street location before using a camera for actual backing-up and parking maneuvers. *Important:* These cameras are no substitute for looking directly at the area into which you are backing.

• Use a spotter. Many older drivers wisely venture out only with a passenger to act as a second set of eyes.

• **Decision.** Thanks to the wisdom that comes with years of driving, seniors actually have a leg up on younger drivers when it comes to decision-making. They recognize threats, anticipate the moves of other motorists and know how to react effectively. *Still, those skills can be maintained throughout your life…*

• Stay up to date. All drivers—not just seniors—should consider taking a classroom-based refresher course every few years. These are available from AAA, AARP, National Safety Council and driving schools around the country, with courses typically taking six-to-eight hours total. Traffic laws, vehicle technology, signage, roadway design and driving techniques continue to evolve.

Examples: Roundabouts used to be rare in the US but now are springing up in many areas. While they're much safer than traditional intersections—because all drivers are moving in the same direction, and no drivers are turning left in front of others—many drivers panic the first few times they encounter them. Even basics such as how to hold the steering wheel have changed—driving instructors used to train people to grasp the wheel at the 2:00 and 10:00 positions, but

---

GOOD TO KNOW...

Cataract Surgery Lowers Risk for Dementia

Study participants who had their cataracts removed were nearly 30% less likely to develop dementia compared with participants with cataracts who did not have the surgery. The restored vision improves stimuli to the brain by allowing higher-quality sensory input and light to reach the retina. Better engagement with the world also might be brain protective.

Cecilia S. Lee, MD, is the Klorfine family associate professor of ophthalmology at University of Washington, Seattle, and lead researcher for a study of 3,000 people with cataracts published in *JAMA Internal Medicine*.

---

now the safest grip is considered to be the 9:00 and 3:00 positions.

There are refresher courses specifically for seniors that focus on maneuvers that have proven statistically problematic for older drivers, including left turns, merges, right turns from a dedicated lane and lane changes.

• **Action.** It's no secret that our reflexes get slower with time, and a loss of flexibility and mobility make it more difficult to maneuver a vehicle. *Steps to keep your mobility in top shape…*

• Modify. Make your vehicle as comfortable as possible so that you will feel confident when driving. Adjust the height of your seat and steering wheel and also your seatbelt. Add a seat cushion that allows you to easily swivel your legs when you need to look over your shoulder. Wrap an ergonomic grip around the steering wheel.

• Maintain. Keep your car in top running order. Spongy brakes, bald tires and poor acceleration are just a few of the maintenance issues that can severely disrupt your ability to drive safely. If your budget allows, consider buying or leasing a latest-model vehicle that will provide you with the newest safety features.

• Practice. If you do get a new vehicle with unfamiliar safety technologies, spend time with the salesperson becoming familiar with the features. Then take the car to an empty parking lot and drive around to get used to the new bells and whistles.

Caution: Don't become overly reliant on safety tech—it could make you less vigilant over time. Instead, continue to drive as if the vehicle did not have these new technologies—and use them to back you up if needed.

MORE WAYS TO STAY SAFE

• **Exercise your body and your brain.** A fit person is a fit driver. Whether it's pickleball, Ping-Pong or yoga, any activity that helps you maintain balance, strength and flexibility also will help you behind the wheel.

Also: Computer games can keep your mind sharp and help your hand-eye coordination.

• **Watch your meds.** Senior drivers are less likely to fall asleep behind the wheel than younger drivers. But many older drivers take prescription drugs, some of which can cause drowsiness or brain fog. Ask your doctors which of your medications have such side effects and arrange your schedule so you do not need to drive after taking them.

FACE CHANGE HEAD ON

Older drivers don't deserve their reputation for being dangerous. Statistically speaking, per mile driven, teens are more likely to be involved in a crash than older drivers. But around age 75, crash rates involving seniors start to rise.

Instead of waiting for loved ones to intervene or until you have an accident, monitor your own driving habits. Have you noticed other drivers honking at you a lot lately? Have you gotten a ticket for driving too slowly? Have you had some near misses? If so, that doesn't necessarily mean you need to hang up your keys, but it does mean that you should take an honest look at your situation.

Start with a professional in-car assessment of your driving skills. Your local driving school or AAA should be able to help you find one. Someone will ride with you for about 45 minutes, noting any deficits, and then will make recommendations that might include taking a class, in-car training or, if your situation warrants it, a clinical evaluation by a physician.

If you feel like your driving career is nearing its end, start planning now for how you'll get around.

How to Deal with Age-Related Night-Vision Problems

Get *regular eye exams* to keep prescriptions current and identify any diseases. Get treatment for other vision issues, such as dry eyes and cataracts. *Use a flashlight or flashlight app* on a smartphone when out walking in dark areas. Turn on more lights indoors, and consider installing night-lights throughout your house. *Keep eyeglass lenses clear*—wash the lenses regularly, and have an optician buff out any small scratches. *Keep your car's windshield and headlights clean*—that will help with driving at night and when the sun hits your windshield during the day. Keep windshield-washer levels topped up. *Adapt to night driving by dimming dashboard lights* and using the night setting on your rearview mirror.

Harvard Health Letter. Health.Harvard.edu

New and Improved Cataract Care

Ravi Goel, MD, a comprehensive ophthalmologist, cataract, and refractive surgeon at Regional Eye Associates in Cherry Hill, New Jersey, an instructor at Wills Eye Hospital, Philadelphia, and a spokesperson for the American Academy of Ophthalmology.

For hundreds of years, cataract removal surgery was only that—removal of the clouded lens that impaired vision. In 1949, Sir Harold Ridley invented the first artificial lens to replace the one that was removed in surgery, but it wasn't a widely accepted practice for decades.

Boost Your Vision

If your eye doctor diagnoses cataracts, it doesn't mean you need surgery right away. *You may be able to use these stopgap measures to significantly boost vision…*

●**Use brighter lights or a magnifying glass to read, knit, or do other detailed tasks.**

●**Wear anti-glare sunglasses.** Protecting your eyes from sunlight can also slow cataract progression.

●**Ask your doctor if dry eye might be aggravating your symptoms.** With 70% of the power to bring an image into focus relying on healthy tear film in your eyes, dry eye can significantly cut vision clarity. Over-the-counter or prescription tear replacement drops might help.

—Dr. Ravi Goel

Now, not only are lenses replaced, but patients aren't limited to a basic, one-size-fits-all approach: Several lens choices offer the opportunity to improve vision. (You might even be able to ditch those reading glasses you've needed for years.)

EARLY CATARACTS

About half of all people will develop cataracts by age 80, but the process starts sooner than you think. Proteins can begin to build up on the lens in your 40s, though they likely won't cause any noticeable effects until your 60s or later. If you notice that colors seem faded, lights look too bright or have haloes, or your night vision is declining, make an appointment with an ophthalmologist. A comprehensive eye exam can identify cataracts as well as other dangerous eye conditions that become more common with age.

WHEN IT'S TIME FOR SURGERY

In the early stages of cataracts, you can try a variety of stopgap measures to improve your vision (see sidebar above). When those measures are no longer sufficient, it's time to have your cloudy lenses replaced with clear ones.

Cataract surgery is an outpatient procedure. Your eye will be numbed, so you won't feel any discomfort, and you may also be given medication to help you relax. In the most common procedure, the surgeon will make a tiny incision and use ultrasound waves to break the cataract apart, remove it, and then replace it with an intraocular lens (IOL). *There are several options…*

●**Fixed-focus monofocal IOLs.** These lenses will give you clear vision at a distance, but you'll still need reading glasses to see up close. If you have cataract surgery in both eyes, you might choose a lens that provides near vision in one eye and a lens that provides far vision in the other, a combination called monovision.

●**Accommodating monofocal IOLs.** Using the natural musculature around the eye, you can shift these lenses from near to far vision. Distance and middle-distance vision are typically excellent with this newer choice, but close-up vision may not improve.

●**Toric IOLs.** These lenses are used for people with astigmatism, a flaw in the eye's curvature that causes blurred distance and near vision. By bending light more efficiently, toric lenses provide focused vision at a single distance, correcting astigmatism so distance glasses are no longer needed.

●**Multifocal IOLs.** These lenses work like progressive or bifocal glasses, with different sections geared for distance, middle, and near vision. Your brain and eyes work together to decide which part of the lens you need at any given time. Multifocal lenses are the most versatile.

WHAT TO EXPECT

If you have cataracts in both eyes, expect to have two separate surgeries. Two procedures separated by mere weeks may seem inconvenient and even wasteful, but there are distinct advantages to this approach. By staging your second surgery once the first eye has healed and vision is stable, you can determine how the new lens behaves. If tweaking seems appropriate, the power of the second lens can then be fine-tuned. Most health insurers cover cataract surgery, though your out-of-pocket costs will vary.

Want to ensure you're among the nine in 10 people for whom cataract surgery spells success? While the odds of complications such as infection, pain, or vision loss are low, your actions in the days and weeks after the procedure influence the outcome. The main goal is preventing infection. You'll need to use antibiotic eye drops several times a day and keep water out of your eyes. You may also need to wear a bandage or shield to stop yourself from rubbing and keep specks of dust or debris from getting in your eye.

Light daily activities are fine as your eyes heal, but avoid bending over, jogging, or lifting heavy objects. You'll schedule follow-up visits with your eye surgeon for the day after the procedure, as well as a week or two later and a month after that.

TAKE NOTE...

Eyedrops Could Replace Your Reading Glasses

According to a recent study, Pilocarpine HCL ophthalmic solution (Vuity), a prescription eyedrop medication recently approved by the FDA for people whose near vision has become blurry with age (presbyopia), helped 35% of participants read three additional lines on a vision chart. Vuity works by constricting pupil size, increasing depth of focus without disrupting distance focus.

Cost: About $100 for a month's supply. Check with your eye doctor whether Vuity is appropriate for you.

Eric Donnenfeld, MD, ophthalmologist and eye surgeon, Ophthalmic Consultants of Long Island, Garden City, New York, commenting on studies of 750 participants presented to the American Academy of Ophthalmology.

Sight Stealer: Ocular Hypertension

Michael A. Kass, MD, Bernard Becker Professor of Ophthalmology and Visual Sciences at Washington University School of Medicine in St. Louis, Missouri.

Glaucoma is called the silent thief of sight. Open-angle glaucoma, the most common type, doesn't have symptoms until late in its course. The key risk factor for glaucoma is ocular hypertension, or elevated eye pressure.

At the start of a study, 46% of participants had evidence of glaucoma in one or both eyes, but only 25% had vision loss when examined 20 years after the study's launch. So not everyone needs preventive treatment—monitoring may be enough.

A prediction model that takes a set of variables into account can help determine if your risk is low, medium or high. The variables are age...level of intraocular pressure...thickness of the cornea...thickness of the rim of the optic nerve (glaucoma causes changes in the rim)...and the results of standard eye exam tests. If needed, an imaging test called *optical coherence tomography* (OCT) can provide information or a baseline from which to look for changes in the future.

Using this approach allows the eye doctor to outline a patient's potential risk for glaucoma and make an informed decision about whether or not to begin treatment to lower eye pressure.

If you choose to monitor ocular hypertension at first, eye-exam frequency will depend on your risk—for low risk, you might see the doctor yearly...for high risk, two or three times a year. Other factors that make more frequent exams necessary are having diabetes, having cataracts at a younger-than-usual age and your age—eye diseases, in general, are more common in people after age 60.

Connection between glaucoma and sleep: A separate study presented at the 2021 Annual Meeting of The Association for Research in Vision and Ophthalmology highlighted the high prevalence of sleep disorders among people with glaucoma. The exact connection between the two conditions isn't fully understood, but one theory is that glaucoma can impair certain cells involved in the body's sleep-regulating system, throwing off circadian rhythms. If you suspect that you have a sleep disorder, talk to your doctor about doing a sleep study to find out if a CPAP machine or cognitive behavioral therapy would help.

The Leading Cause of Vision Loss

Chris Iliades, MD, retired ear, nose, throat, head, and neck surgeon who now dedicates his time to patient education through medical writing.

A ge-related macular degeneration (AMD) is more common than glaucoma and cataracts put together, and it's the leading cause of vision loss in people over age 50. Once you have it, there is no cure, but you can take steps now to reduce your risk.

The macula is the central part of the retina at the back of the eye. Light-sensitive cells in your macula are responsible for central vision, what you see in front of your face. When your macula starts to degenerate, you begin to lose your central vision: what you need to drive, read, see faces, and work with your hands. AMD does not affect your peripheral vision, so you will not be completely blind, but loss of central vision is a handicap.

CONTROLLABLE RISK FACTORS

The biggest risk factor for AMD, as you might expect from the name, is age. AMD starts to occur after age 50. After age 75, about one-third of people will have some amount of AMD.

Genes appear to play a role, too. Researchers estimate that 75% of people carry the genes for AMD, which can be passed down through families. But many people never get AMD, so we know that there are clearly other contributing factors. *Controlling these is the key to reducing your chances of developing AMD...*

• **Quit smoking.** If you smoke, you are up to five times more likely to get AMD.

• **Exercise and maintain a healthy weight.** Being obese doubles your risk of AMD.

• **Get high blood sugar, high blood pressure, or high cholesterol under control.**

• **Wear sunglasses.** There is some evidence that ultraviolet rays from the sun can cause AMD, especially if you have blue eyes. Sunglasses also reduce your risk of cataracts.

• **Eat a healthy diet rich in antioxidants,** such as leafy green vegetables and other colorful vegetables and fruits. Oxidative stress,

The Stages of AMD

AMD has three stages...

• **Early stage.** Your vision is still normal, but an eye specialist can look into your eye with a special lens and see early changes of AMD.

• **Intermediate stage.** You start to have symptoms, such as blurred vision, blank or dark spots in your central vision, or seeing straight lines as wavy or curvy. One way to test for early symptoms of AMD is with a visual test called the Amsler Grid, which you can find on the American Macular Degeneration Foundation website at Macular.org/amsler-chart. If you see any dark, blank, blurry, or wavy areas on the grid, let your doctor know.

• **Late stage.** You have complete loss of central vision. AMD does not affect your peripheral vision.

which occurs when unstable molecules called free radicals damage cells, may play a role in causing AMD. Antioxidants capture these free radicals and prevent cell damage.

THE ROLE OF SUPPLEMENTS

Two National Eye Institute studies, called the Age-Related Eye Disease Studies (AREDS and AREDS2), found that high doses of antioxidant supplements could delay and possibly prevent the progression of AMD. The recommended supplements are vitamins C and E, the minerals zinc and copper, and the antioxidants lutein and zeaxanthin. These supplements are combined into a product called AREDS2 that you can get at drug or health food stores. The National Eye Institute recommends taking AREDS2 if you have intermediate AMD in one or both eyes to help slow down the vision loss.

TYPES OF AMD

There are two types of AMD, and the cause and treatment for each type is different...

• **Dry AMD is the most common type.** It happens when a type of protein builds up beneath the macula, causing the macula to become thin and dry. Symptoms of central vision loss are gradual, and complete loss of central vision rarely occurs. The only treatment for dry AMD is AREDS2. Treatment may slow down dry AMD, but it does not cure it.

•**Wet AMD is less common.** In this type, abnormal blood vessels grow under the macula and leak, causing rapid degeneration of the macula and a rapid loss of vision. The main treatment for wet AMD is an injection of a substance called anti-vascular endothelial growth factor directly into the macula. This treatment may reduce the growth of the abnormal blood vessels or even stop the growth for a while, but the injections need to be repeated. Like dry AMD, wet AMD cannot be cured.

REGULAR CHECKS LOWER RISK

You can reduce your risk of AMD, but you can't completely prevent it. That's why the most important step is to get regular eye exams. The American Academy of Ophthalmology recommends a complete eye exam that includes looking at your retina and macula for everyone at age 40. If you are over age 65, you should get the exam every one or two years. An eye doctor can diagnose AMD before you have symptoms. Starting treatment at the early stage is your best bet for preventing the progression of AMD.

Caffeine Can Increase Glaucoma Risk

Caffeine increases glaucoma risk if there is a genetic predisposition for high intraocular pressure (IOP).

Recent finding: Compared with people who had low genetic propensity for high IOP and who consumed little caffeine, those who had the highest genetic tendency for high IOP and consumed more than 320 mg of caffeine daily (about three cups of coffee) had a 3.9-fold increased risk for glaucoma. If glaucoma runs in your family, limit coffee to two cups a day.

Louis Pasquale, MD, is professor of ophthalmology at Icahn School of Medicine at Mount Sinai, New York City, and leader of a study of more than 120,000 adults, published in *Ophthalmology*.

EASY TO DO...

To Reduce Undereye Bags and Other Facial Swelling

Freeze your daily facial toner into cubes, then rub a cube on your face after cleansing—start at your forehead and work down. The cold will help reduce swelling, including bags under eyes. You also can chill face masks—in the refrigerator, not the freezer—for a similar effect.

Caution: Freezing may reduce the potency of toners that contain retinol, vitamin C, salicylic acid and glycolic acid.

Real Simple.

Gardening May Lead to a Longer Life

In communities worldwide where many people are age 100 or older, residents have been consistently found to do gardening well into old age. Gardening may increase well-being and longevity by keeping people connected with sunlight, fresh air and plant life...providing an ongoing form of physical activity... giving people who grow fruits and vegetables a source of super-fresh, high-nutrition plant foods...keeping the mind sharp by requiring planning and problem-solving...and establishing a form of meditative mindfulness by keeping gardeners centered in the moment.

Roundup of studies by environmental and health researchers in the UK, the US and the Netherlands, reported at CNBC.com.

Signs of Hearing Loss You Shouldn't Ignore

*Buzzing or ringing that comes and goes—*this can indicate nerve damage, often caused by using headphones at too-high volumes. *Balance problems—*the inner ear sends signals to the brain to help the body balance, so stumbling more often could indicate ear damage. *Forgetfulness*—difficulty hearing makes remembering harder. The brain uses more energy to process sound and devotes less to thinking and memory. *Pain from loud noises*—some irritation caused by sirens, car horns and similar loud sounds is normal, but actual pain may indicate hearing loss. *Trouble hearing in places with background noise*—this could be caused by poor acoustics or by the ear's decreased ability to differentiate among sounds. If you have any of these worrisome symptoms, talk to your doctor.

Roundup of otolaryngologists reported on The Healthy.com.

Online Support If You're Losing Your Hearing

SayWhatClub.org is a support group where you can connect with others who have hearing loss. HearingLossHelp.com has more than 1,000 posts answering questions about hearing loss, plus a section on assistive listening devices. HISHearingLoops.com specializes in installing hearing loops, a sound system that can connect to your hearing aid via Bluetooth to deliver music customized to your hearing loss.

Tom Yaxley, YG Financial Group, PC, Champaign, Illinois, and a subscriber to *Bottom Line Personal*.

Not Enough Americans Are Getting Their Hearing Checked

Among Americans over age 50, 80% have not been asked about their hearing by their primary doctors within the past two years, and 77% have not been checked by a hearing specialist.

But: Research shows that around half of older adults have some degree of hearing loss, which has physical and mental health reper-

cussions, including higher rates of depression, falls and cognitive decline.

Michael McKee, MD, is associate professor, department of family medicine at University of Michigan, Ann Arbor, and leader of research published as part of the National Poll on Healthy Aging.

Anti-Aging Skin Care— Hope or Hype?

Jessica Weiser, MD, a board-certified dermatologist in New York City and assistant clinical professor of dermatology at Columbia University.

When it comes to skin care, fantastic promises are everywhere. Creams that range from $10 to several hundred dollars promise sunny, youthful faces, while procedures that can cost thousands offer relief from fine lines, wrinkles, and scars.

The vast array of products and procedures can leave you with more questions than answers. Here's a quick guide to what you can realistically expect in the world of anti-aging skin care.

OVER-THE-COUNTER PRODUCTS

Products that you buy at the drugstore or beauty counter may soften fine lines, reduce pore size, and lessen crepe-like texture to the skin, but they won't do anything for deep lines and folds. *Here are the ingredients you're likely to see...*

•**Antioxidants.** Just as a diet filled with antioxidant-rich fruits and vegetables is good for overall health, antioxidants applied to the skin can help reduce signs of aging caused by unstable molecules (free radicals) that damage collagen, the protein that keeps skin plump. This process is called oxidative stress. Antioxidants stabilize free radicals by giving them an extra electron. Some of the antioxidants that you'll see in skin-care products include vitamin C, green tea extracts, polyphenols, niacinamide, and coenzyme Q10.

•**Alpha hydroxy and other acids.** In nonprescription strengths, these acids, which also include lactic, glycolic, and salicylic acids, are mild exfoliating chemicals. They're designed to create some skin-cell turnover, so you'll see some improvement in skin quality over a period of months when used twice a week. But because you're not abrading a layer of skin, you're not getting a true peel with these products. The strength required to abrade skin would be dangerous to use at home and is only available professionally.

- **Peptides.** When formulated as small molecules, these proteins can penetrate skin and stimulate cell turnover, often with less irritation than retinols.

- **Retinols.** These vitamin A derivatives, when found in OTC products, are milder than the prescription tretinoin, which means they provide both milder improvement and milder side effects. Keep in mind that there are different types of retinol and it's hard to tell what you're getting in typical products.

The products you choose and when you use them depends on what you're trying to accomplish.

If you want to combat wrinkling, use an antioxidant product in the morning to shield skin and a retinol-based one at night for skin renewal. (Retinol makes skin vulnerable to the sun, so you don't want to use it during the day.) If you want to soothe dry and sensitive skin, use a product with glycerin or hyaluronic acid to help skin retain moisture.

More expensive does not guarantee more effective when it comes to skin-care products. The key is finding the active ingredients that create the best results on your skin type, which will vary significantly from person to person. Oily skin will be more tolerant of retinol and acid treatments, while dry, sensitive skin will respond better to humectants and heavier emollients to help restore the skin barrier.

LIGHT THERAPY

Another way to get some mild skin firming and cell turnover is to try LED therapy. This treatment uses different wavelengths of light to reduce inflammation, heal wounds, and promote anti-aging effects. The strongest devices are limited to dermatologists' offices, but the U.S. Food and Drug Administration has approved several LED light devices for home use. The verdict is still out on their effective-

Healthful Skin Habits

Lifestyle habits can have a big impact on skin quality. Think of these steps as part of your anti-aging skincare.

- **Use sunscreen daily.** The ideal product is a true sunscreen, rather than a tinted moisturizer or foundation with SPF. To get the full SPF protection from makeup, you'd need to apply an amount equal to a nickel, and that's more than most people are willing to put on their face. Choose a physical barrier sunscreen with at least 10% zinc oxide and/or titanium dioxide. There are many health reasons to avoid chemical-based sunscreens, including that they can increase the risk for oxidative skin damage.

- **Do not sunbathe.** The less sun you get, the longer your skin will stay youthful. There's still no such thing as a healthy tan.

- **Don't smoke.** The smoke itself triggers the destruction of collagen and, on a surface level, the repeated squinting reaction creates or deepens lines around eyes and lips.

- **Avoid home peel kits that include micro-needling rollers.** Designed to help active ingredients in products get deeper into the skin, professional-quality devices can be effective in the hands of a dermatologist. However, the needles in home products are not long enough to achieve that goal yet are long enough to break the skin and cause infection and scarring. Never use anything that breaks the surface of your skin.

—Dr. Jessica Weiser

ness, but the American Academy of Dermatology considers the therapy to be safe as long as you are not on any medication that makes you sensitive to sunlight.

PROFESSIONAL-GRADE RESULTS

To get more noticeable results, you'll need to visit a dermatologist who can determine your skin type and its needs, listen to what bothers you most about your appearance, and know what products and procedures will be most effective. You might be surprised by all the possible treatments that exist.

Not only can you get stronger light therapy, but you'll also unlock access to creams like tretinoin (Retin-A), a form of vitamin A that can boost collagen production when applied at least two times per week, leading to smoother, younger-looking skin. Tretinoin can cause redness and flaking as it starts to work and is not a replacement for all other skin products.

For both daily care and rejuvenation, there are now many specialty skin-care formulas that have gone through rigorous clinical testing. They're made with slightly different active ingredients and often more effective combinations than what you'll find in drug- or beauty-store brands, so some of them can travel down pores and help activate stem cells to get robust skin turnover. While these medical-grade brands are not prescription items, you can buy them only from a dermatologist.

FILLERS AND PROCEDURES

Among the most visible and immediate skin-rejuvenating treatments are injectable dermal fillers that build volume where tissue has been lost, such as in deep creases or hollow cheeks. They can soften folds, enhance the jawline, and bring back body to the lips. Fillers are usually injected in the doctor's office and don't require surgery or downtime. *They can be made of a variety of substances…*

• **Those made from hyaluronic acid** last for six to 12 months before the body dissolves the molecules.

• **Fillers made of calcium hydroxylapatite** are calcium-based molecules that may last for about 12 months for most patients.

• **Poly-L-lactic acid** has been used for many years in medical devices, such as dissolvable stitches. It is a small particle suspended in sterile water that stimulates the production of collagen to smooth fine lines. The water is resorbed a few days after treatment, leaving a matrix of particles to stimulate collagen production over a period of many weeks.

Your dermatologist may suggest a range of other nonsurgical options as well…

• **Chemical peels.** In this procedure, the doctor will apply a solution to your skin to remove the top layers. Peels may be used to treat wrinkles, discolored skin, and scars.

• **Radiofrequency micro-needling.** These devices use insulated needles that deliver high-intensity radiofrequency energy into the skin to stimulate new collagen growth and re-texture all skin types safely.

• **Laser therapy.** In this therapy, the doctor will apply a low-level laser to the skin. Many types of lasers can be used to address fine lines and wrinkles, uneven pigmentation such as age spots or rosacea, acne scars, and skin tightening.

RESULTS MAY VARY

Word of mouth is a great way to find a dermatologist, but keep in mind that a specific procedure that worked for a friend or colleague might not be the right one for you. Research the doctor's credentials—he or she should be board certified in dermatology—and investigate what's offered at a practice. Generally, more options are better. Having just one type of laser, for instance, often indicates that the doctor isn't as tech-savvy as he or she could be.

You want to establish a rapport with someone you can trust and who will educate you about choices rather than just tossing names of procedures at you. Also, looking at a dermatologist's personal aesthetic may help you decide who you feel comfortable with. According to research published in the *Journal of Cosmetic Dermatology*, a dermatologist's appearance, which can be very natural or very dramatic, often reflects their approach to rejuvenation.

A Few Extra Pounds Are OK

Older adults who have gained a little weight live longest. People who live longest enter their 50s with a normal body-mass index (BMI, 18.5 to 24.9) but then take on an overweight but not obese BMI (25.0 to 29.9) over the next few decades. Next longest lived are those who stay at a normal BMI throughout their lives…followed by those who are overweight throughout their lives. Not surprisingly, the least long-lived are those who started out obese (BMI of 30.0 and above) and gained more weight through the years.

Study of more than 8,000 adults ages 31 to 80 by researchers at The Ohio State University, Columbus, published in *Annals of Epidemiology*.

Varicose Veins Can Be Repaired Instead of Removed

In severe varicose vein disease, damaged veins are usually removed or destroyed, but that means that those large blood vessels can no longer be used if patients later need coronary artery bypass surgery.

Recent development: a thin sheath placed around a defective vein can alleviate symptoms and save the vein in 95% of cases.

Dominic Mühlberger, MD, attending physician, vascular surgery department, St. Josef Hospital, Ruhr-Universität, Bochum, Germany.

You Can Golf After Knee Replacement

Swinging a club requires significant knee rotation, and knee replacement is common among golfers. But golfers often worry that having the surgery may affect their ability to play golf.

Recent finding: Among patients who had total knee replacement, 81.5% were able to return to golf—resuming play an average of five months after surgery. Golfers reported significant postsurgical improvement in knee pain, regardless of the type of implant they received. Most said they had fewer limitations while golfing and no decline in performance.

Study of 1,900 golfers who had total knee replacement by researchers at Henry Ford Health System, Detroit, published in *Sports Health*.

7

Private and Personal

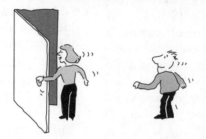

Beyond Diet and Exercise: Treating Obesity Like a Disease

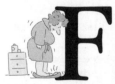For decades, people with obesity have been told, "Eat less and move more." While those are undeniably helpful behavioral changes, they're rarely sufficient to help people with obesity lose significant amounts of weight.

In 2013, the American Medical Association officially recognized obesity as a disease. This was an important leap forward, helping to open the public's and the medical community's eyes to the fact that obesity is not a choice but rather the result of complex factors, including genetics…socioeconomic status (which impacts access to healthy food)…medications a person may be taking for other conditions…sleep…and more.

A NEW MEDICINE THAT WORKS

The Food and Drug Administration recently approved the anti-obesity medication (AOM) *semaglutide* (Wegovy)—the first such treatment to receive approval since 2014. Originally used to treat type 2 diabetes under the brand name Ozempic, this drug works in the brain to reduce hunger and cravings. Like other AOMs, semaglutide is for patients with a body mass index (BMI) of 30 or higher…or for those with a BMI of 27 or greater who have at least one weight-related condition, such as high blood pressure, high cholesterol or type 2 diabetes.

Recent study: In a 2021 *New England Journal of Medicine* study, 1,961 adults were

Robert F. Kushner, MD, medical director of Center for Lifestyle Medicine at Northwestern Medicine in Chicago. He is author of several books including *Six Factors to Fit: Weight Loss That Works for You!* Dr. Kushner was the corresponding author for the 2021 *New England Journal of Medicine* "Semaglutide Treatment Effect in People with Obesity (STEP) 1" study group. *Disclosure:* Dr. Kushner is on the advisory board for Novo Nordisk (manufacturer of semaglutide) and receives honoraria.

injected weekly with 2.4 mg of semaglutide or received a placebo for 68 weeks. All the participants also received individual counseling on diet and physical activity every four weeks. Less than 5% of those in the placebo group lost 15% of their weight via diet and exercise alone compared with 50% for the semaglutide group. These results are far superior to those seen with other weight-management medications, which tend to lead to a loss of 6% to 11% of one's body weight. This means semaglutide is about 1.5 to two times more effective than other AOMs such as Contrave (*naltrexone/bupropion*) and Qsymia (*phentermine/topiramate ER*).

The fact that so many of the study participants taking semaglutide lost 15% of their weight is noteworthy because that benchmark is where we often see obesity-related conditions such as high blood pressure and type 2 diabetes begin to reverse or even go into remission. And despite what weight-loss companies and gyms claim, it is very difficult to achieve this degree of weight loss with diet and exercise alone.

TREATING OBESITY AS A DISEASE

People who struggle with their weight have historically resisted using AOMs and surgeries for a variety of reasons...

•**Stigma.** There's ample stigma surrounding obesity in general and medication for obesity specifically. People trying to lose weight feel as if they should be able to "do it on their own" by working out and cutting calories. There's no shame in needing chemotherapy to treat cancer, but many individuals with obesity feel shame over needing medication.

A person with obesity doesn't just take medicine and instantly lose weight. It needs to be combined with regular physical activity and a healthful, calorie-controlled diet. Most AOMs help dampen appetite...reduce cravings and thoughts about food...and make you feel more content between meals. With those reinforcements, people are better able to adhere to a healthy lifestyle.

•**Lack of coverage.** Medicare explicitly rules out coverage for AOMs. But Medicare Advantage plans provide Part A and Part B coverage along with extra benefits and may offer expanded coverage for weight-loss treatment plans. Medicaid may cover them, depending on the state in which you reside. Coverage from private insurers varies from no coverage at all to limited coverage, meaning there still is a substantial copay. Insurers may not cover these drugs the way that they cover other medications because they do not view obesity as a chronic disease (as opposed to an aesthetic and thus elective issue)...and/or perhaps they realize that with millions of potential candidates, the cost could be astronomical. Certain drugs may be affordable for some people—Contrave and Qsymia may cost about $100 a month after insurance if you work with a mail-order pharmacy. Semaglutide costs about $1,000 a month, rendering it out of reach for most patients.

SHOULD YOU TRY AN AOM?

If your insurer covers semaglutide or you can afford the $12,000 out of pocket annually, ask your primary care provider if you are a candidate. Many doctors don't mention AOMs, primarily because they haven't been trained to do so.

Semaglutide comes in two versions. The 2.4-mg version, used in the *NEJM* study, is branded Wegovy and is approved for chronic weight management. The lower, 1-mg dose Ozempic, is approved for type 2 diabetes.

Important: If you have diabetes, the lower dose of semaglutide likely will be covered by insurance.

Semaglutide is self-administered via a weekly injection in the belly, just under the skin. You will start at a lower dose and gradually build up to the full dose over four months. You should notice a reduction in appetite more or less immediately. Side effects include nausea and/or diarrhea, but these tend to dissipate with continued use. The medication should not be used by patients with a personal or family history of medullary thyroid cancer or in patients with the rare condition multiple endocrine neoplasia syndrome type 2 (MEN-2). Your health-care provider will be able to tell you if you are a candidate for its use.

AOMs need to be taken long term. Be sure you have reasonable expectations about how effective the medicine will be. Work with a counselor or registered dietitian to understand these medications and craft a nutrition and exercise plan.

If cost is a barrier: Semaglutide and other AOMs are costly. Ask your doctor for a referral to an obesity medicine specialist, who can determine if you are a good candidate for any of them. Some are available in generic form, which increases affordability.

If you are employed, contact your human resources department to encourage your employer to include AOMs as part of its group health insurance plan. You also can join the Obesity Action Coalition (ObesityAction.org), a national advocacy group composed of like-minded people that provides educational resources and advocates for more access to treatments.

Hemorrhoid Fundamentals

Nimalan A. Jeganathan, MD, a colorectal surgeon and assistant professor of surgery at Penn State Health in Hershey, Pennsylvania.

I t's the most common medical problem that no one likes to talk about. But, with millions of people experiencing discomfort from hemorrhoids every year, it's also a problem that doctors are very familiar with. Fortunately, there are straightforward ways of getting relief.

Though people often use the term hemorrhoids to describe a medical condition, hemorrhoids are actually just another part of the human anatomy: Everyone has these veins inside the anal canal that help support the sphincter muscles and maintain continence. When they become enlarged, and the tissues that support them weaken, people develop the condition of the same name.

WHAT'S GOING ON

There are two types of hemorrhoids: internal and external.

• **Internal hemorrhoids originate in the anal canal.** You may find out you have them only from a colonoscopy report. If you strain on the toilet, one may create a small amount of bleeding that you'll see on the toilet paper or in the water. (Keep in mind that a single drop of blood can turn the whole toilet bowl red, so it's important not to panic.)

If a hemorrhoid gets larger and starts to bleed more, however, you should not ignore it. An internal hemorrhoid can grow and develop a stalk that gets longer until it actually protrudes from the anus. This prolapsed hemorrhoid can cause discomfort or pain, irritation, and possibly itching as well.

• **Exterior hemorrhoids form outside the rectum.** (You can see them with a mirror.) These veins can be irritated and/or painful if the area is inflamed and swollen. Typically, there isn't much bleeding, but an external hemorrhoid can swell suddenly to the size of a walnut in a condition called thrombosis. That can lead to increased pain, inflammation, and swelling, and needs to be evaluated by your doctor.

Besides being a natural consequence of aging, hemorrhoids can develop from everyday habits that increase pressure in the anal canal. Constipation because of a low-fiber diet, heavy lifting, straining to pass stool or simply sitting for long periods on the toilet, not getting enough exercise, and being overweight all contribute to their formation.

WHEN TO SEEK TREATMENT

Hemorrhoids are treated only when symptoms like bleeding or pain become bothersome, not just because a hemorrhoid is enlarged. If you have bleeding during bowel movements or discomfort that doesn't improve after a week of home care, talk to your doctor. Don't let any feeling of embarrassment stand in your way—hemorrhoids are a condition that colorectal specialists see every day.

For 90% of patients, hemorrhoid treatment is focused on adding fiber to the diet and other lifestyle remedies to prevent progression, encourage regular bowel movements, and avoid straining.

Some people swear by topical treatments, like *phenylephrine* (Preparation H) or witch hazel. While these may provide temporary relief, they are usually not a good long-term solution. *To address the underlying problem, follow some simple guidelines...*

●**Increase fiber.** Getting more fiber in your diet with fruits, vegetables, and whole grains helps soften stool, increase its bulk, and reduce constipation, which in turn prevents the straining that leads to hemorrhoids.

As a bonus, fiber also has other tremendous health benefits, including weight loss and reduced risk of diabetes, stroke, heart attack, and high blood pressure. The recommended daily fiber intake is between 25 grams for women and 38 grams for men. Consuming enough from your diet can be difficult and usually requires taking over-the-counter fiber supplements.

●**Drink plenty of fluids.** Aim for the often-suggested eight glasses of water to help keep stool soft and help fiber supplements do their job.

●**Rethink bathroom habits.** Stop scrolling on your phone and doing other types of reading on the toilet. This extra sitting time leads to extra straining and more intra-anal pressure. It's also important to go to the bathroom

Don't let a feeling of embarrassment stand in your way: Hemorrhoids are a condition that colorectal specialists see every day.

as soon as you feel the need to go. If you delay, stool can actually harden and become difficult to pass.

●**Lose weight if needed.** Extra pounds put a strain on anal veins. In addition to changes in diet, try to move more. Sitting all day isn't good for health or hemorrhoids, and regular exercise also helps you stay regular.

●**DIY.** If you have a protruding internal hemorrhoid, you can push it back into the anus yourself. This isn't dangerous to do and may help alleviate some swelling.

NEXT STEPS

When lifestyle changes aren't enough to alleviate hemorrhoids, the next step is in-office procedures, such as rubber-band ligation, which involves tying the hemorrhoid off, and sclerotherapy, which involves injecting a liquid agent into the vein. Both usually involve several office visits. The procedures carry a small risk of a local infection, usually in the first few days, and your doctor will alert you to red flags to watch for, such as severe pain, fever, and the inability to urinate.

Sometimes surgery is needed. A hemorrhoidectomy can reach the very base of the hemorrhoid and remove it along with any affected surrounding tissue. Improvements in surgical techniques have gone a long way toward reducing the pain associated with the procedure, but there is a lengthy recovery: It may take up to four weeks for all pain and bleeding to resolve.

The first few days can be especially difficult, though anesthetics injected in the area during surgery should help in the immediate aftermath. Nonsteroidal anti-inflammatory drugs are the first-line medication for managing pain. Doctors try to avoid prescribing opioids, not only because of the risk of addiction, but because constipation is a major side effect—and that's the last thing you want when recovering from anal surgery. Soaking in a tub and applying warm compresses help some people, while others find relief with a cold pack.

Is It Really a Hemorrhoid?

Don't always assume that rectal bleeding and/or pain is due to hemorrhoids. *Two conditions are often confused with hemorrhoids...*

●**Anal fissure.** This is a tear in the anal canal, similar to getting a paper cut on a finger. It may burn or cause bleeding when having a bowel movement. It can often heal on its own, but any straining will slow down the process. A topical agent like lidocaine ointment may ease the burning sensation. Increasing dietary fiber will usually result in healing.

●**A more serious condition, though less common, is a colorectal polyp or cancer.** Increasing age (greater than 45 years) and a family history of colorectal cancer should be a reason to get a colonoscopy before assuming bleeding is from hemorrhoids.

Safe and Easy Way to Treat Anal Fissures

Anal fissures are small tears in the inner lining of the rectum. They can cause blood in the stool and pain during bowel movements, but they're generally not dangerous and are easy to treat by getting a lot more fiber, either as a supplement or by eating more fruits and vegetables. Also increase how much water you drink.

Helpful: An over-the-counter stool softener and soaking in a warm tub for 10 to 20 minutes, especially after a bowel movement. If the above steps don't help sufficiently or for recurrent fissures, talk to your doctor.

UniversityHealthNews.com

What You Need to Know About Diverticulitis

Anne Peery MD, a gastroenterologist and associate professor of medicine at the University of North Carolina Chapel Hill School of Medicine.

One day, seemingly out of nowhere, you're hit with intense lower abdominal pain. It's difficult to stand up straight.

You have a fever and, as you think about the things you've eaten or people you've spent time with the past few days, the pain refuses to budge. You may also have nausea, constipation, diarrhea, or symptoms reminiscent of a urinary tract infection, such as an increased urge to urinate or burning while doing so. Gastroenterologists see this constellation of symptoms quite often, and a singular diagnosis usually springs to mind: diverticulitis.

WHAT IS DIVERTICULITIS?

One of the most common gastrointestinal diseases, diverticulitis is an inflammation of tiny sac-like protrusions that form in the wall of the colon. These marble-sized pouches, called diverticula, are found in more than half of Americans over age 60, but most of the time, they don't cause trouble. But for about 5% of people with diverticulosis, those pouches will become inflamed or infected. When that happens, the condition progresses to diverticulitis, which demands immediate medical attention.

WHO DEVELOPS DIVERTICULITIS?

We are just now starting to truly understand why people get diverticulitis. It has long been blamed on a low-fiber diet, but while a high-quality diet is associated with reduced diverticulitis risk, the truth is that genetics, not diet, are responsible for about 50% of one's risk. Siblings of patients with diverticulitis, for instance, are believed to have a threefold higher risk of developing it themselves.

That said, nutrition does have an impact, with a diet high in fruits, vegetables, whole grains, poultry, and fish linked with reduced diverticulitis risk, and vegetarians enjoying some protection over carnivores. A high-fiber diet is important to manage diverticulitis or possibly even avoid it in the first place. Fiber should come from foods, not supplements.

Vigorous physical activity is also associated with a reduced risk. Diverticulitis is more common among men than women at younger ages, but over age 60, rates are higher for women. Regular use (at least twice a week) of aspirin or nonsteroidal anti-inflammatory drugs such as ibuprofen increases risk, as does obesity, smoking, and the use of hormone replacement therapy for menopause.

Immunocompromised patients—those with cancer or rheumatological conditions, for example—tend to experience diverticulitis at higher rates than the general population, possibly due to chronic steroid use. Interestingly, these patients often present with milder symptoms, delaying diagnosis. They also experience more complications.

PAIN IS THE NUMBER ONE SYMPTOM

The pain usually appears suddenly, most often in the left lower quadrant of the abdo-

> The pain usually appears suddenly, most often in the left lower quadrant of the abdomen. Patients often describe it as the worst pain they've ever had.

Myths and Controversies

•**Seeds and nuts.** Patients with diverticulitis are often told to avoid eating nuts, popcorn, and seeds to reduce the risk of complications, but this is largely an old wives' tale. A *JAMA* study debunked this guideline nearly two decades ago. There's no reason to think these foods will lodge in diverticula, causing inflammation. On the contrary, they're anti-inflammatory in nature and high in fiber, promoting healthy stool formation.

•**Antibiotics were used for decades to treat acute uncomplicated diverticulitis,** but increasing evidence, including a 2020 review sponsored by the Agency for Healthcare Research and Quality, indicates that there isn't enough evidence to support the practice. Antibiotic treatment is strongly recommended in immunocompromised patients; those with other chronic conditions or who are frail; those who have a fever, vomiting, or other signs of infection; and everyone with complicated diverticulitis.

•**Stress.** Research cannot yet prove a rock-solid link between stress and diverticulitis, but we do know that stress and anxiety can exacerbate gastrointestinal symptoms in general. Anything you can do to improve your global mental health is going to improve GI symptoms and outcomes.

—Dr. Anne Peery

men. Patients often describe it as the worst pain they've ever had. Other symptoms can include fever, constipation (excess inflammation may prevent stool from moving through the colon), diarrhea, and urinary symptoms because an inflamed colon is sitting atop the bladder.

Most people see their primary care physician or visit an emergency room when the pain begins. Your doctor will draw blood to see if you have an elevated white blood cell count, which indicates possible infection. He or she may also run blood tests to confirm inflammation and will rule out a urinary tract infection. An abdominal CT scan is also strongly recommended with the first episode to identify and diagnose diverticulitis and also help determine severity.

About 5% of people with acute uncomplicated diverticulitis will go on to develop complicated diverticulitis, involving an abscess or hole in the wall of the colon, through which gas and fluid escape. These patients are almost always hospitalized, require antibiotics, and may need to have a temporary drain inserted in their abdomen to promote healing. Surgery to remove part of the colon may be necessary in some cases.

WHAT HAPPENS AFTER A FLARE-UP?

Your gastroenterologist will tell you when to progress from a clear liquid diet (during an episode) to low-fiber solid foods (eggs, cooked fruit, pasta, dairy foods) and then, once all symptoms have subsided, to a high-fiber routine (produce, beans, brown rice, bran and whole-grain cereals). It's important to maintain communication with your doctor during the clear liquid diet phase to ensure you don't lose too much weight.

Some people with diverticulitis will experience chronic gastrointestinal (GI) pain and, eventually, be diagnosed with irritable bowel syndrome (IBS). In a Swedish trial, periodic abdominal pain was reported by nearly half of uncomplicated diverticulitis patients at one-year follow-up. This IBS pain is sometimes treated with a low dose of a tricyclic antidepressant such as *amitriptyline*, *imipramine* (Tofranil), or *nortriptyline* (Pamelor). These drugs help reduce stomach sensitivity by blocking pain signals sent from the GI tract to the brain.

Six to eight weeks after diverticulitis symptoms resolve, you should have a colonoscopy to rule out malignancy, as colon cancer can resemble diverticulitis on a CT scan. The risk is higher in patients with complicated diverticulitis.

Rosacea May Signal a Deeper Problem

Rajani Katta, MD, a board-certified dermatologist and volunteer clinical faculty member at Baylor College of Medicine and University of Texas Houston Health Science Center. Dr. Katta is the author of seven books and more than 80 medical journal articles and book chapters. Her latest book is *Glow: The Dermatologist's Guide to a Whole Foods, Younger Skin Diet.*

To the casual observer, rosacea—a condition marked by facial flushing, pesky bumps, and broken blood vessels centered on the nose and cheeks—might seem to be a skin-deep problem. But many of the estimated 16 million Americans who cope with it are highly aware that what they put in their bellies directly influences the symptoms on their faces.

Rosacea patients routinely experience flare-ups in response to specific foods (see sidebar) and eliminating those foods can reduce symptoms. Now researchers are digging deeper and finding that what's happening in the gut itself may play a role in this chronic condition.

FOOD AND THE MICROBIOME

What we eat directly affects the bacteria, fungi, and other organisms that thrive in the gut microbiome. Within 24 hours of eating a high-fat, high-sugar diet, for example, there are markedly fewer good gut microbes and more plentiful bad ones inhabiting what's commonly referred to as your "gut biome."

The good microbes play many roles: They act as police officers who battle invading germs, teachers who train the immune system to know the difference between good and bad substances, and factory workers who take what we eat, particularly fiber, and turn it into short-chain fatty acids that strengthen the inner lining of the gut as well as the skin.

Bad gut microbes outnumbering good gut microbes causes an unbalanced gut microbiome (dysbiosis), which has been linked to gastrointestinal conditions such as celiac disease, Crohn's disease, ulcerative colitis, and irritable bowel syndrome—all of which are

Food and Rosacea

Avoid these common triggers…

●**Hot temperature foods or drinks,** like coffee and tea

●**Spicy foods,** such as hot sauce, cayenne, jalapeno, and red peppers

●**Alcoholic beverages of any kind**

●**Cinnamaldehyde foods,** such as citrus, tomatoes, cinnamon, and chocolate

Eat more of these…

●**Prebiotics** from fruits, vegetables, and whole grains

●**Probiotics,** from yogurt, kefir, tempeh, sauerkraut, miso, and kombucha

also more common in people with rosacea. In one study, researchers found that people with rosacea were 13 times more likely to have small intestinal bacterial overgrowth (SIBO), and that treating the SIBO with antibiotics also resolved the rosacea.

TREAT THE GUT TO TREAT THE SKIN

Think of it this way: Your gut is essentially a garden. For more good microbes to thrive, you need to "fertilize" them with the right foods in addition to avoiding your trigger foods. That means eating more probiotics, also known as good gut microbes, and prebiotics, which nourishes them.

Prebiotics comes from the fiber in fruits, vegetables, and whole grains. Stick with real foods, since supplements offer only questionable benefits.

Probiotics come from foods like yogurt, kefir, tempeh, sauerkraut, miso, and kombucha, all of which contain live microbes that have long demonstrated numerous health benefits. While food sources are best, you can also get probiotics in supplement form. While there are many species of probiotics, look for a supplement with at least 1 billion colony-forming units (CFU) of *lactobacillus* or *bifidobacterium.*

Hidradenitis Suppurativa: Help for a Mysterious Skin Condition

Patrick Zito, DO, PharmD, a board-certified dermatologist and voluntary assistant professor of dermatology at the University of Miami Miller School of Medicine Dr. Phillip Frost Department of Dermatology & Cutaneous Surgery.

Hidradenitis suppurativa can be an unpredictable disease. One person may have an occasional small, painful bump in the armpit, while another may have chronic pain, severe scarring, and inflammatory bowel disease. But there is one thing that many people with HS have in common: a long, frustrating road filled with misdiagnoses and failed treatments. On average, it takes seven to 10 years after symptoms appear to get an HS diagnosis, researchers reported in the journal *Dermatology*.

UNDERSTANDING HS

HS begins when a hair follicle becomes blocked and forms a small, painful bump. It most often strikes in areas with apocrine sweat glands—such as the armpits and the groin—as well as under and around the breasts. It can progress through three stages and can become severe enough to interfere with normal functioning and movement, even causing disability.

People with HS also have a higher risk of a variety of other conditions, including diabetes, squamous cell carcinoma, obesity, metabolic disorders, spondyloarthritis, PAPA syndrome (pyogenic arthritis, pyoderma gangrenosum and acne), polycystic ovarian syndrome, hypertension, dyslipidemia, inflammatory bowel disease, and spondyloarthropathy.

PREVENTION AND TREATMENT

While there is no cure for HS, early diagnosis and treatment can limit inflammation and skin damage, and lower the risk of systemic conditions. *Management takes a multipronged approach...*

• **Lose weight if necessary.** While HS strikes people of any body weight, it is more prevalent among people with obesity. While the relationship is complicated—obesity may occur with HS but not cause it—researchers in Denmark found that the number of patients reporting HS symptoms after weight loss from bariatric surgery decreased by 35%. They concluded that a weight loss of more than 15% was associated with a significant reduction in disease severity.

• **Don't smoke.** Researchers recently discovered that deficiency in a cell-communication system called the Notch pathway likely plays a causal role in HS. Smoking suppresses Notch signaling, which is why smokers with HS have more affected body areas than non-smokers.

• **Use antibacterial washes.** HS nodules are highly prone to infections. To reduce the risk, use antimicrobial washes such as *chlorhexidine* (Peridex, Hibiclens) or benzoyl peroxide (an ingredient in a wide variety of anti-acne products). Some dermatologists recommend bleach baths, where you soak in a 0.005% diluted bleach solution for five to 10 minutes twice per week. (Never put full-strength bleach on your skin.)

• **Lifestyle.** Avoid irritating your skin by keeping high-risk areas cool and dry, wearing loose-fitting clothing, and replacing shaving with clippers, waxing, or laser hair removal.

IN-OFFICE PROCEDURES

Depending on your specific condition, your dermatologist may suggest an in-office procedure to address the nodules or abscesses...

• **Steroid injections** can reduce inflammation and the size of non-infected nodules.

• **Abscesses** can be drained in the office, but there is a high rate of recurrence.

• **Your dermatologist or a plastic surgeon may "deroof" an abscess** by removing the skin that covers it or may excise the whole lesion and any tunnel.

• **Laser surgery** can help treat lesions and scars in some patients whose disease is otherwise stable and medically managed.

• **Laser hair removal** can prevent outbreaks by destroying the hair follicles in high-risk areas.

While these procedures can address the disease in a particular location, they don't prevent flares from appearing on other parts of

Home Remedies

Many people with HS report success with home remedies that haven't been studied in clinical trials. *Here are the most commonly recommended products on the Facebook Hidradenitis Suppurativa Support Group...*

●**To prevent infection.** Dial antibacterial body, apple cider vinegar, honey

●**For pain.** Boilease (over-the-counter), Vicks VapoRub, warm compresses

●**To help a lesion drain.** Ichthammol (drawing-out-salve), hydrocolloid bandages, Vicks VapoRub

●**To reduce odor.** White vinegar

●**To reduce inflammation.** Turmeric, used as a topical treatment or taken as a supplement, zinc, eliminating dairy and yeast from the diet.

the body or address underlying inflammation, so medical management is important even when these are successful.

MEDICATIONS FOR HS

A variety of medications show promise in managing HS...

•**Creams.** Topical antibiotics such as *clindamycin* (Cleocin T, Clindagel) and *dapsone* (Aczone) can help treat infection and reduce inflammation. A topical corticosteroid such as *triamcinolone* (Kenalog, Triderm) can reduce local inflammation, but it should be used only for short periods of time (up to two weeks) to avoid damaging the skin. Topical *resorcinol* (Resinol, R A Acne) can open clogged hair follicles and reduce inflammation.

•**Oral antibiotics.** A class of drugs called tetracyclines have both antibacterial and anti-inflammatory properties. A common first choice is *doxycycline* (Vibramycin, Doryx, Oracea, Acticlate, Doxy). This medication can cause severe nausea, so let your doctor know if you need to try a different drug.

•**Hormonal medications.** HS strikes follicles with associated apocrine glands. Apocrine glands are inactive until hormonal changes at puberty. Drugs that block the effects of androgens such as testosterone help many people with HS.

These include *spironolactone* (Aldactone) and *finasteride* (Proscar, Propecia). Birth control pills can also help women who have menstrual-related flares.

•***Metformin***, which is commonly used to treat diabetes, can reduce HS-related inflammation. One small study found that about 70% of people who took metformin had improvement in their symptoms and quality of life.

•**Biologics.** For moderate to severe disease, biologic medications are very promising. In fact, the only medication specifically approved to treat HS is *adalimumab* (Humira). Studies show that people who received adalimumab injections have "noticeably fewer abscesses (lumps with pus) and nodules (hard, deep lumps)," the American Academy of Dermatology reports.

ACCESS TO QUALITY CARE

Not all dermatologists treat HS, so you may need to shop around. Look for a board-certified dermatologist who is familiar with the latest advances in HS. (Doctors who have more recently completed medical school may be more up-to-date on the latest advances in treating this disease.)

Poor Fitness Is Linked to Higher Psoriasis Risk

According to a recent study, men with the lowest levels of physical fitness during their youth had a 35% higher risk of developing psoriasis when they reached ages 37 to 51.

Psoriasis is a chronic, systemic inflammatory disease that can manifest as plaque psoriasis (reddened, flaky, itchy skin lesions) or the joint condition psoriatic arthritis. The increased risk for psoriatic arthritis was 44% among the low-fitness men.

Study of 1.2 million men conscripted into the Swedish Army by researchers at University of Gothenburg, Sweden, published in *PLOS One*.

Natural Breakthroughs in Breast Cancer Prevention

Tara Scott, MD, chief medical officer at Revitalize Medical Group in Akron, Ohio, clinical assistant professor at Northeast Ohio Medical University in Rootstown, Ohio. RevitalizeMed.com

The statistics are well-known but still shocking: Every year, more than 330,000 women are diagnosed with breast cancer, and more than 43,000 die from it.

Those frightening numbers are a relatively recent development: Breast cancer rates have more than doubled over the last few decades.

MODERN LIFESTYLE, RISING CASES

During my more than 20 years as a practicing gynecologist, I've seen a growing number of cases among my patients. *I think there are several reasons for this steady rise…*

•**There is an increasing level of exposure to chemicals** such as bisphenol A (BPA) found in many water bottles, and phthalates, found in soaps and shampoos, that interfere with our hormones (the body's endocrine system). Exposure to these endocrine disruptors can upset the balance of the female sex hormone *estrogen*—a leading trigger of breast cancer.

•**Our highly processed diets alter the gut microbiome**—the trillions of friendly and unfriendly bacteria in the gastrointestinal tract. When there are more "unfriendly" bacteria, there are higher levels of the enzyme beta-glucuronidase, which prevents the intestinal breakdown of estrogen, resulting in the reactivation of estrogen and an increase in the risk of breast cancer.

•**Non-stop stress generates excess** *cortisol,* a hormone that interferes with the breakdown of estrogen and increases inflammation (another risk factor for cancer).

•**A sedentary lifestyle has been linked to an increased risk of breast cancer,** perhaps because of increased body fat, poor blood sugar regulation, and inflammation.

•**There are several hormonally driven gynecological conditions that indicate a woman has excess levels of estrogen**—a leading risk factor for breast cancer, including endometriosis, uterine fibroids, heavy menstrual bleeding, and polycystic ovary syndrome (PCOS). If you have any of these conditions (or a family history of breast cancer), prevention is extra important for you.

These and other lifestyle factors, such as being overweight or having more than one alcoholic drink a day, can nearly double your risk of breast cancer, according to a new study published in *JAMA Network Open.* But that means that healthy lifestyle factors can do the opposite. Recent scientific studies show that the following steps can help you prevent breast cancer and, if you've already had it, keep it from coming back.

EAT MORE FIBER

Researchers at Harvard Medical School analyzed data from 20 studies on fiber and breast cancer and found that people who ate the most fiber lowered their risk of breast cancer by 18%.

Why it works: Higher fiber intake feeds the friendly bacteria in your gut, crowding out unfriendly bacteria. It also bulks up your stool and helps counter constipation, both of which help with estrogen detoxification.

What to do: Increase your intake of high-fiber fruits, vegetables, and whole grains. To ensure maximum fiber intake, consider taking a fiber supplement, too. Psyllium husk works great.

SPICE WITH ONION AND GARLIC

In a study published in the journal *Nutrition and Cancer,* women who ate a dish spiced with onion and garlic more than once a day had a 67% lower risk of breast cancer than women who never ate onions or garlic.

Why it works: Onions and garlic are loaded with *prebiotics,* a type of fiber that feeds probiotics, allowing them to flourish in your gut. Probiotics may help increase levels of estrobolome, a type of bacteria that specifically metabolizes estrogen.

What to do: Make sure you eat a dish containing onion or garlic at least five days a week.

EAT LESS RED MEAT AND MORE POULTRY

In a seven-year study published in the International *Journal of Cancer*, researchers analyzed health data from more than 40,000 women. They found that women who ate the most red meat had a 23% higher risk of breast cancer than those who ate the least. However, those who ate the most poultry had a 15% lower risk of breast cancer compared with those who ate the least. Women who substituted poultry for red meat had a 28% lower risk of breast cancer.

Why it works: Red meat typically delivers high levels of fat and growth hormones, both of which have been linked to breast cancer.

What to do: Eat red meat no more than a few times a month. Increase your intake of organic poultry. You might also want to eat more wild-caught fatty fish like salmon and sardines. They are rich in omega-3 fatty acids, and studies link a higher intake of omega-3s with a lower risk of breast cancer.

EXERCISE REGULARLY

Many studies link regular exercise to a lower risk of breast cancer. Now, a new study published in the *Journal of the National Cancer Institute* shows the unique power of exercise for secondary prevention, too. Looking at more than 1,300 women diagnosed with breast cancer, the study found that women who exercised at a moderate intensity for at least 2.5 hours per week before and after their cancer diagnosis were 55% less likely to have their cancer return and 68% less likely to die of the disease. Even women who started exercising *after* the diagnosis were 46% less likely to have a recurrence and 43% less likely to die of the disease.

Why it works: Regular exercise helps improve and regulate nearly every cell, tissue, system, and organ—including strengthening your immune system, your main defense against cancer. Regular exercise also reduces circulating estrogen.

What to do: Aim for a weekly minimum of 2.5 hours of moderate aerobic exercise like brisk walking, biking, water aerobics, dancing, doubles tennis, or hiking.

LOSE WEIGHT

A study of more than 180,000 women published in the *Journal of the National Cancer Institute* found that women who lost weight after the age of 50 and kept it off had a lower risk of breast cancer. And the more weight they lost, the lower the risk. Women who lost 20 pounds or more decreased risk by 26%. But even women who lost 5 to 10 pounds decreased their risk by 13%.

Why it works: Fat cells generate *estrone*, the type of estrogen generated after menopause. It is even a more stimulatory hormone than estradiol, which is generated by the ovaries, and can cause growth in breast tissue that leads to cancer.

What to do: Look at the main cause of your overweight. It's different for each person. Are you eating too much? Are you an emotional eater? Are you not exercising enough? Is your thyroid out of whack? Is your stress too high?

Explore and address the causes of your weight gain—ideally, with the help of a physician, health coach, or weight loss program.

SKIP HAIR DYES AND STRAIGHTENERS

An eight-year study published in the *International Journal of Cancer* looked at more than 46,000 women and their use of permanent hair dyes and straighteners. *The researchers found a consistent pattern of increased risk for breast cancer in women who used the products in the year before the study began…*

- **African American women who used permanent hair dye every five to eight weeks or more had a 60% increased risk.** (In general, the higher the frequency of use, the higher the risk, said the researchers.)
- **Caucasian women who used permanent hair dye every five to eight weeks or more had an 8% increased risk.**
- **Women who used chemical hair straighteners every five to eight weeks had a 30% increased risk.**
- **Women who used semipermanent or temporary hair dye had very little increase in risk.**

What happens: Hair dye and straighteners contain endocrine disruptors, and the latter also contains formaldehyde, a carcinogen.

119

What to do: It's best to just avoid these products.

AI Spots Prostate Cancer

A newly developed artificial intelligence program can spot signs of prostate cancer in routine CT scans better than radiologists who viewed the same images, a study found. The more scans it saw, the more skilled it became.

Royal Melbourne Institute of Technology.

Exercise Helps Kill Cancer Cells

According to a recent study, men with prostate cancer who exercised daily for three months had increased blood levels of myokines, proteins secreted by muscles that help suppress tumor growth and trigger immune cells to kill cancer cells. And post-exercise myokines significantly suppressed growth of live prostate cancer cells. Researchers believe exercise, especially high-intensity resistance training—ideally, every day—should be included in treatment for any type of cancer.

Robert Newton, PhD, professor of exercise medicine at Edith Cowan University in Australia and lead author of a study published in *Medicine & Science in Sports & Exercise.*

A Painful Issue for Men

Petar Bajic, MD, a urologist at the Glickman Urological and Kidney Institute in Cleveland, Ohio, and assistant professor of urology at the Cleveland Clinic Lerner College of Medicine of Case Western Reserve University. He specializes in men's health and sexual medicine.

Most men probably couldn't tell you where their epididymides are, but they may become uncomfortably aware of this bit of anatomy when they develop a painful condition called epididymitis—inflammation of coiled microscopic tubes that lie

Sexually Transmitted Infections on the Rise

While most epididymitis cases in older men are not linked to sex, such cases are becoming more common. That's because STIs are on the rise among older Americans. The U.S. Centers for Disease Control and Prevention reported a doubling of sexually transmitted infections in people over age 65 between 2007 and 2017. The two STIs most often associated with epididymitis are chlamydia and gonorrhea. Both can be cured with antibiotics. If you learn that one of these infections is causing your symptoms, it's important to let recent sexual partners know, so that they, too, can seek testing.

—Dr. Petar Bajic

at the back of each testicle, inside the scrotum. Each tube, or epididymis, stores sperm as it matures and then transports it to its next destination in the male reproductive tract. In older men, it's most commonly caused by prostate problems, infections in the bladder or kidneys that spread to the epididymis, or a sexually transmitted infection (STI). (See sidebar above.)

If you have swelling and pain at the back of one of your testicles, it's important to see a doctor to get a definite diagnosis and the fastest possible relief. Here are a few things to know.

GETTING A DIAGNOSIS

A typical man with pain and swelling in his scrotum doesn't show up at a doctor's office saying, "I think I have epididymitis." The doctor won't immediately jump to that conclusion either. *That's because such symptoms can have many different causes and the exact location of the discomfort can be hard to pinpoint...*

•**Sudden, severe pain in the scrotum could be caused by testicular torsion,** a twisted testicle that can quickly lose its blood supply. Delayed treatment can lead to loss of the testicle.

•**Pain and a lump in a testicle might raise concerns about testicular cancer,** but most testicular cancers don't cause pain.

•**Men who have recently had vasectomies** often develop a feeling of fullness or congestion in the testes and epididymides, but this usually is temporary, not painful, and does not involve inflammation.

The doctor will strongly consider epididymitis if pain and swelling radiating from the back of one testicle have developed over the course of a few days. The testicle itself may or may not be swollen. A man with suspected epididymitis also might have a fever, painful urination, or other urinary symptoms, such as needing to urinate frequently or having trouble getting a stream of urine started. Some will also have discharge from the urethra.

If you have possible symptoms of epididymitis, expect your health-care provider to conduct a physical exam that will include checking to see if the area around the epididymis is swollen and tender to the touch. You should also expect a digital rectal exam, in which the doctor inserts a lubricated gloved finger in the rectum to check the prostate.

DIFFERENT TREATMENTS FOR DIFFERENT CAUSES

The exam and initial tests usually give the doctor a good idea of what's causing the epididymitis. If a bacterial infection seems likely, the doctor may prescribe antibiotics right away while awaiting results to confirm the infection. You might be asked to take antibiotic pills for as long as two to four weeks, longer than is usual for many common infections. That's because the medication can take some extra time to work on hard-to-reach tissues.

If the doctor sees no clear signs of infection, you might start your treatment with anti-inflammatory medications, such as ibuprofen or naproxen. Those should help soothe inflamed tissues and relieve pain. You also might be advised to rest with your scrotum raised and to apply ice to the area for short periods. If those treatments don't work, the doctor may prescribe an antibiotic after all, in case a hidden infection is at work.

If an enlarged prostate is thought to be the underlying cause of the epididymitis, treatment of that problem will also be part of the plan.

TREATING CHRONIC EPIDIDYMITIS

While most men get better after a few weeks of treatment, others develop chronic or recurring pain. When symptoms persist for more than three months, your doctor may suggest a test called a diagnostic spermatic cord block. In this test, a doctor injects a local anesthetic into the spermatic cord, the bundle of nerves, ducts, and blood vessels that connects the testicles to the abdominal cavity. If the numbing medicine does not stop the pain, it's likely that the epididymis is not the source after all.

If the cord block does temporarily relieve your pain and nothing else is working, your doctor might offer you a surgery called microscopic denervation of the spermatic cord. In that procedure, a surgeon makes a small incision and uses a microscope to locate and permanently cut the nerves causing the pain. Another surgical option is the removal of the epididymis. Like any surgery, these procedures carry small risks of infection and other complications, so they should be considered only as last resorts after less invasive treatments have failed.

Best Way to Pee at a Urinal

Research involving a water tank and nozzles to mimic a stream of urine found that the best way to prevent splash-back is to stand as close to the urinal as possible and direct the stream to hit the back of the urinal at a downward angle—don't aim directly into the pool that forms at the bottom of the urinal. An even less splashy way to relieve oneself is to sit on the toilet.

Study by researchers at Brigham Young University, Provo, Utah, presented at a meeting of the American Physical Society Division of Fluid Dynamics.

ED and Your Heart

Chris Iliades, MD, retired ear, nose, throat, head, and neck surgeon who now dedicates his time to educating patients through his medical writing. He is a regular contributor to Bottom Line Heath.

We've all seen the advertisements that show a good-looking, middle-aged man smiling from ear to ear because an erectile dysfunction (ED) drug saved his sex life.

What the ads don't show, though, is that he may have a much more serious problem to worry about: a higher risk of heart disease.

A 2020 review published in the journal *BJU International* looked at seven studies and found that, compared with men without ED, those with the condition have a 45% higher risk of developing cardiovascular disease, a 50% higher risk of being diagnosed with coronary heart disease, and a 55% higher risk of having a heart attack. A 2021 review of 14 studies including over 90,000 men found that the risk of heart attack is even higher: 62%. ED ranks as high as having a family history of heart disease or being a smoker when it comes to heart disease risk.

BLOOD VESSELS EXPLAIN THE LINK

To get an erection, you need good blood flow into the corpora cavernosa, the spongy tissue inside the penis that fills with blood. Most cases of ED arise when narrowed blood vessels limit blood flow to the penis, called vascular ED.

One of the causes of narrowed blood vessels is a disorder called endothelial dysfunction, a type of coronary artery disease that decreases the amount of blood that can flow through arteries.

It doesn't affect only sexual performance: The same arterial narrowing occurs on the surface of the heart as well.

In some people, it can cause chest pain (or angina), but for many men, ED is the only symptom—one that serves as an important warning that the heart may be at risk. Researchers believe that endothelial dysfunction appears about five years before the onset of atherosclerosis—a condition in which plaques made of fats and cholesterol stick inside blood vessels. While both endothelial dysfunction and atherosclerosis narrow blood vessels, the latter can cause blockages, too, which can lead to heart attacks, heart failure, and ischemic stroke.

TAKE ACTION NOW

The risk factors for ED, endothelial dysfunction, and atherosclerotic heart disease are all the same, so some basic lifestyle tweaks can lower your risk of all three...

• **Stop smoking.** Smoking is a major risk factor for both heart disease and ED.

• **Drink alcohol only in moderation.** Moderation for a man is no more than two drinks per day.

• **Follow a Mediterranean-style diet.** According to the American Heart Association (AHA), this diet features fruits, vegetables, whole grains, olive oil, and fish or poultry. It limits solid fats, red meat, processed foods, and sweets.

• **Get enough exercise.** The AHA recommends at least 150 minutes of moderate-intensity aerobic exercise every week, muscle-strengthening exercises on at least two days per week, and spending less time sitting. Getting up and moving instead of sitting, even for just five hours a week, improves cardiovascular health.

• **Work with your doctor to lose weight if you are overweight.**

• **If you have high cholesterol, high blood pressure, or diabetes,** work with your doctor to get these conditions under the best control possible.

TALK TO YOUR DOCTOR

ED is not a normal part of aging, so if you begin to experience it—at any age—let your doctor know. He or she will want to rule out reversible causes of ED, such as depression, drug use, or low testosterone, and may look for diseases that cause ED, such as diabetes, multiple sclerosis, kidney disease, prostate disease, Parkinson's disease, and Alzheimer's disease.

If you still experience ED after you've made lifestyle changes, the usual next step is to take an ED medication like *sildenafil* (Viagra), *avanafil* (Stendra), *tadalafil* (Cialis), or *vardenafil*. Common side effects include headache, facial flushing, nasal congestion, diarrhea, and backache. Sildenafil and tadalafil can induce temporary impaired color vision. These drugs can cause blood pressure to temporarily drop by five to eight points in healthy men, but in men who take nitrate drugs, such as nitroglycerin, they can lead to a dangerous reduction of 25 to 51 points and should be avoided. The

FDA also urges caution for men with a history of congestive heart failure, unstable angina, low blood pressure, uncontrolled high blood pressure, or a history of stroke, heart attack, or serious disturbances of the heart's pumping rhythm within six months.

Even if these drugs solve your ED, it's still important to follow up with a cardiologist to monitor your heart health. ED is a serious red flag, and ignoring it can endanger much more than your intimacy.

Is Sex OK After a Recent Heart Attack?

Barry A. Franklin, PhD, director of preventive cardiology/cardiac rehabilitation at Beaumont Health in Royal Oak, Michigan. He is a member of the Bottom Line Health advisory board. DrBarryFranklin.com

This question is commonly asked by middle-aged and older heart patients. Fortunately, numerous studies now provide reassurance to those who have such concerns.

Sexual activity is associated with a very light to moderate energy expenditure and associated transient increases in heart rate and blood pressure. I often counsel patients that if they can exercise at a 3 METs workload, such as walking at 3 miles per hour (mph) on a level treadmill or walking at 2 mph on a 3.5% grade or higher without adverse signs or symptoms, they can safely resume sexual activity.

Studies show that sexual activity is a probable contributor to heart attacks in fewer than 1% of all cases. In the hour after sexual activity, the relative risk of a heart attack does increase two- to fourfold, but it rapidly returns to baseline. An intriguing finding from these studies is that regular physical activity reduces the risk of sex precipitating a heart attack. Individuals in the studies who exercise vigorously three or more times each week had no increased risk of having a heart attack triggered by sex.

Extramarital sex appears to be more demanding from a cardiovascular perspective for men with known or suspected heart dis-ease. Most coital deaths occur with mistresses or prostitutes. Researchers believe that excess alcohol intake, cigarette smoking, and other stressors may further increase arousal and the demands on the heart.

GOOD TO KNOW...

Surprising Benefits of Sex

Studies have found that sex boosts your body's ability to create antibodies, which help fight off viruses and bacteria...lowers heart attack risk...lessens pain...lowers blood pressure...boosts brainpower...and helps you live longer.

MedicineNet.com

New Advances in Hair-Loss Treatment

Sara Wasserbauer, MD, ABHRS, FISHRS, a hair restoration expert in private practice with offices throughout the San Francisco Bay area.

About half of women and even more men experience age-related thinning of the hair, but recent advances can slow the loss and, in some cases, even help hair regrow.

The most common type of hair loss is called androgenetic alopecia, a.k.a. male-pattern baldness (a receding, M-shaped hairline plus thinning at the top of the head) or female-pattern baldness (all-over thinning). It's caused by age, hormones, and genetics. Chronic underlying illnesses such as untreated thyroid disorders or anemia can accelerate hair loss, but when the illness is treated, that hair loss usually reverses.

MEDICAL THERAPIES

When it comes to slowing or reversing hair loss, therapies fall into two main categories: medical and surgical. Here are the most common medical treatments...

•Minoxidil (Rogaine). Applied twice daily to thinning areas, topical minoxidil keeps hair in the growing phase, which means that treated hairs don't shed as frequently as they normally would. It also stimulates regrowth.

For patients who experience scalp irritation, there is an oral formulation. Oral minoxidil was originally used as a high blood pressure medication, but when used in very low doses (around 1 milligram [mg]/day or less, versus the standard 10 to 30 mg/day dose for blood pressure), it stimulates hair regrowth and reduces shedding. It can improve existing high blood pressure, too. Patients with heart failure should avoid oral minoxidil.

• **Dandruff shampoo.** When lathered into hair and left on for five minutes a day, two to three times a week, dandruff shampoo may calm hair-damaging inflammation while killing a common yeast, *Malassezia*, that causes hair loss, itching, and dandruff. Ask your doctor for a prescription for an antifungal shampoo containing 2% ketoconazole, which a 2019 *Biomedical Dermatology* study found to be as effective as 2% minoxidil in women with female-pattern hair loss. (*Ketoconazole* is the active ingredient in the OTC dandruff shampoo Nizoral AD, but it contains only 1% ketoconazole.) Other options include Head & Shoulders, Selsun Blue, and Neutrogena TGel, which contain different active ingredients with similar effects.

• *Finasteride* **(Propecia) and** *dutasteride* **(Avodart).** These daily oral medications are a mainstay of treatment for male-pattern hair loss. They block dihydrotestosterone, a naturally occurring steroid that promotes hair thinning. Like minoxidil, they can help maintain and possibly regrow existing hair, but they won't work with complete baldness. Combining Propecia or Avodart with Rogaine can enhance effects. Postmenopausal women may be candidates for use, but women of childbearing age shouldn't even touch these drugs, let alone use them, as they can cause fetal abnormalities during pregnancy.

• **Scalp micropigmentation (SMP).** This camouflage technique uses medical-grade ink to create hundreds of tiny dots on the scalp, mimicking the look of individual hairs. SMP differs from tattooing in that the pigment is different and isn't deposited as deeply.

In someone with complete baldness, this can be done in a way that resembles a buzz cut, almost like a permanent 5-o'clock shadow on the skull. For all-over or patchy thinning, it creates the illusion of fullness. Results are instant and last five to 10 years. No recovery is needed. Because UV light breaks down the pigment, wearing a hat when outdoors can reduce the need for touchups. Depending on the area treated, expect to spend one to three hours with your SMP specialist, with a total cost of $3,000 to $6,000.

SURGICAL THERAPIES

If medical management isn't effective, there are two surgical procedures: follicular unit extraction (FUE) and follicular unit transplantation (FUT or "strip method"). In both, hair is surgically removed from the back and sides of a patient's head (the "horseshoe" region) and strategically transplanted to areas of baldness or thinning. The patient is under local anesthesia. This hair in this area is genetically different from the hair on the top of the head in that it rarely thins with age, so once it's moved to the top, it can grow there for decades.

In FUE, the donor site is shaved before individual follicles (each follicle usually contains one to four hairs) are removed and transplanted. You can expect small scars where follicles are removed, which usually end up concealed by existing hair. Recovery takes three to five days.

With FUT, which doesn't require shaving, a long, thin strip of scalp is removed before individual follicles are harvested and transplanted. The donor area is stitched back up, leaving a barely visible scar (unless you buzz your hair shorter than a #2 on a pair of standard clippers or razor shave your head), and stitches are removed after seven to 10 days. FUE may be better suited to patients with moderate hair loss and FUT for more significant loss.

Both FUE and FUT are day-long procedures that typically cost between $10,000 and $20,000, depending on where you live and the amount of hair transplanted. Results are permanent and, with a skilled surgeon, appear very natural. There is no more "hair plugs" look.

8

Investment Insight

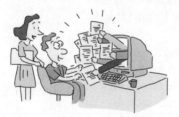

Join or Start an Investment Club for Fun and Profit

Could joining or starting an investment club jump-start your finances? Nearly half of American households have no exposure to the stock market and lacking the money to invest isn't the only reason why. Many Americans find investing in the stock market scary—even more intimidating than doing their taxes, applying for a mortgage or paying off credit card debt, according to a 2020 JP Morgan Chase survey.

In an investment club, members pool money and select investments by voting during monthly meetings. It's a social way to learn about the stock market and can help overcome investing fears.

But starting or joining an investment club has its own challenges. Clubs must file tax returns, establish rules and bear the pressure of trying to select profitable investments—and if you've ever been part of a committee, you probably already know that acting as a group does not always guarantee intelligent decisions. *Here's how to do it right…*

JOINING AN INVESTMENT CLUB

Joining an investment club isn't like joining a bridge club or a gym. It's important to choose one that matches your investment approach and has members you can trust and feel comfortable interacting with.

BetterInvesting, the nonprofit organization formerly known as the National Association of Investment Clubs, has a "Visit-A-Club" program (https://bit.ly/3mKKzvi) that points prospects to clubs in their areas that let outsiders visit and potentially join. Or ask friends who belong to investment clubs whether their

Douglas Gerlach, president of ICLUB-central, a provider of accounting and tax tools for investment clubs. He also produces a monthly webinar for investment clubs. He is author of *Investment Clubs for Dummies*. ICLUB.com

clubs are accepting new members and whether they would recommend joining.

Warning: Clubs that openly solicit new members often are not true member-operated clubs, but instead investment funds run by a money manager.

Before agreeing to join an existing investment club…

•**Attend a few meetings to get a sense of the personalities.** If you won't enjoy socializing with the other members, the experience isn't likely to be positive. Or if one or two members dominate, your investment ideas might not be considered. Most investment clubs are close-knit groups of friends, family members, church members or coworkers. It can be difficult for outsiders to fit in and find a voice if you're not in this "clique."

•**Ask to see the club's current portfolio.** Does it seek blue-chip stocks? Aggressive small-company stocks? A mix of the two? Does it hold stocks for multiple years or trade frequently? Is its investing in line with your goals and risk tolerance? Also ask to see the club's "Investment Policy Statement," and confirm that its investments and recent performance are in line with its investment philosophy.

•**Ask about contributions.** How much would you have to invest if you joined? Are penalties assessed for late payments? Also ask to see the club's "operating documents"—that is, its partnership agreement and bylaws—to learn other potentially important rules, such as the procedure for withdrawing money.

•**Ask to see the club's recent tax filings.** The IRS requires all investment club partnerships to file an annual return, and many states do as well—more on this below. Confirm that the club files its taxes by the deadline each year. Fines for late or missed filings can be severe and would be paid by members—including members who had not yet joined at the time of the infraction.

LAUNCHING A CLUB

If you launch your own investment club, the choices you make at the outset could shape the club's long-term financial results—and have tax and legal complications.

•**Form a general partnership.** You don't have to pay a lawyer to set this up—free forms are available at my website, ICLUB.com, or at BetterInvesting.org. There might be a state filing fee, but it usually does not exceed $100.

General partnership arrangements are the most common investment club structure. Lawyers sometimes voice concerns that general partnerships do not provide liability protection—in theory, one partner could be held legally responsible for another partner's debts. But in practice, tens of thousands of investment clubs have been structured this way without any known liability issues arising. Still, if liability risk is a major concern, you could structure your club as a limited liability company (LLC).

Once the partnership or LLC is established, it can request a tax ID number by filing Form SS-4, *Application for Employer Identification Number*, with the IRS…open a checking account in the partnership's name…and open a brokerage account with a discount broker.

•**Create a checks-and-balances system and monitor the club's books.** One member of the club should be elected treasurer and take primary control of its checking and investment accounts. A different club member should be named secretary and receive and review the club's bank and brokerage account statements. This makes it much harder for any one person to embezzle the group's money. Arrange things this way even if the club treasurer is a close friend—the next person elected treasurer might be someone you don't know well. Clubs also should elect a president to preside over meetings and a vice president to step in when the president is not available.

Transparency: During one monthly meeting each year, all the members of the club should scan the account transaction histories together in search of any unexplained withdrawals or missing deposits.

•**Allow different members to invest different amounts.** Many investment clubs insist that every member contribute the same amount—often $50 to $100 per month. That's a mistake. Some members might be forced to drop out when they can't afford to make contributions…while other members who wish to invest more will be prohibited from doing so.

Result: The club has fewer members and less money than it could, which hurts its performance by increasing the impact of fixed costs, such as tax-reporting expenses. Instead, let club members invest different amounts and weight each member's voting power accordingly.

• **Draft a club investment policy statement.** It should summarize the types of investments the club will or won't consider—a club might restrict itself to investing in domestic stocks, for example…the specific types of stocks it will favor, such as dividend-producing stocks or stocks over a certain market capitalization…risk levels, time horizons and turnover rates it is targeting…and/or its annual return goal. Having this policy statement in place will help focus club members on the sorts of investment ideas they should be bringing to club meetings. It also could prevent an overly aggressive club member from talking the group into an inappropriate investment.

• **File Form 1065 with the IRS each year—***US Return of Partnership Income.* General partnerships are "pass-through tax entities"—rather than pay taxes themselves, they simply divide up those taxes for partners to report on their own returns. Also provide a Schedule K-1 to partners and the IRS.

MAKING INVESTMENTS

The goals are largely the same whether you're selecting investments for a club or for your own portfolio, but there are some nuances worth noting when it comes to investment club investing.

• **Use a slow-and-steady approach to portfolio construction with a new investment club.** It's tempting to ask club members to make a big initial contribution so that the club has a sizable pot of money available from day one to build a diversified portfolio. But demanding a significant up-front investment will prevent many potential members from joining…and investing in multiple stocks right at the start forces club members who might be totally new to investing to make multiple stock picks. Instead, ask for monthly investments of $50 to $100…put off making any investments until the club has been meeting for three to five months…and then invest all the money that has accumulated in the club's coffers in a single stock. The portfolio won't be diversified at first, but you also won't have very much money on the line at this point. Choose a second stock three to five months later when the club's account balance has built up again and continue this pattern.

• **Don't blame members for poor investments.** Once the club votes on a stock, the responsibility is shared equally, no matter who proposed a struggling stock.

• **Resist the urge to hold emergency or weekly meetings.** Monthly club meetings reduce the odds of emotion-driven panic selling when the markets have a very bad day. This advantage can be lost when clubs hold emergency meetings following market routs.

• **Avoid the temptation to lock in winners and hang onto losers.** When investors sell a stock that has increased in value, they feel like they've made a smart financial move because they've earned a profit. When they sell one that has lost money, they feel exactly the opposite—and if they don't sell these struggling investments, they don't have to admit they've made a mistake. Deciding to sell off winners and hang onto losers results in portfolios full of the worst ideas.

When Complex Is Better Than Simple

Craig L. Israelsen, PhD, personal financial planning program executive in residence at Utah Valley University, Orem, and author of *7Twelve: A Diversified Investment Portfolio With a Plan.* 7TwelvePortfolio.com

M ost fund investors want to simplify their portfolios, but sometimes complicated pays. My research has found that investors willing to hold three index funds/exchange-traded funds (ETFs), which focus on components of the total stock market including large-caps, mid-caps and small-caps, can earn thousands of dollars more in the long run than a single index fund or ETF that tracks the US stock market.

Example: Over the past 20 years (through year-end 2020), a $10,000 investment in the Vanguard Total Stock Market Index Fund produced an annualized return of 7.05%, or $41,787. By holding three funds with the same market-cap weighting—70% in the Vanguard 500 Index Fund…20% in the Vanguard Mid-Cap Index Fund…and 10% in the Vanguard Small-Cap Index Fund—and rebalancing once a year, you would have gotten a 7.58% return, or $46,353. And you would have done even better if you accepted more volatility and held these funds in equal amounts, rebalancing annually—an 8.61% annualized return, or $56,712.

Reason: Three funds allow you more meaningful exposure to smaller companies, which tend to grow faster.

Also: If you need money and the stock market has a bad year, a one-fund portfolio leaves you no choice but to sell shares and lock in losses. With three funds, you can be strategic about which shares to liquidate since different asset classes don't always move in unison.

Important: Use the three-fund strategy in tax-deferred accounts. Otherwise, annual rebalancing leaves you on the hook for capital-gains taxes.

---

10 Best Dividend Stocks for the Next 10 Years

Kelley Wright, managing editor of the *Investment Quality Trends* newsletter, San Juan Capistrano, California, and author of *Dividends Still Don't Lie.* IQTrends.com

---

With bonds facing an extended bear market, fixed-income investors are increasingly turning to dividend-paying stocks to generate regular cash flow. Picking dividend-payers used to be easy. You invested in "widow-and-orphan" stocks—iconic blue-chips that treated dividends as sacrosanct, such as AT&T, Ford and Walt Disney. But over the course of the pandemic, each of those companies announced dividend cuts and/or suspensions.

Dividend-stock expert Kelley Wright says that to stay safe and prosper in this environment, income investors will need to tweak their approach to picking dividend stocks in the years ahead. The stocks he favors today are not only fundamentally sound but have proven to thrive even in a pandemic.

We asked Wright what criteria he uses to choose those stocks and the most attractive investments he's finding now…

DIVIDEND STOCKS FOR CHANGING TIMES

The coming decade will look very different from the last one for income investors. Expect to see higher inflation and interest rates…a new bull market that has much greater volatility…and more economic uncertainty. As the economy continues to reopen, the key isn't just to chase the most well-known dividend stocks or the highest-yielding ones or the best stock performers. *Instead, I use five criteria to find rock-solid stocks that can continue to pay dividends through good times and bad…*

• **Bulletproof dividends**—at least 20 years in a row of uninterrupted dividends including 2020.

• **Decent dividend yields**—a high annual yield can be deceptive because it's hard to sustain. But the yield should be substantially higher than benchmark dividend sources such as the S&P 500 (recently 1.55%) and the 10-year US Treasury bond yield (recently 3%).

• **Dividend growth**—to stay ahead of inflation, I look for increased payouts over many years.

• **Catalysts for the next decade that can generate strong earnings growth.**

• **Attractive valuations relative to the stock's own long-term history using measurements such as price-to-earnings ratio (P/E).**

MY FAVORITE DIVIDEND-PAYERS NOW

Adding one or more of the following stocks to your portfolio can increase stability and improve your income and chances for solid returns…

• **AbbVie (ABBV).** This giant drug company has increased its dividend payouts for 50 consecutive years. The stock has potential due to its acquisition of Allergan (maker of Botox), and a strong pipeline of new immunological drugs. Warren Buffett scooped up about $1.8 billion worth of AbbVie stock in 2020.

Recent yield: 3.7%.

• **Aflac (AFL).** You've seen the light-hearted TV ads with the quacking duck, but the company is a global juggernaut, underwriting supplemental health and life insurance policies for more than 50 million people. AFLAC has made a big bet on pet insurance, which should pay off in the next decade because cats and dogs are increasingly seen as family members that need health-care protection, too.

Recent yield: 2.8%.

• **Consolidated Water Co.** (CWCO) operates seawater-desalination and water-treatment plants in the Caribbean, Indonesia and the US to produce up to 70 million gallons of water daily. The company, which is expanding into more global markets, will benefit from the chronic shortage of drinkable water. By 2025, half of the world's population is expected to be living in water-stressed areas.

Recent yield: 3.2%.

• **M&T Bank Corp (MTB).** This mid-Atlantic regional bank, founded in the 1850s, now has more than 1,100 branches in 12 states stretching from Maine to West Virginia. The February 2021 acquisition of Connecticut-based People's United Financial makes M&T the 11th largest bank in the country with more than $200 billion in assets.

Recent yield: 2.9%.

• **Omnicom Group (OMC),** the world's second-largest advertising agency, has paid uninterrupted dividends since it was formed in 1986. It is benefiting from the massive shift from analog advertising, such as print, TV and billboards, to digital advertising and marketing. Omnicom's Fortune 500 clients increasingly need to reach consumers through e-mail, social media and other digital means.

Recent yield: 3.6%.

• **PepsiCo (PEP).** Twenty-three of the company's brands including Doritos, Lay's and Quaker Oats garner more than $1 billion in revenues a year. During the pandemic, PepsiCo added to its burgeoning energy-drink empire with the acquisition of Rockstar Energy Beverages. It also has partnered with the alternative meat company Beyond Meat to create plant-based protein snacks. PepsiCo raised its quarterly dividend by 5% in 2022, making 50 straight years with an increase.

Recent yield: 2.7%.

• **Phillip Morris International (PM).** Many investors shun companies involved in manufacturing cigarettes. But for those who don't mind, this leading international tobacco company, which was spun off the US company Altria in 2008 to protect its assets from federal and civil lawsuits, sells more than 130 different brands abroad including Marlboro and Parliament. About one-quarter of the company's total revenue now comes from reduced-risk, smoke-free tobacco products such as IQOS, which heats tobacco to create a vapor instead of burning it, reducing the release of harmful chemicals. Sales of heated tobacco products were up nearly 40% in Europe in the first quarter of 2022 year over year.

Recent yield: 5.1%.

• **Public Storage (PSA)** is the undisputed market leader in self-storage facilities, operating more than 170 million square feet of space in 40 states. The long-term need for self-storage accelerated during the pandemic as millions of people relocated or downsized their possessions to accommodate working at home. Performance should continue to be especially strong in West Coast markets where zoning laws and high-priced land restrict new supply of storage facilities.

Recent yield: 2.6%.

• **Texas Instruments (TXN)** is a world leader in "dumb tech." The 92-year-old company manufactures 80,000 different types of basic analog semiconductor chips, which are designed to control simple processes such as on-off power management and sound and thermal control in consumer electronics and automotive and industrial products. It's not as exciting as the sophisticated digital semiconductors such as processors made by Intel, but it is immensely profitable. Texas Instruments churns out tens of billions of chips annually. That number is likely to increase because analog chips are key components in the massive array of new electronic devices ranging from door locks to high-tech clothing.

Recent yield: 2.8%.

•**Tyson Foods (TSN)** produces one-fifth of all the beef, pork and chicken in the US, including popular store brands such as Jimmy Dean and Hillshire Farm. Tyson has two major catalysts for growth in the next decade—a plant-based chicken line made from pea protein called Raised & Rooted that currently sells in 10,000 US grocery stores. Tyson recently received approval from the Chinese government to sell chicken and pork to mainland China, where meat production has been hurt by bird and swine flus.

Recent yield: 2%.

Any Tech-Stock Bargains Left?

Brian Colello, CPA, director of technology equity research at Morningstar Inc., Chicago, which tracks 621,000 investment offerings. Morningstar.com

After dominating the stock market for a decade, that's no longer the case with tech stocks, which are weighed down by sky-high valuations, rising interest rates and investor fears that the remote-work trend that has boosted profits for tech companies will fade. Through April 30, 2022, the S&P 500's tech sector returned 11% versus 61% for the leading sector—energy. That doesn't mean investors should abandon tech. Over the coming decade, tech businesses will grow far faster than the overall economy. But you can no longer simply buy what's hot, regardless of price, and expect to make money.

Three tech stocks with attractive valuations, including two beaten-down companies selling

at bargain prices and a reasonably priced tech giant…

•**Intel (INTC)** is a leading manufacturer of semiconductor chips and microprocessors. Its stock was knocked down last year after delays in product upgrades. But it is spending $20 billion to build manufacturing facilities in Arizona and is expanding into lucrative new markets for chips including self-driving cars and smart-home devices.

Recent share price: $44.01.

•**Microsoft (MSFT).** The $2 trillion company can no longer count on robust growth from its Windows operating systems and Office productivity software. But it has diversified into fast-growing areas such as cloud computing, social media and video gaming.

Recent share price: $269.50.

•**Splunk (SPLK).** The software maker provides more than 15,000 companies with powerful tools to spot opportunities in the vast amount of customer data they collect. The recent stock price doesn't reflect Splunk's enormous growth potential due to recent operational challenges as it switches its business model to deliver software through subscriptions over the Internet.

Recent share price: $94.89.

Create Your Own Target-Date Fund Customized Just for You

Paul Merriman, founder of The Merriman Financial Education Foundation, dedicated to educating do-it-yourself investors, Bainbridge Island, Washington. He is author of *We're Talking Millions! 12 Simple Ways to Supercharge Your Retirement*, available for free at PaulMerriman.com/signup, and creator of the weekly podcast "Sound Investing." PaulMerriman.com

About 40 million Americans have invested in target-date funds (TDFs), those ready-made, all-weather portfolios of stock and bond funds that automatically grow more conservative as you age toward a specific retirement date. TDFs have attracted more than $1.7 trillion in assets because they are simple to use, offer wide diversification in tumultuous times and provide solid returns even if you have no interest or expertise in managing your nest egg.

But top financial educator Paul Merriman thinks you can do better—with just a little effort. He says you can replicate your own version of a TDF using low-cost exchange-traded funds (ETFs) and reap several benefits, including saving tens of thousands of dollars in fees…customizing your fund to improve performance…and tailoring it to your own personal time horizon and risk tolerance.

Below, Merriman shares with us the hidden drawbacks of conventional TDFs…and he provides a step-by-step guide to building your own TDF.

TDF DRAWBACKS

Conventional TDFs have been around for more than 25 years, but investors still are in the dark about how much they cost and their risks and shortcomings. *Here's why I think they are not the best solution for many small investors…*

•**TDF fees often are too high.** Conventional TDFs charge an average annual expense ratio of 0.55%, or $550 per $100,000 investment. Many fund families use in-house actively managed funds that drive up costs, such as Capital Group's American funds (annual expense ratios range from 0.61% to 0.81%)…Fidelity's Freedom funds (from 0.49% to 0.75%)…and T. Rowe Price (0.34% to 0.64%). By contrast, you could construct a do-it-yourself (DIY) TDF with an expense ratio of just 0.09%, or $90 per $100,000.

•**They are too generic.** Conventional TDFs cater to millions of investors so they're forced to take a one-size-fits-all approach, and that may not align with your individual needs.

Example: Most TDFs are offered in five-year intervals, and each fund family has a proprietary "glide path"—the rate at which portfolio allocations grow less risky, gradually shifting from stocks to bonds as you age. So if you plan to retire in 2027, you would have to use a 2025 fund or a 2030 fund, neither of which may be right for you.

•**They are too conservative.** Most TDFs keep a minimum of 10% of their portfolios in bond funds. This reduces volatility but hurts young investors who have decades to go before retirement by creating an unnecessary drag on long-term performance. Also, many conventional TDFs drop their stock exposure too much during your working years so that you end up with a 50% stock–50% bond allocation at age 65. While your portfolio should grow less daring as you get closer to needing the money, a 50%–50% allocation may not provide enough growth to make your money last another 30 years once you stop working.

•**They rebalance too frequently.** Many TDFs buy or sell stocks and bonds on a regular basis in order to maintain their desired asset allocation. Frequent rebalancing lowers the short-term volatility of your portfolio and keeps it targeted to the appropriate level of risk—but it also curtails positive momentum and decreases long-term performance.

THREE STEPS TO BUILD YOUR OWN TDF

You can correct many of the shortcomings of conventional TDFs by putting together and managing one on your own. This may sound intimidating, but it's relatively easy to set up and, once established, takes little annual oversight.

Note: I typically recommend DIY TDFs for IRAs because they offer a variety of investments. However, it may be possible to build one in a 401(k) account, too, using mutual funds.

STEP #1: **Decide on your asset-class allocation.** Until age 40, you are best-served by having a 100% stock allocation in your portfolio and no bonds. This maximizes your returns, and you will have plenty of time to recover from any bear markets. Depending on your situation, split the stock portion of the portfolio by putting 50% in a total US stock market ETF and 50% in a total international stock market ETF.

If you are a moderate or aggressive investor, put one-third of your portfolio in both the total US and international ETFs and the remaining one-third in a small-cap value ETF. Why own small, undervalued companies? Because they have the best long-term performance records of any stock asset class. In the past century, small-cap value stocks have returned approximately an annualized 13% versus 10% for large-cap stocks.

Once you are over age 40, begin adding a fixed-income component to your portfolio to tone down volatility. Split your fixed-income allocation among three different types of bonds in the following proportions—an intermediate-term bond ETF (50%)…a short-term bond ETF (30%)…and an inflation-protected government bond ETF (20%).

STEP #2: **Choose your glide path from age 40 to 65.** I recommend that a moderate investor shift 8% of his/her stock allocation into bonds every five years. If you start with a 100% stock allocation at age 40, you would have 60% in stocks and 40% in bonds by age 65. A more aggressive investor could shift 6%, which produces a 70% stock/30% bond allocation at retirement age. A very conservative investor should raise bond allocations and lower stock allocations by 10% every five years, leading to a 50% stock/50% bond makeup at age 65.

STEP #3: **Choose the actual investments for your TDF.** *Here are the six allocation categories I use and a variety of low-cost funds I like in each category…*

• **Total US Stock Market.** Avantis US Equity ETF (AVUS)…iShares Core S&P 500 (IVV)…Vanguard Total Stock Market ETF (VTI).

• **Total International Stock Market.** Avantis International Equity ETF (AVDE)…SPDR Developed World ex-US ETF (SPDW)…Vanguard Total International Stock ETF (VXUS).

• **US Small-Cap Value.** Avantis US Small Cap Value ETF (AVUV)…SPDR S&P 600 Small Cap Value ETF (SLYV)…Vanguard S&P 600 Small-Cap Value ETF (VIOV).

• **Intermediate-Term Government Bonds.** iShares 7-10 Year Treasury Bond ETF (IEF)… SPDR Portfolio Intermediate Term Treasury ETF (SPTI)…Vanguard Intermediate-Term Treasury ETF (VGIT).

• **Short-Term Government Bonds.** iShares 1-3 Year Treasury Bond ETF (SHY)…Schwab Short-Term US Treasury ETF (SCHO)…Vanguard Short-Term Treasury ETF (VGSH).

• **Inflation-Protected Government Bonds.** iShares 0-5 Year TIPS Bond ETF (STIP)… Schwab US TIPS ETF (SCHP)…Vanguard Short-Term Inflation-Protected Securities ETF (VTIP).

GET THE MOST OUT OF YOUR DIY TDF…

• **Rebalance no more than once a year— once every 18 months is even better.** In addition to making glide path changes to your stock-bond allocations every five years, rejigger holdings back to your current allocation over shorter time periods. In a conventional ETF, you have little control over when your manager rebalances, but you can set your own schedule with a DIY fund. While less frequent rebalancing will raise your portfolio's short-term volatility, it tends to raise long-term performance also.

• **Be realistic about how much investment discipline you have.** By far, the greatest challenge of a DIY TDF is sticking to your investment plan consistently year after year. That's relatively easy to do when you own a conventional TDF because you can't fiddle with the fund's underlying ETFs. The danger of a DIY fund is thinking that you are smarter than the market or panicking in down markets and making shortsighted moves that hurt your long-term performance. If you don't think you can stick with it, you are better off owning a conventional TDF from a low-cost provider such as Charles Schwab or Vanguard.

• **Get help from a financial advisor when you reach age 65 (or retire).** TDFs are designed to deliver you to your desired retirement age. But finding a suitable asset allocation for your portfolio in retirement is a lot trickier and more individualized. You need to limit portfolio ups and downs because you now are drawing money from it—but you also need to generate enough growth to make your nest egg last another 30 years.

Direct Indexing: Customize Your Fund

Larry Swedroe, chief research officer at Buckingham Strategic Wealth, which oversees more than $26 billion in assets, St. Louis. BuckinghamStrategicWealth.com

I ndex funds and exchange-traded funds (ETFs) revolutionized investing by providing a simple way to get instant diversification. Now, brokerage firms like Fidelity, Vanguard and Wealthfront are taking the next step—direct indexing, which allows you to replicate a major index identically or customize one to reflect your personal preferences by eliminating particular stocks or industries.

Examples: You could invest in the stocks of the S&P 500 Index but remove tobacco stocks.

How it works: Instead of buying shares in a fund that tracks a major index, your broker purchases the underlying individual stocks in that index, minus the companies you don't want. In taxable accounts, direct indexing also can produce better after-tax returns because your broker monitors your portfolio for losing positions. Those stocks are sold, and shares of similar companies are purchased as replacements. That allows your portfolio to replicate the returns of the benchmark index plus capture capital losses without running afoul of the IRS wash-sale rule, which states that you cannot buy the same or substantially identical security within 30 days before or after selling one at a loss. Using capital losses to offset capital gains this way can earn direct indexers 1% to 1.5% more in after-tax returns annually. If capital losses exceed gains in a given year, you can apply them in future years, or use them to offset up to $3,000 of ordinary income per year.

Drawbacks: Higher fees—Fidelity Managed FidFolios carry a 0.4% annual expense ratio versus just 0.03% for a conventional fund such as the iShares Core S&P 500 ETF.

Keep in mind—direct indexing is most effective when using indexes that track highly liquid US and international large-cap stocks.

Investing in the Next Big Thing: Finding Tomorrow's Blockbusters

David Mazza, managing director and head of product at Direxion, an asset-management company with $26.6 billion in assets offering mutual funds and exchange-traded funds, New York City. He oversees the Direxion Moonshot Innovators ETF (MOON), launched in November 2020. Direxion.com

W ouldn't it be great if you had purchased Bitcoin when it was selling for $320 instead of $32,000? Or in electric-vehicle maker Tesla's stock just a few years ago, before it soared 1,800%?

The fund that investment expert David Mazza oversees specializes in investing in "moonshots"—high-risk companies that offer visionary products and services that change the world and the way we live...and make their investors a fortune!

Betting on moonshots isn't for everyone. Owning these stocks can be a white-knuckle roller-coaster ride with the possibility of steep losses. Valuing these companies has less to do with price-to-earnings ratios and return on equity than faith and imagination.

Still, today's world is transforming so quickly that if you get in early on these stocks—before the big money is made—you may need only a small amount of exposure to boost your overall portfolio returns for years. *We asked David Mazza how investors can identify moonshot stocks and which ones his fund currently owns…*

FINDING THE NEXT BIG THING

To identify moonshot potential, investors should focus on nascent industries and trends where disruptive technology is creating vast consumer markets and needs that never existed before.

Next, look at small and medium-sized companies that are still in the early stages of their earnings cycles. Make sure these young companies are innovation industry leaders. My team and I do this by first comparing how much companies stress innovation in their annual reports and other SEC filings…and then by comparing how much they spend on research and development relative to their sales versus their peers.

PROMISING MOONSHOT TRENDS

The following companies have market capitalizations ranging from $90 million to $3.2 billion, and all have the potential for massive expansion...

•**Hydrogen economy.** The race to wean the world off polluting fossil fuels and to power the next generation of vehicles has hydrogen fuel cells poised to take off. A fuel cell is an electrochemical device that combines colorless, odorless hydrogen fuel with oxygen to produce electricity. During the process, water vapor is generated but no carbon dioxide, the culprit blamed for climate change. Hydrogen vehicles can go farther between fill-ups than battery-powered cars, and refueling time is similar to gasoline-powered cars. *Stock we own now...*

•Ballard Power Systems (BLDP). The Canadian company makes hydrogen fuel cells for commercial vehicles including buses, forklifts, ferry boats and trains. About 80% of the hydrogen buses in Europe use Ballard fuel cells, and Volkswagen has an $80 million deal with Ballard aimed at manufacturing Audi hydrogen cars. *Market capitalization:* $2 billion. *Recent share price:* $6.66.

•**Natural killers.** Immunotherapy treatments are tailored to strengthen your own immune system to combat cancer and infectious diseases. Scientists have focused on enhancing "natural killer" (NK) cells produced in the body's bone marrow. New technology allows NK cells to target proteins in cancerous tumors without harming healthy tissue. The global cancer immunotherapy market is growing 10% annually and likely will reach $175 billion by 2027. *Stock we own now...*

•ImmunityBio (IBRX) has no existing products on the market, but it boasts a pipeline of 25 immunotherapy drugs in late-stage clinical trials, including one for bladder cancer designated a breakthrough therapy by the FDA. The company's CEO, Patrick Soon-Shiong, MD, a billionaire South African transplant surgeon, previously invented and sold the rights to the blockbuster cancer drug Abraxane. *Market capitalization:* $1.14 billion. *Recent share price:* $3.45.

•**Hack attack.** For years, the threat from ransomware—criminals breaking into computer networks and locking up digital information until victims pay a ransom—was broadly discussed. But the threat seemed distant, and the cost of the necessary security steps was high. Now, hacking has become a national security threat, crippling food and energy providers and shutting down hospitals and big municipalities. A ransomware attack is expected to occur every 11 seconds. *Stock we own now...*

•Varonis Systems (VRNS). Governments and national-defense agencies rely on this cybersecurity company's software to protect sensitive data stored on premises and in the cloud. Varonis specializes in insider-threat detection. Most cyberattacks are caused by insiders or involve the hijacking of an insider's credentials. If Varonis detects a threat, it can limit the damage from breaches by automatically locking down sensitive data. *Market capitalization:* $3.2 billion. *Recent share price:* $30.19.

•**The final frontier.** Outer space is an integral part of our lives with orbiting satellites that allow us to connect to the Internet and get GPS directions. Only about 600 people have been to space. New scientific and technological advancements, such as smaller, reusable rockets, have ignited a space race that will yield commercial ventures ranging from manufacturing computer chips in zero gravity to mining on the moon and space tourism. Spending on space ventures is expected to triple to $1.1 trillion by 2040. *Stock we own now...*

•Virgin Galactic Holdings (SPCE). Billionaire entrepreneur Richard Branson made history this past summer when he became the first space "tourist" to reach suborbital space more than 50 miles above the New Mexico desert on the company's VSS Unity rocket-powered spaceplane. Virgin Galactic Holdings, which designs, develops and produces its own vehicles, is the first to receive a commercial license and FAA approval to carry passengers into space. It has collected $80 million in ticket sales and deposits. Branson wants to complete 400 space flights per year, generating $1 billion in revenue per spaceport in coming years, with the potential to build dozens of spaceports around the world. *Market capitalization:* $1.5 billion. *Recent share price:* $5.85.

nology and talent from the studio that created visual effects for movies and TV shows such as *The Lord of the Rings* and *Game of Thrones*.

Investing in the Metaverse

Mario Stefanidis, CFA, vice president of research at Roundhill Investments, which launched the Roundhill Ball Metaverse ETF (META), New York City. Roundhill Investments.com

What if you didn't just go online to buy clothes but could actually shop inside the Internet? Like in an immersive video game, you would wear virtual-reality (VR) goggles and your avatar would walk through a three-dimensional store, trying on and buying stuff. Thanks to advancements in VR equipment and computing power, this disruptive virtual space—the Metaverse—will allow people to increasingly spend time in digital worlds, shopping, holding meetings, touring houses for sale and watching concerts. Analysts estimate the global Metaverse market could reach $800 billion by 2024.

How to invest: Many investors have exposure to global technology giants that are developing Metaverse devices and online platforms, including Apple, Microsoft and Meta Platforms (formerly Facebook). *Here are three smaller software and gaming companies that aren't yet household names but offer applications that will form the Metaverse's building blocks in the next few years…*

•**Matterport (MTTR)** is a spatial-data company that makes specialized cameras and software to take 3-D images of real places such as real estate for sale, then re-creates them in the virtual world.

•**Roblox Corp. (RBLX)** provides an online video-game platform used by about 43 million daily visitors to play immersive 3-D games and participate in live digital concerts and fashion shows.

•**Unity Software (U)** is used by designers in the video-game industry to build digital worlds. It recently acquired digital tools, tech-

The Death of Cash: The Digital-Payment Revolution

Lisa Ellis, partner and senior analyst overseeing the digital-payment, processing and IT services industry for MoffettNathanson, an independent equity research firm, New York City. Barron's ranked Ellis as one of the 100 most influential women in US finance in 2020. MoffettNathanson.com

While the use of paper bills and coins has waned for years, fears about the physical transmission of coronavirus encouraged millions of consumers to embrace alternatives to exchanging cash, including ordering groceries online…using "digital wallets" to store and access money electronically…and carrying "contactless" credit cards and smartphone apps to transmit payment information. And with each transaction, the service providers receive a fee.

The result is a digital payment system that could reach $10.5 trillion by 2025.

Another reason to invest in the accelerating death of cash: The winners have already emerged. While there will continue to be startups, the digital-payment market is dominated by a handful of companies that are likely to grow larger and more profitable in the coming years as using cash grows increasingly rare, not just in the US but all over the world.

We asked digital-payment expert Lisa Ellis for her thoughts on this revolution and the types of companies she covers if investors are interested in doing further research…

3 WAYS TO GAIN EXPOSURE

For growth-oriented investors…

•**Pure-play payment processors.** These businesses exist mostly as apps on your computer, laptop or mobile phone and are used for Internet commerce and digital-cash exchange. They allow you to buy items online with a click

135

of a button or in physical locations by scanning a QR code with your mobile phone. You also can make "peer to peer" (P2P) payments using a digital wallet to send and receive money to and from friends, family members and businesses with just a cell-phone number or an e-mail address. Some pure-play companies also enable small businesses to accept credit card and digital payments from consumers.

Outlook: These companies are among the industry's most exciting and fastest-growing players. They were ideally positioned at the start of the pandemic to benefit from housebound consumers flocking to e-commerce and P2P payments. Their stocks soared last year but have relatively high valuations now and will experience ups and downs going forward because expectations are so high.

Examples of pure-play payment processors that I cover...

• PayPal (PYPL) is the leader in online payments with more than 390 million active users. Its P2P service—Venmo—and PayPal Checkout button on almost every top retailer's website led to $1.25 trillion in total payment volume in 2021. PayPal recently started offering specialty services including Honey, a deal-finding tool to help shoppers seek low prices and earn rewards for online purchases.

• Block (SQ). Founded by Twitter CEO Jack Dorsey, the company, formerly known as Square, is best known for its pocket-sized, white card reader that plugs into laptops or smartphones, allowing small merchants to process credit card payments face-to-face or over the Internet. Block software also helps merchants collect payments, manage invoices, offer gift cards and prepare their taxes. But it's Block's second business, Cash App—an innovative P2P payment network of more than 30 million users—that sent the company's stock rocketing upward in 2020. Cash App offers a wide array of services, including its popular Boost rewards program and the ability to buy and sell stocks.

For investors looking to add blue-chip global giants to their portfolios...

• **Credit and debit card processors.** Most investors are familiar with these global companies, which perform the authorization, clearance and settlement functions for transactions between banks that issue plastic cards and banks of merchants that accept the cards. Technology such as contactless cards embedded with radio chips is enhancing the volume and frequency of purchases that consumers charge. The companies also sell many related business services ranging from data analytics to fraud prevention.

Outlook: These companies should see strong, steady post-pandemic growth, and their valuations still are reasonable. While credit and debit card processors got a boost in business from e-commerce purchases during the pandemic, that didn't offset the dramatic slowdowns in entertainment and overseas travel spending. I expect those areas to begin to rebound strongly, as well as show continued future expansion in emerging markets, where credit and debit card penetration still is low.

Examples of credit and debit card processors that I cover...

• Mastercard (MA) is the second-largest payment processor in the world. It is likely to grow modestly faster over time than Visa due to its smaller size and relatively higher presence in underpenetrated overseas markets, especially Europe.

• Visa (V) processes about $13 trillion in transactions a year, linking 100 million sellers with 3.8 billion credit and debit cards. The stock is suffering short-term headwinds, including a US Justice Department investigation for anticompetitive behavior in the debit card space. But I don't think that hurts its long-term potential, which includes upside from Visa's new payment product Visa Direct.

For value-oriented investors...

• **Traditional merchant and bank payment processors.** These companies focus on processing payments for financial institutions and traditional brick-and-mortar merchants rather than online consumers. They process transactions behind the scenes at fast-food restaurants and clothing and grocery stores... and they provide payment solutions and software technology for banks processing bill-payment, lending and Automated Clearing House (ACH) transfers, the electronic network in which money moves between banks.

Outlook: These companies don't have the spectacular growth or services of other digital-payment industry players, but they will play a vital role in the future and their stocks trade at attractive valuations. Recovery will be gradual as brick-and-mortar sales bounce back and the mergers add revenue and cost synergies.

Example of a merchant and bank payment processor that I cover…

• Fiserv (FISV) controls about one-third of the US market share for traditional merchant and bank processing, including many top quick-service restaurants such as McDonald's and Burger King and hundreds of small and midsize banks. The company's $22 billion acquisition of payment processor First Data in 2019 will broaden its exposure to brick-and-mortar merchants and should result in cost savings of hundreds of millions of dollars annually.

Invest in High-End Collectibles with Fractional Shares

Michael Fox-Rabinovitz, CFA, partner with the investment management firm Chartwell Capital, New York City. He is author of *Own a Fraction, Earn a Fortune* and *Unlock the Vault: A Blueprint for Building Wealth With Fractional Ownership.*

Many online investment startups now specialize in acquiring high-priced collectibles that only millionaires can afford, then allow small investors to buy shares in those collectibles, ranging from fine artwork and sports memorabilia to rare comic books and historical documents. Demand for collectibles has surged during the pandemic as people stuck at home and flush with cash make investments they feel more passionate about than plain-vanilla stocks and bonds.

Advantages of buying fractional shares: Prices for collectibles have little correlation with the stock market's movements so they can act as useful—albeit unusual—alternative assets to diversify your portfolio. Investing in the right collectible also can yield explosive profits when it's eventually sold at auction or to a private collector. In 2020, thousands of investors paid $50 per share for a $140,000 vintage copy of Nintendo's *Super Mario Bros.* videogame. It sold in August 2021 for $2 million, or about $667 per share.

Firms that offer fractional investing are regulated by the SEC, and they make collectible investing as easy as trading stocks online at Fidelity or Robinhood.

But it's not right for everyone—collectibles can take a long time to sell, tying up your money for years. And they don't generate earnings or dividends as stocks do, so they can be high-risk, unpredictable investments.

To help you decide what's right for you and how to profit from fractional investing, we spoke to collectibles investment expert Michael Fox-Rabinovitz, CFA…

HOW IT WORKS

Online collectible firms typically purchase items ranging in price from $10,000 to more than $5 million, often relying on software algorithms and historical databases of sales to try to outsmart the market and find collectibles that will have the best returns.

A set number of fractional shares, usually priced at $10 or $25 per share, are registered with the SEC. The firm holds an initial public offering (IPO) online. To invest, you download the company's app, open an account, then wire money from your bank to fund your account and purchase fractional shares of the collectible. You can view detailed descriptions of the collectibles through the app, including prices, number of shares offered, comparable asset value and certificates of authenticity and other documents.

After the IPO shares are all sold and following the 90-day SEC-mandated lock-up period, you can buy or sell shares on the secondary market through a trading platform on the firm's website.

The investment firm insures and physically stores your Monet painting or Lamborghini. Some firms take a cut of the eventual profits once the collectible is sold. Others take their fee as a percentage of the IPO and/or charge investors an ongoing fee.

Most firms aim to hold the collectibles for five years or longer. However, if a majority of the shareholders agree, they can be sold at any time after the SEC holding period. *Caveats for investors…*

● **Keep investments to 5% or less of your overall portfolio.** Spread your bets around instead of focusing on a single item. Since prices for individual fractional shares tend to be low, put money in multiple baseball trading cards or different pieces of artwork, depending on your interests.

● **Plan to hold your shares long term.** Technically, you don't have to wait for a collectible to be sold in order to cash in. You can buy or sell fractional shares on the website of the firm that owns the collectible. But this is a relatively tiny secondary market, so the price you get on your shares may not be desirable.

BEST COLLECTIBLES FIRMS NOW

I look for areas of the collectibles market with the following characteristics—items with significant historical and/or cultural importance…extensive history of past sales and benchmark data to help determine market value…clear provenances of ownership with extensive documentation so you don't have to worry about fakes. Areas that meet these criteria now include sports memorabilia, art, vintage comic books and videogames, and antique cars. *Here are the best firms and what they specialize in…*

● **Collectable (Collectable.com).**

Specialty: Sports memorabilia. The site offers more than 100 collectibles from baseball, basketball, golf and other sports.

Why invest in sports memorabilia: Over the past decade, the PWCC, the largest trading-card marketplace in the world, reports that its 2500 index (PWCC 2500 Trading Card List), which tracks the increase in value of the 2,500 sports cards with the highest market value, rose almost 400% versus 197% for the S&P 500. *Examples…*

● 1952 Jackie Robinson trading baseball card. The first Topps trading card issued of the immortal Brooklyn second baseman.

● Kareem Abdul-Jabbar's NBA record basketball. Jabbar used this ball to score the final

point of his career, number 38,387, the most in basketball history.

● Tiger Woods's Titleist Te I3 putter. Woods used the club during his late 1990's tournament wins.

● **Masterworks (Masterworks.io).**

Specialty: About 60 works of fine art valued at more than $200 million and ranging from 19th-century Impressionists to contemporary artists.

Why invest in art: Art collectors hold more than $1.7 trillion in assets. Although returns on art have underperformed the stock market in the past decade, from 2000 to 2021 the Artprice100 Index, which monitors auction prices of the works of 100 top artists, is expected to have increased 400%. *Examples…*

● Andy Warhol's "1 Colored Marilyn (Reversal Series)," a dramatic 1979 oil-and-silkscreen ink portrait of Marilyn Monroe in swirls of turquoise and hot pink.

● Claude Monet's "Coup de Vent," an 1881 oil painting depicting the windswept Normandy coast on a summer's day.

● **Otis (WithOtis.com).**

Specialty: Vintage comic books. The site also sells shares in more than 100 small pop-culture collectibles including designer sneakers, toy action figures and vintage videogames.

Why invest in comic books: The value of comic books has exploded in recent years driven by the prevalence of top-grossing movies featuring comic book superheroes. The Nostomania 500 Comic Book Stock Index, which measures the performance of 500 of the most desired and valuable comic books, was up nearly 800% over the past decade, including a more than 200% jump just this year. *Examples…*

● Avengers #1 comic book. One of the most sought-after items in comic book publishing, this premiere issue from Marvel was published in 1963.

● Pokémon Yellow. The 1999 videogame, published by Nintendo for the Game Boy player, helped kickstart one of the most popular franchises ever.

● **Rally (RallyRD.com).**

Specialty: Antique cars. Rally offers Porsches, Ferraris and Ford Mustangs from the 1950s to the 2000s, some of which are on display at the firm's New York City location. And now Rally is branching out into other unique collectibles.

Why invest in vintage cars: The market has a history of stable returns and low volatility. Over the past decade, the Historical Automobile Group International (HAGI) Top Index, which tracks the value of 50 representative classic cars, has returned about 160%. *Examples…*

• 1985 Ferrari Testarossa. 12-cylinder model with flying mirror and center-lock wheels.

• 1955 Porsche 356 Speedster. One of just 193 cars in the "Speedster Blue" color with original engine and door panels.

Investing in Semiconductor Chips

John Buckingham, principal and portfolio manager for Kovitz Investment Group, which manages $7 billion, Aliso Viejo, California, and editor of *The Prudent Speculator* newsletter. ThePrudentSpeculator.com

Semiconductor chips, which power everything from Apple Watches to refrigerators to Teslas, are a hot commodity now. Investors can make big profits—but they also can get burned. A shortage of these chips due to 2020's manufacturing shutdowns, coupled with post-pandemic demand from automakers and electronics manufacturers, has sent prices soaring. The shortage is expected to extend into 2023—great news for semiconductor stocks. But semiconductors are a boom-and-bust industry. In good times, chip makers initiate expansions—Intel is spending nearly $25 billion on plants in Arizona and New Mexico…Samsung Electronics is investing $116 billion in its foundry and chip-design businesses. But expansions often lead to a supply glut…and investors who pay sky-high prices for these stocks now can wind up with losses later.

Take advantage of the chip boom…

• **Look at equipment makers for chip manufacturers.** The federal government is subsidizing efforts to do more US-based chip manufacturing, while the Internet of Things is seeing semiconductors included in just about anything imaginable.

Consider: Lam Research (LRCX) and Cohu (COHU), which are reasonably priced.

• **Invest in undervalued chip makers.**

Consider: Micron Technology (MU), specializing in memory chips, which have catalysts for long-term demand including 5G smartphones, graphic cards for video games and solid-state hard drives in PCs and laptops.

Use Real-Return ETFs to Protect Against Inflation

They provide a real return above the rate of inflation and are easier than choosing a variety of assets that thrive in rising-price environments.

Worth considering: SPDR SSgA Multi-Asset Real Return ETF (RLY), a fund of funds that owns 11 other SPDR ETFs focusing on areas such as agribusiness, metals and mining, and REITs… IQ Real Return ETF (CPI), a more conservative fund that uses US Treasuries, ultra-short corporate bonds and foreign currencies.

Neena Mishra, CFA, is ETF research director at Zacks Investment Research, Chicago. Zacks.com

REIT Investors: Be Cautious About Work from Home

Uncertainty remains as to how much of the workforce will make a physical return to their offices. Office buildings and business districts aren't headed for extinction, but changes appear inevitable. Commercial real estate investors should seek out financially strong, well-diversified companies.

Examples: Boston Properties (BXP)... and, to a lesser extent, Kilroy Realty Corporation (KRC). But be prepared to play a long game as the market sorts itself out.

Reuben Gregg Brewer is an investment journalist for *The Motley Fool*, Alexandria, Virginia. Fool.com

Robo-Picks for Your Investments?

Neena Mishra, CFA, ETF research director at Zacks Investment Research, Chicago. Zacks.com

There are more than 20 exchange-traded funds (ETFs) run by artificial intelligence (AI)—software that can think for itself and learn from past experiences. The funds range from AI Powered Equity ETF (AIEQ), run by Watson (the IBM supercomputer that has bested two *Jeopardy* champions)...to offerings from giant firms such as BlackRock and State Street. The supercomputers analyze economic and market patterns and sort through vast amounts of stock data at speeds that would take a thousand human analysts to match.

But: The performance of many AI-run funds hasn't significantly beaten that of the stock market. AIEQ, launched in 2017 and focused on large-cap stocks, has three-year annualized returns of 7% versus 11% for the S&P 500 Index.

Reality: It's hard for even a supercomputer algorithm to gain an edge investing in big companies that are widely scrutinized. One-quarter of AIEQ's assets are devoted to giant tech stocks that you may already own or could find in a cheaper ETF that tracks the S&P 500 Index.

There is a compelling case, however, for using supercomputers in niche areas that typically get less attention from Wall Street. *Two funds that track indexes using AI to select stocks...*

•**SPDR S&P Kensho Clean Power ETF (CNRG)** invests in 40 to 45 smaller companies driving innovation in the clean-energy sector, including solar, wind and hydroelectric power.

Annualized performance since its October 2018 inception: 29.23%.

•**SPDR S&P Kensho New Economies Composite ETF (KOMP)** owns nearly 500 stocks of companies that are disrupting industries using advancements in AI, robotics and automation.

Annualized performance since its October 2018 inception: 10.4%.

9

Money Management

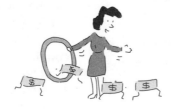

Go Rogue! Using Unconventional Wisdom for Financial Decisions

Top economist and Wall Street gadfly Laurence J. Kotlikoff, PhD, believes that the way most of us go about planning our finances is all wrong. We let emotions and irrational fears sway us and, even worse, rely on conventional wisdom about personal finances, which often benefits only the financial industry. Instead, Kotlikoff—who doesn't hesitate to chide financial-firm executives for bilking customers with misleading advice—says you will have greater security and a better life if you make choices about money the way a hard-nosed economist does—focus on how your financial choices will impact your long-term standard of living. After all, once you have established the lifestyle and level of income you enjoy each

year, it's immensely painful to be forced to scale back.

We asked Kotlikoff for his unconventional advice about housing, retirement, debt and investing…

HOUSING

***CONVENTIONAL WISDOM:* Pay off your mortgage as soon as possible if you are near or in retirement—but don't use IRA or 401(k) money.** That money should continue to grow tax-deferred.

***UNCONVENTIONAL WISDOM:* Consider tapping your tax-deferred accounts to pay off your mortgage.** For most retirees today, retiring mortgage debt is the equivalent of earning a guaranteed 3% to 4% return. That will support your standard of living better

Laurence J. Kotlikoff, PhD, professor of economics at Boston University. He is president of Economic Security Planning, which offers financial-planning software, and author of 20 books including *Money Magic: An Economist's Secrets to More Money, Less Risk, and a Better Life.* Kotlikoff.net

141

than the fixed-income part of your retirement portfolio. Sure, you have to pay taxes on traditional IRA or 401(k) withdrawals, but you still can come out ahead, especially if you are in a lower tax bracket than you'll be in down the road when you start taking Social Security. Once you own your home, your monthly bills drop significantly, and that makes it easier to ride out stock market turbulence with your remaining investments.

Caveats: There's less incentive to pay off your mortgage in retirement if you have a mortgage rate below 3% or if your itemizable deductions are high enough so that you don't take the standard deduction on your taxes and need the mortgage interest payments for deductions.

RETIREMENT

CONVENTIONAL WISDOM: **Take Social Security benefits as soon as you are eligible.** Most of us start taking payments as soon as we retire.

Why: You hope to get back what you paid into the system before you die or before the Social Security trust fund is depleted and the government reduces everyone's payouts.

UNCONVENTIONAL WISDOM: **Postpone taking Social Security payments as long as possible.** Unless you have serious health concerns that will likely shorten your life or you have no other assets to live on, the advantages of delaying Social Security are too good to ignore. This is true even if benefits are cut by up to one-quarter down the road (an unlikely outcome). Each year you put off receiving your benefits increases your monthly lifetime payouts from 7% to 8%. And if you delay until age 70 (when annual increases in benefits stop), your monthly payout is about 75% higher than at age 62.

Delaying also allows you to maximize widow(er)s and eligible divorced widow(er)s benefits. If you die, your spouse—and your ex-spouses married to you for a decade or longer—are entitled to receive the higher of their own retirement benefit or your retirement benefit for life. And by spending down your tax-deferred accounts before age 70, the taxes

you eventually will pay on your Social Security benefits will be smaller.

Also: It would take an act of Congress to reduce future Social Security payouts. Washington is unlikely to shortchange more than 70 million baby boomer constituents.

More likely: The fund will be bailed out by raising taxes that the rich pay on their Social Security benefits.

CONVENTIONAL WISDOM: **Beware of annuities**—contracts that typically allow you to make a lump-sum payment now to an insurance company in exchange for eventually receiving a guaranteed monthly payout for the rest of your life. They are complex and have high fees. Plus, if you die right after paying the lump sum, you get nothing.

UNCONVENTIONAL WISDOM: **Even people who are annuity-averse may want to consider a Qualified Longevity Annuity Contract (QLAC).** QLACs are deferred annuities that let you delay payouts until you reach advanced old age. That allows you to avoid living like a miser because you fear running out of money later on. QLACs are easy to understand and have no annual fees, and your payout amount is fixed and guaranteed for life. You can invest up to 25% of your tax-deferred retirement accounts (up to $145,000 in 2022) in a QLAC. In exchange, you'll get an annuity that can start paying out as late as age 85. The amount will depend on your age when you purchased the QLAC, how much money you paid for it, your gender and how high interest rates were when you bought it. Wait to purchase a QLAC at least until age 72 when you are otherwise forced to take required minimum distributions (RMDs) from your taxable (non-Roth) retirement accounts. Payouts typically are bigger than what you could earn from a long-term bond portfolio that you might invest in on your own.

Even better: The IRS allows you to exclude the QLAC when calculating your RMDs, which start at age 72, allowing those taxable distributions to be smaller. You can add riders to your QLAC for "cost-of-living adjustments" to keep pace with inflation…and "return-of-premium" so that your spouse and other heirs will receive the initial amount that you invested in the QLAC if you die before you get any payouts.

INVESTING

***CONVENTIONAL WISDOM:* The older you get, the more conservative your portfolio should be—more bonds and less stock.** Traditional formula to figure out your stock allocation: Subtract your age from 100. So a 65-year-old should have no more than 35% in the stock market. A 75-year-old, just 25%.

***UNCONVENTIONAL WISDOM:* Increase your allocation to stocks as you age throughout your retirement.** As you age and eat up your assets, more of your total resources become tied up in Social Security benefits. But receiving these benefits are akin to inflation-indexed bonds.

To maintain a proper overall balance of risky and safe resources: Invest an ever larger share of your ever-declining investable assets in stocks.

Unclaimed Assets: How to Find Them

Mark Kantrowitz who maintains the "Unclaimed Property" page at UnclaimedProperty.info. He is publisher of the student-loan information website PrivateStudentLoans.guru and author of *How to Appeal for More College Financial Aid.*

Tens of billions of dollars are just waiting to be claimed—and you could be the winner. That may sound like a come-on for a sweepstakes promotion, but it's the reality of unclaimed assets hiding in the coffers of state and federal government agencies. To be a winner, you have to know where to look for the assets.

WHERE THEY COME FROM

The assets include retirement plan proceeds from former employers…security deposits released by long-ago landlords…bank and financial accounts sitting dormant for years…insurance policy proceeds…matured savings bonds…and much more.

"Escheatment" laws that cover unclaimed assets require that financial institutions and other businesses hand over assets to state governments if the proper owners cannot be located, and some federal agencies have unclaimed assets, too. These laws vary by state but are growing stricter as governments increasingly view unclaimed assets as a source of revenue. In many states, financial institutions are required to turn over money simply because they have had no contact with the account holder in as little as two or three years.

Generally, the assets can be reclaimed without time limits or penalties (although also without further interest payments once they become unclaimed assets).

WHERE AND HOW TO SEARCH

•**Search state unclaimed-asset databases in every state where you have lived or worked.** For most states, you can do this by entering your name and other basic info into the master search page on the website Missing Money.com. Eleven states do not share their unclaimed asset data with that site, however —California, Connecticut, Delaware, Georgia, Hawaii, Kansas, New Jersey, Oregon, Pennsylvania, Washington and Wyoming. For these states, click "states" on MissingMoney.com, then click the appropriate state on the map to go to its unclaimed-assets online database. Search states even if you haven't lived or worked in them for decades. These sites and searches are free.

If you find a listing for money that seems to be owed to you, follow the directions to reclaim it. The process varies by state but usually requires filling out a form available on the state website.

Helpful: With these state sites—and with the other databases listed below—also search any former names you have used, such as maiden names…common misspellings of your name—Smith if your name is Smyth, for example…and your name flip-flopped, with first name last and last first if your last name is one that's commonly used as a first name, such as Patrick or Thomas. Typos such as these are one reason why money might have failed to reach you and became lost in the first place.

•**Search the names of any businesses you owned over the years.** And search the names of any now-deceased relatives for whom you were an heir or estate executor. Claiming money that previously belonged to a deceased relative or to a now-closed business can be challenging. The state is likely to request extensive documentation to establish that you are the proper owner. If the state still does not accept that you are the proper recipient and the amount involved is worth the expense, it might be necessary to hire a probate attorney to help recover the money.

•**Search for missing retirement plan money if you might have forgotten to roll over a 401(k)** from a long-ago employer or you worked for a company that had a traditional pension plan. The Pension Benefit Guaranty Corporation, the federal agency that guarantees traditional pension plans, maintains a searchable database of unclaimed traditional pension benefits at Search.PBGC.gov.

Also check the National Registry of Unclaimed Retirement Benefits (UnclaimedRetire mentBenefits.com), a free service offered by PenChecks, the largest processor of retirement plan benefits. It lists both unclaimed 401(k) assets and traditional pension assets. Widows and widowers should search for pension assets in their deceased spouse's name as well.

If these searches come up empty but you're concerned that you've lost track of retirement benefits from a particular past employer, additional options include contacting that former employer's human resources department… and/or PensionHelpAmerica (PensionHelp. org), which provides free assistance with pension problems and is run by the nonprofit Pension Rights Center.

•**Search for unpaid life insurance benefits.** The National Association of Insurance Commissioners offers a free policy-locator service (https://EApps.naic.org/life-policy-locator) that could help you track down life insurance policies and annuity contracts of deceased relatives that name you as a beneficiary. This isn't a searchable database—you'll have to complete and submit an online form and then wait up to 90 days to see if any participating insurance companies find unclaimed benefits for you.

•**Search for unredeemed savings bonds. It's very common for people to lose track of US savings bonds**—these often are given as gifts to children, then forgotten before the bonds reach maturity. To track them down, complete Treasury Department Form 1048, *Claim for Lost, Stolen, or Destroyed United States Savings Bonds* (TreasuryDirect.gov/ forms/sav1048.pdf). This form asks for details that most people don't have, such as the missing bond's issue date and serial number, but file anyway. Include as much detail as you can and leave the rest blank. The most important details to include are your name and Social Security number and—if the bond was a gift—the name and Social Security number of the gift giver.

•**Search for federal income tax refunds due to you.** If you were owed a tax refund but didn't file a return, the IRS might owe you money. The catch is that, unlike most unclaimed assets, this type has a deadline. You must file a return within three years of the date of the original deadline.

Example: If you were due a refund in 2020 but didn't file, you must file by May 17, 2024—three years after the original 2020 filing deadline of May 17, 2021.

You also might be owed money by the IRS if you filed a return but the refund was returned to the IRS as undeliverable or did not make it into your bank account as an electronic deposit. On IRS.gov/refunds, click "Check My Refund Status" to track a refund filed for during the current year (or final six months of the prior year) or call the IRS at 800-829-1954 to initiate a refund trace.

•**Search for money you're owed from old FHA-insured mortgages.** If you paid Federal Housing Administration insurance on a mortgage, there are two situations where the US Department of Housing and Urban Development (HUD) might have money for you…

•You acquired a mortgage loan after September 1, 1983…paid an up-front FHA mortgage insurance premium at closing…*and* did not default on your mortgage payment. If this is true, you might be owed a refund on a portion of the FHA insurance premiums you paid.

•Your loan originated before September 1, 1983…you made payments on that loan for more than seven years…*and* your FHA insurance terminated before November 5, 1990. If this is true, you might be eligible for a share of the earnings from the Mutual Mortgage Insurance Fund.

There's an online search tool at https://ENTP.hud.gov/dsrs/refunds that can tell you if there's FHA money due to you.

BEWARE FEES AND SCAMS

Some people make a living tracking down other people's unclaimed assets. They search online databases, contact people they find listed there and offer to reunite them with their money in exchange for a cut of the proceeds—

GOOD TO KNOW...

Checking and Savings Tips

Everyone Should Have Two Bank Accounts

A checking account for paying bills…and a savings account for emergencies, such as healthcare needs or job loss. Couples need at least three accounts—one for each partner and one combined account. Partners should discuss how much money each of them should put into the comingled account. If you use a debit card, open a separate account tied to it—that way, if the card gets stolen, your entire checking account is not at risk.

Clark.com

How Much Money to Keep On Hand

Do you have enough—or too much—cash in your bank accounts?

Checking: Since it is meant for paying everyday expenses and recurring bills, keep enough money for at least one month's worth of expenses in this account, plus the overdraft fee if you have one.

Savings: This is where to keep cash for emergencies—set aside three to six months' worth of your expenses. You also can use a savings account to save for special purposes, such as a planned trip or the down payment on a house.

Lifehacker.com

---

from 10% to more than half. Some states, but not all, have laws limiting the amount these asset finders can charge.

Don't agree to this. The person may be a scammer who is trying to get you to reveal personal information such as your Social Security number to steal your identity and/or who tries to convince you to pay an up-front fee and then disappears with your money.

And even if this lost-asset finder is not a scammer, he/she isn't doing anything that you couldn't do yourself in just a few minutes. If you receive a call or an e-mail along these lines, that's a tip-off that you should check the databases for yourself. If you don't find any assets under your name, wait a few months and try again—sometimes these professional finders pay fees to obtain advance access to new listings that haven't yet found their way into the databases.

Bank Overdraft Fees on Their Way Out

Capital One and Ally Bank have eliminated fees for having insufficient funds in an account. Other banks, including Bank of America and First Citizens, are lowering fees due to pressure from government regulators and competition from low-fee online banks.

If your bank charges overdraft fees: Ask if there's a way to link your checking account to your savings account to reduce overdraft risk, or ask to have the fees waived.

Ken Tumin, cofounder of the bank-review website DepositAccounts.com.

Credit Unions Anybody Can Join

DepositAccounts.com

Credit unions often pay more for deposits, charge less for loans and offer better terms than banks do—even Internet banks. Required to have a field of membership, which used to be a company or community, credit unions now often are open to members of associations that can be joined by anyone, usually at low cost. Many credit unions have online applications, and almost all make it easy to do business no matter where you live.

Examples: Boeing Employees Credit Union, based in Tukwila, Washington...PenFed in McLean, Virginia...First Technology Federal in San Jose, California...Alliant in Chicago... Mountain America in Sandy, Utah...Lake Mich-

igan in Grand Rapids...Digital Federal in Marlborough, Massachusetts...Patelco in Dublin, California...Teachers Federal in Hauppauge, New York. For a complete list, updated daily, visit DepositAccounts.com/credit-unions/any one-can-join.

Fight Rising Inflation with Series I Bonds

These US government savings bonds, available commission-free at TreasuryDirect. gov, can help protect your cash's purchasing power. They pay a combined fixed interest rate for the life of the bond (recently 0%), plus a variable inflation rate (recently 4.81%), which adjusts in May and November.

Drawbacks: The maximum purchase is $10,000 annually per person...bonds can be redeemed only after 12 months...there is an early-withdrawal penalty of three months' interest within the first five years.

Ken Tumin, founder of DepositAccounts.com, a website owned by LendingTree that monitors bank interest rates, based in Longwood, Florida.

"NeoBanks" Aren't Worth the Hassle

Ken Tumin, cofounder of DepositAccounts, a website now owned by LendingTree that provides bank rates, reviews and news. DepositAccounts.com

A new breed of financial company —"neobanks," such as Affirm, Betterment, Chime, M1 Finance, T-Mobile Money and Wealthfront—tout attractive interest rates, low fees and speedy access to money that arrives via direct deposit.

But: They come with hidden dangers...

•**Most neobanks lack bank charters from state or federal regulators authorizing them to operate as banks.** They often partner with chartered banks that hold their customers' money. Thanks to these partnerships, most—though not all—neobank accounts are FDIC-insured, and customers likely would get their money back if the neobank fails.

●**Customer service is lacking.** Customer service generally is provided only via e-mail or online chat.

●**Joint accounts often aren't available.** Many neobanks allow only one owner per account. Others don't let account owners designate beneficiaries, which can render money inaccessible for months when an account holder dies.

●**ATM networks and bank services are lacking.** Some neobanks offer low-cost or free access to ATM networks, but many don't. And most offer only a limited range of accounts and services.

●**Their eye-catching interest rates often are temporary.** New neobanks frequently pay relatively high rates on checking and savings accounts to attract customers—but those rates tend to drop within one or two years.

●**Not all neobanks operate the same way.** Many, including Affirm, M1 Finance and T-Mobile Money, partner with chartered, FDIC-insured banks. Others, including Betterment and Wealthfront, partner with networks that spread account holders' deposits among several chartered, FDIC-insured banks. And some, including BlockFi and Celsius, don't partner with FDIC-insured banks—so their customers risk losing their money if the neobank fails. Recently a few neobanks, including Varo and LendingClub Bank, have obtained charters and become true online banks with their own FDIC insurance.

What to do: Consider an established online bank, such as Ally or Discover, instead of a neobank. These offer higher interest rates and lower fees than bricks-and-mortar banks...and provide customer service via 800-numbers, fee-free access to ATMs and FDIC insurance.

If you're willing to endure the neobank hassles: Consider these neobank accounts with appealing rates, low fees and FDIC insurance...

●**T-Mobile Money checking**—no-fee access to more than 55,000 ATMs and 1% interest that climbs to 4% on up to $3,000 in deposits for eligible T-Mobile customers. T-MobileMoney.com

●**LendingClub Bank High-Yield Savings** —0.85% interest on balances $2,500 and above. Bank.LendingClub.com

●**Affirm Savings pays 0.65% interest.** Affirm.com/savings

Worst Time to Ask for a Loan

Because of decision fatigue, bank credit officers are more likely to turn down a loan-restructuring request at midday than earlier or later in the day. Decision fatigue—tiredness from continuously making difficult decisions over an extended period—inclines people to take the easiest or safest option. Loan restructuring for a customer having difficulty making payments involves balancing a customer's needs against the risk for repayment failure. According to a recent study, such requests were more often granted early in the day...and after credit officers' lunch break.

Study by researchers at University of Cambridge, UK, published in *Royal Society Open Science.*

Using a Reverse Mortgage to Tap Home Equity

Keith Gumbinger, vice president of New Jersey-based HSH Associates, which publishes mortgage and consumer loan information. HSH.com

The recent run-up in real estate values is great news for home sellers—but what if you don't want to sell? Reverse mortgages offer a way for homeowners age 62 and up to tap home equity without moving or locking themselves into monthly debt payments.

Reverse mortgages haven't always had a stellar reputation—detractors pointed to huge costs and horror stories of seniors evicted from their homes. But virtually all reverse mortgages issued today are federal-government–insured "Home Equity Conversion Mortgages" (HECMs) offered through Federal Housing Administration–approved lenders, which have reasonable terms and solid consumer protections. *What to know if you're considering a reverse mortgage...*

•**No monthly payments does not mean no interest.** While the money borrowed doesn't need to be paid back until the borrower sells the home, moves out or dies—when proceeds from selling the home can be used to repay the debt—interest does accumulate until the loan is paid, eroding home equity.

•**Only you and your spouse can defer repayment and remain in the home as long as you like.** Adult children, nonspousal partners or others living in the home might be forced to pay off the loan or move out when you move or die. A nonborrowing spouse must be disclosed to the lender and named in the loan document in order to remain in the home.

•**Fees remain significant.** Reverse mortgage fees are likely to total 6% to 8% of your "potential equity draw"—the total amount of home equity you could tap. That's steeper than the 2% to 5% of a typical mortgage.

Sign up for quarterly rewards—keep track of what they are and whether there are any stipulations such as spending limits. *Read the fine print*—for example, rewards for groceries may exclude superstore purchases. *Take advantage of perks*—for instance, travel-focused cards may give airport-lounge access and lost-luggage insurance. *Plan large purchases carefully*—if you're planning to purchase something costly, sign up for a card with a good bonus for that type of item first. *Don't carry a balance*—it can easily cancel the value of any rewards.

Bankrate.com

Best Ways to Maximize Credit Card Rewards

Consider your spending habits—choose a card with higher rewards in those areas, such as shopping or travel, and a separate card that gives rewards for everyday spending if the first one does not. *Look for a sign-up bonus*—read the terms carefully, and make sure you scrupulously comply, such as by spending a certain amount within a certain time frame.

Rejected for a Credit Card Application? Take These Steps

Find out why—the issuer must mail you an "adverse action report" detailing the reason for the rejection. *Review your credit history*—get a free copy of the credit report that the issuer used and check for errors. *Try the lender's "reconsideration line"*—where you call to have your application reviewed. *Repair your credit*—pay down debt and avoid maxing out cards. *Find a card that's a better fit*—look for credit cards that are more likely to lend to someone with your credit score.

LifeHacker.com

Monthly Credit Checks Boost Your Score

People who review their scores at least every month are more likely to improve their credit behavior and borrowing habits and their score.

Recent example: More than one-third of subprime consumers who regularly monitored their credit raised their credit scores to a near-prime level or better (good and excellent credit). Among consumers who did not monitor their scores, only 18% increased them.

Amy Thomann, head of consumer credit education at TransUnion, one of the three major credit bureaus, in Chicago, quoted in USA Today.

Consider Adding a Note to Your Credit Report

If you lost your job because of the coronavirus pandemic and have been unable to keep up with your bills. The note—called a "consumer statement"—explains missed or late payments to potential lenders and may help offset negative information if you apply for a loan or credit card. Be sure to remove the note when your financial situation improves and you are again able to meet all your payment obligations.

Beverly Anderson, president, global consumer solutions, Equifax, credit bureau based in Atlanta, quoted at BusinessInsider.com.

Closing Unused Credit Card Accounts Hurts Your Credit Score

John Ulzheimer, president of The Ulzheimer Group and a credit expert who has held positions with Equifax and Fair Isaac, which created the most popular credit score. JohnUlzheimer.com

Did you know that closing credit cards—even ones that are rarely used—can actually lower your credit score?

Why would that be? Your "credit-utilization ratio"—the percentage of your available credit that you currently are using—is a significant component of your credit score, and lower is better. When you close a card, your available credit declines...which means that the percentage of your available credit you're currently using climbs—and that can cost you points on your credit score.

On balance, not closing unused credit cards is the smart move—or, better yet, make purchases with otherwise unused cards every few months to dissuade their issuers from canceling them.

Exceptions: Consider closing an unused card if it has a high annual fee and a low credit limit—that low limit means it probably isn't helping your credit-utilization ratio enough to justify its cost. And strongly consider canceling any joint credit cards you have with your spouse if the relationship appears headed toward divorce.

GOOD TO KNOW...

Best FICO Credit Score

Best FICO credit score to have—760. That is the level at which you will get the most benefits and best deals on mortgages, car loans, credit card rewards and more.

Bottom line: A perfect score of 850—which about 1.6% of the US population has—is not likely to get you significantly better deals or better rates than a score of 760.

Roundup of experts on credit scores reported at CNBC.com.

Fix Your Financial Relationship with Your Partner

Kathleen Burns Kingsbury, founder of KBK Wealth Connection, a wealth psychology coaching and consulting firm, Waitsfield, Vermont. She is author of several books, including *Breaking Money Silence: How to Shatter Money Taboos, Talk Openly About Finances, and Live a Richer Life*. BreakingMoneySilence.com

Evaluating money roles within a relationship allows you to set more effective boundaries with each other, decrease tensions and uncertainty, and perhaps even deepen your sense of intimacy and teamwork in the relationship.

Wealth psychology expert Kathleen Burns Kingsbury shares here her favorite strategies for couples…

FOSTERING TEAMWORK

Improving your financial relationship doesn't mean that you need to change who you are as a person or split all financial tasks 50-50. Often, major improvements come from minor adjustments such as making sure both partners participate in big money decisions and talking regularly to get a clearer picture of one another's money goals.

What you should do together…

• **Assemble a file with a master checklist or spreadsheet of all financial accounts and documents.** Include information about how they can be accessed—passwords, locations, account numbers. This is a low-conflict, easy task that brings peace of mind to both partners. *The file should include…*

• Names, addresses, phone numbers and e-mail addresses of financial advisers—attorney, broker, insurance agent and accountant

• Auto titles and maintenance records

• Bank and brokerage investment accounts (taxable and retirement)

• Contracts (legal, etc.)

• Estate-planning documents (wills, trusts, etc.)

• Home mortgage and other loan documents

• Insurance policies

• Recurring bills, outstanding debts

• Social Security records

• Tax records

As you build the spreadsheet and put together the file, create a list of issues that you want to discuss and financial chores you can do together or take on separately.

Examples: Change passwords that are too simple…update your wills…make sure beneficiary forms in investment accounts have been filled out.

• **Use a personal-finance app for couples.** The software typically allows couples to sync various accounts online to better collaborate on financial transactions…set up monthly bill-payment reminders…and automatically categorize and track spending so you can see how you're progressing. *Recommended apps…*

• Mint is one of the most comprehensive personal-finance apps with nearly 30 million users. *Cost:* Free. Mint.com

• Honeydue offers unique features for couples such as the ability to directly message each other through the app if, for instance, a recent charge doesn't look familiar. *Cost:* Free. Honeydue.com

Important: While couples should strive to be transparent about their finances and activities, no one likes to be micromanaged. I suggest that partners agree to have individual accounts for discretionary spending up to an agreed-upon amount each month without needing to consult one another.

• **Conduct a monthly financial meeting.** These should be no longer than 30 minutes. Start each one by focusing on a small, positive financial accomplishment such as staying within budget for the month or lowering credit card debt. Check in to make sure you're making progress toward financial goals, and review upcoming tasks or events. End the meeting by discussing one area of your financial relationship you want to work on. Afterward, reward yourselves with an activity you both like to do.

• **Use Kingsbury's Rules of Engagement.** *You need to treat each other thoughtfully when you discuss finances because disagreements over money and money roles have the potential to escalate into full-blown power struggles...*

• Be respectful. Listen without interrupting. Reflect back what you've heard to ensure accuracy before you make your own point. Recognize that both viewpoints are valid.

• Use "I" statements to communicate how you feel and what specific action triggered those feelings. Otherwise, you come across as scolding or nagging. Instead of saying, "How could you bounce another check?" try, "It's upsetting to me when a check bounces because we get hit with late fees."

• Don't mind read. Couples tend to jump to conclusions about each other's motives. Instead of being judgmental, be curious. Trying to increase mutual understanding about the other person's experiences and values will yield more effective resolutions than trying to convince your partner that you are right.

IF YOU ARE THE MONEY PERSON...

• **Find ways to reinforce your partner's involvement in financial matters.** Include him/her in all conversations and e-mails with advisers, even if they seem trivial or perfunctory. Never just hand your partner financial documents to sign without explaining what they are.

IF YOU ARE THE LESS INVOLVED PARTNER...

• **Take responsibility for educating yourself.** If your partner doesn't have the ability to be a good teacher and coach, seek out advisers who can fill in your knowledge gaps or take an adult-learning course in personal finance.

• **Ask for a "great gift."** If your partner likes to be in control and is stubborn about sharing information with you or seeking your participation in financial decisions, say, "The greatest gift you could give me is letting me be more involved. It would alleviate a lot of my fears and stress knowing that we are doing this as a team and as equals."

Steps to Take When a Spouse Has Died

Get certified copies of the death certificate. Ask the funeral home to provide at least a dozen for taking care of paperwork. *Contact your spouse's employer.* The employer may owe you retirement funds or insurance payouts. And if the employer provides your health insurance, you'll need to know how long the coverage will last. *Alert your spouse's life insurance company.* Have all your documentation so you can file a claim. *Probate the estate.* Contact the lawyer who set up the will, and get started settling the estate. *Collect all financial records.* Gather info on banking, taxes, insurance, bills and credit cards—and run a credit report so you know exactly what you're dealing with. *Cancel or switch over accounts.* Cell phones, utilities, etc. *Contact the Social Security Administration.* The sooner you do so, the sooner you can collect benefits.

Kiplinger.com

Suffered a Financial Setback? Reapply for Financial Aid

Apply—or reapply—for college financial aid for your child ASAP if you have had a financial setback. Colleges may increase aid packages under special circumstances, such as a lost job or big medical bills. But schools' contingency funds may run dry, so soon as you have proof of your setback—a termination letter from your employer, for instance—call the financial-aid office or visit its website to apply for aid or an adjustment.

Mark Kantrowitz, financial-aid expert and publisher of PrivateStudentLoans.guru.

Getting Divorced? Protect Yourself from These Financial Surprises

Jacqueline Newman, Esq., managing partner of Berkman Bottger Newman & Schein, LLP, a divorce law firm, New York City, and author of *The New Rules of Divorce: Twelve Secrets to Protecting Your Wealth, Health, and Happiness.* BerkBot.com

Breaking up is hard to do—yet more than 750,000 American marriages will end in divorce this year. And while many of those people saw the end of their marriages coming, most will be taken by surprise by aspects of the divorce process.

Despite what divorcees often expect, few get a chance to denounce their spouses' misdeeds in court—the usual process is more like a financial negotiation than a courtroom drama. And while playing hardball with a soon-to-be-ex is a common—and, in some cases, justified—impulse, it generally results in both spouses suffering more than necessary. Even people who have been through a divorce before may be surprised if they end up divorcing again—divorce court rulings have changed in some significant ways in the past 10 or 20 years. *So before you head to court, be wary of these potential surprises…*

•**Spousal support has become a lot less supportive.** A divorcing spouse who earned little or no income during the marriage often expects to receive a share of his/her former spouse's income sufficient to maintain the lifestyle to which she (or he) had become accustomed, in addition to her share of the marital assets.

Don't count on it! Divorce courts have been moving away from spousal support in recent decades. They reason that virtually every adult is capable of earning a living for himself/herself—even spouses who gave up their careers long ago to raise families. Today's divorcees still might receive some support for a limited number of years—details vary by state and judge—and they'll still receive their share of the marital income and potentially child support for young children, but the era of lifetime spousal support is over. Unless their share of the marital assets is sufficient to pay their bills for the rest of their lives, former stay-at-home spouses often must get jobs when the marriage ends.

•**The primary parent can no longer assume that he/she will receive full custody of the kids.** A decade or two ago, the parent who did most of the child rearing—almost always the mother—would almost certainly get custody of the children in a divorce…but not anymore. In recent years, 50/50 custody has become many courts' default position. Before the pandemic, primary parents could argue that their spouses weren't qualified to share custody because they didn't know the children's preferences and routines. But after a year or two of quarantining together, career-focused parents are more likely to know when little Bobby goes to bed and how he likes his sandwiches sliced.

Also: This shift affects grandparents, too—the share of custody that a parent receives can have a dramatic impact on the amount of time that the parents' parents get with their grandchildren.

•**A single tax return could shape your entire divorce agreement.** A divorcing couple's most recently filed tax return often plays a major role in negotiating the divorce settlement. Divorce attorneys can present other financial information for consideration as well, but that one tax return tends to weigh heavily.

That's especially notable these days—tax returns for many households have been atypical due to the pandemic and the red-hot stock market.

Rule of thumb: If a marriage is ending, the low-earning spouse generally benefits by filing for divorce when investments have been rallying and the most recent tax return shows relatively high income…the high-earning spouse benefits by filing when the opposite is true.

•**Vengeance will cost you.** Instructing a shark of a divorce attorney to rip your spouse to pieces doesn't increase your odds of getting a great settlement. But it does increase the odds that your spouse will hire a shark, too…or that the attorney your spouse hires will respond in kind.

Result: These sharks will fight it out, and you'll end up with more or less the same percentage of the marital assets that you would have received if both spouses hired attorneys focused on working toward a fair settlement… but there will be fewer assets to divide, because those attorneys will end up getting a bigger piece of the pie.

• **A big-city divorce attorney can be a poor choice for a small-town divorcee.** A local attorney will have tried so many divorces before the local judges that he/she usually can predict the outcome if a divorce reaches court. That means he knows whether and for how much to settle—a huge home-field advantage. An out-of-town attorney usually can't do that…plus he likely will charge much more per hour than the local attorney.

• **Your spouse's infidelity doesn't matter.** Divorcees often imagine that providing proof that their spouse was unfaithful will swing the proceedings in their favor. But in most states, it won't even be a consideration—the modern "no fault" divorce process is about dividing up the assets, not assessing blame for the failure of the relationship. Divorce courts also won't care about your spouse's profligate spending, poor work ethic or other unpleasant behavior.

Potential exception: If your spouse feels very guilty about the infidelity or other misbehavior, your attorney might be able to convince him/her to agree to a settlement that's favorable to you.

• **Premarital assets sometimes become marital assets.** Many married people know that the assets they owned before they wed generally will not be divided up as marital property in a divorce. But it is very easy to accidentally transform premarital assets partially or entirely into marital property.

Common misstep: Commingling premarital assets with marital assets—perhaps by using money earned during the marriage to purchase additional shares of stock in a premarital investment account…or to pay for repairs on a rental property that was owned before the marriage. In fact, simply trading stocks within a premarital investment account could partially transform that account into a marital asset even if no money enters or is removed from the account. Divorce courts have ruled that actively managing an asset during a marriage means that it is no longer entirely a premarital asset because the time the married person spent making investment decisions is itself a marital asset.

The value of the assets at the date the marriage began most likely still will be treated as a premarital asset, but any appreciation that occurred during the marriage is likely to be a marital asset. Leaving the management of premarital assets to professional managers could avoid this problem. The challenge of maintaining the status of premarital assets is one reason why prenuptial agreements are such a good idea.

• **It probably doesn't matter that an account is in your name.** If assets in an account were purchased using money accumulated during the marriage, then the account will be treated as a marital asset whether it is in one spouse's name or both names.

Potential exception: If one spouse inherits or is gifted assets during the marriage…keeps those assets in his/her own name…and never commingles them with marital assets, those assets are likely to be considered that spouse's separate assets in many states.

• **Gifts you gave each other while married are marital property.** If a gift was purchased using marital assets, it doesn't matter that your spouse gave it to you—it will be considered a marital asset during the divorce.

This leads to a question—are wedding and engagement rings marital or separate assets? Wedding rings are exchanged during the wedding ceremony, so they generally are treated as gifts given during the marriage and considered marital property. But the bride-to-be received her engagement ring as a "conditional gift" prior to the marriage, so unless marital assets were used to repair or improve the ring during the marriage, it's likely to be considered separate property and therefore is hers to keep. The engagement ring is considered a "conditional gift" because it is given on the condition that the bride follows through on her commitment to wed—if she doesn't, courts generally rule that the giver can reclaim the ring.

How to Choose a Charity Worthy of Your Money

Stacy Steele, director of marketing and communications at Charity Navigator, a New Jersey–based nonprofit that evaluates other nonprofits. CharityNavigator.org

How can givers be sure that a nonprofit deserves their donations? *We asked Stacy Steele of Charity Navigator, the world's largest independent nonprofit evaluator, what donors need to know...*

INVESTIGATING A NONPROFIT

Before writing a check to a charity, take these three steps...

•**Confirm that the charity is a "501(c)(3)" nonprofit.** This means it has been approved by the Internal Revenue Service to be recognized as a tax-exempt, charitable organization, so donations to it are tax-deductible. The best way to confirm this is to use the organization's Employer Identification Number (EIN) to verify its status. Enter the number into the IRS's Tax-Exempt Organization Search tool. (On IRS. gov, choose "Charities & Nonprofits" from the top menu, then "Search for Charities" from the menu on the left.) You also can search by the nonprofit's name, but many nonprofits have similar names, which can cause confusion.

Caution: Don't donate to any charity that doesn't have an EIN. All 501(c)(3) nonprofits must have an EIN officially registered with the IRS.

•**Investigate what the organization actually delivers.** At the heart of any nonprofit is its stated mission. Connected to that mission are its values, goals and a breakdown of its programs and services. These are key bits of information for any donor because they provide a guide to how your money will be used and the impact of your gift.

Short descriptions of nonprofits' missions and key projects often can be found within their Form 990 tax returns, which should

TAKE NOTE...

Often-Overlooked Assets to Watch Out for in a Divorce

Restricted stock units—executive-level corporate jobs often provide these as future income tied to performance or other factors. If you are the non-earning spouse, find out about these units—they cannot be transferred, but something of equivalent value can be, although valuation can be difficult. *Pensions*—if your soon-to-be-ex has one, be sure its value is taken into account. If the company offering the pension has filed for bankruptcy or there are other complicating factors, expect to hire an expert to determine value. *Military benefits*—there are special rules governing military benefits in a divorce, and filling out the right paperwork is crucial. Consult a divorce lawyer with experience in the field. *Bitcoin and other cryptocurrency*—these can be held many ways, and valuations can change rapidly. Consult a professional with valuation knowledge in the field.

Kiplinger.com

be available via the IRS's Tax-Exempt Organization Search tool. The information also is available on some charity-evaluation websites, such as my organization, Charity Navigator (CharityNavigator.org)...and/or on the nonprofit's own website under a heading such as "mission," "financials," "history," "projects" and/or "successes."

•**Determine how effectively the organization puts donors' money to use.** What percentage of each dollar received by the organization goes toward its programs...and what percentage goes to overhead, salaries and attempts to raise more money? How cost-effective are those fund-raising efforts? Some nonprofits are far more efficient than others.

You can find certain financial details in the nonprofit's Form 990. There also are nonprofit evaluators such as Charity Navigator that analyze and share data beyond financials that also consider the importance of good governance, and other core areas of nonprofit effectiveness, including the impact and results of your donations…the organization's approach to strategy, leadership and adaptability…and its culture and relationship to the community it serves. To view available Forms 990 for rated nonprofits, search for and visit the organization's profile on CharityNavigator.org. See the "Additional Information" section, and select "Data Sources (IRS Forms 990)."

TOP NONPROFITS TODAY

At press time, the following organizations appeared within Charity Navigator's Top Ten Lists of "10 of the Best Charities Everyone's Heard Of." These large, well-known nonprofits have budgets exceeding $100 million and at least $65 million in net assets. The Top Ten Lists are electronically selected based on an algorithm built into Charity Navigator's Star Rating system. Value judgments are not made about the missions that nonprofits pursue—it's up to donors to decide which causes matter most to them.

•**Direct Relief** focuses on disaster response, emergency preparedness and the prevention and treatment of disease. Direct Relief.org

•**Enterprise Community Partners** works to increase the supply of affordable housing, advance racial equity and promote upward mobility. EnterpriseCommunity.com

•**MAP International** is a Christian organization providing medicine and health supplies to people in need. MAP.org

•**Matthew 25: Ministries** is an international humanitarian aid and disaster relief organization. M25M.org

•**The Rotary Foundation of Rotary International** makes grants intended to promote peace, fight disease, provide clean water and sanitation, support mothers and children, improve education and strengthen local economies. On Rotary.org, select "Our Foundation" from the "About Rotary" menu.

•**Vitamin Angels** provides vitamins and minerals to pregnant women, new mothers and young children in need. VitaminAngels. org

•**World Resources Institute** seeks to protect the environment and its capacity to provide for current and future generations. WRI.org

•**Americares** provides medicine, supplies, health care, emergency preparation and recovery assistance to people and communities in need. Americares.org

•**Feeding America** operates a nationwide network of 200 food banks that provide food to more than 46 million people through 60,000 food pantries and meal programs. FeedingAmerica.org

•**DonorsChoose** allows citizen philanthropists to fund specific project requests from teachers in US public schools. Donors Choose.org

How to Get Rid of Your Timeshare

Brian Rogers, owner of Timeshare Users Group, the premier source of help and advice for timeshare owners. TUG2.com

Getting out from under a timeshare that you no longer want can be inexpensive and simple. *Here's how to do it…*

•**Adjust your expectations.** Many people assume that a timeshare will have gained value over time or that they'll be able to sell it for around what they paid for it.

Reality: Your purchase loses most of its value the minute you sign the contract—whether you've purchased a deeded week (a specific week and unit size at one resort) or bought into a points system (which allows more flexibility about timing and location). It's almost a guarantee that the very thing you just paid $20,000 for is being offered for free online because that is the actual value of the product and there are far more people looking to sell than are browsing for resale timeshares. Asking for any amount more than "free" will attract only scammers.

If you're still paying off the loan for your timeshare, you have almost no good options—nobody is going to take on that debt when they could get a timeshare for free.

If you still owe on the loan: Transfer the balance of the loan to a line of credit that has a better interest rate.

If you no longer have a loan, here are three options…

1. See if the resort will take it back. Most resorts have what's called a "deed-back" program, in which you can sign the timeshare back over to the resort for free or for a small fee. Looking into the deed-back program always should be your first step, even if you believe that you can sell your timeshare on the resale market. If you simply want to be free of your maintenance fees, sign the timeshare over and be done with it.

2. Try to sell it. Go on eBay or my site (TUG2.com) to see what similar properties are selling for and price accordingly. Unless you possess a rare gem, you'll be effectively giving away the timeshare. You can make your ad more attractive by agreeing to pay the closing costs (it's usually just a few hundred dollars).

3. Stop paying maintenance fees. Eventually the resort will foreclose, and you no longer will own the timeshare. And yes, this foreclosure likely will show up on your credit report.

Important: Never stop paying on a loan, which will significantly harm your credit.

What you shouldn't do: Never pay an exit company to dispose of your timeshare. Their methods are the same options as above. The exit company will charge you $5,000 simply to call the resort and use the same deed-back program you could have used for free. Or it will charge you thousands to instruct you to stop paying your maintenance fees, which will result in the same foreclosure. There's no circumstance in which an exit company makes more sense than attempting the steps laid out here by yourself first.

Debt Collectors Can Use Social Media

Debt collectors can use social media to contact you. A new rule from the Consumer Financial Protection Bureau, which went into effect November 30, 2021, will allow debt collectors to contact consumers by e-mail, text and direct messages on social-media sites. There is no limit as to the number of times they can reach out.

Small plus: No more than seven phone calls per debt can be made each week.

Rachel Gittleman, CFA, financial services and membership outreach manager at Consumer Federation of America, Washington, DC. ConsumerFed.org

10

Insurance Insider

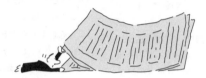

Avoid These 5 Costly Medicare Mistakes

Medicare covers a lot of health problems—and causes a lot of headaches. The complex program features four parts …10 supplemental coverage options…hundreds of drug plans…and a virtually endless list of rules. *Here are big mistakes to avoid…*

***MISTAKE:* Enrolling at the wrong time.** When should you first sign up for Medicare? The short answer is that you become eligible at age 65—there's a seven-month "initial enrollment period" that includes the month of your 65th birthday plus the three months before and the three months after.

The longer answer is…complicated. It might make sense for you to delay enrolling in certain parts of Medicare beyond age 65 if you're covered by an employer's group health insurance plan. But it depends on the size of the employer.

If the employer providing your coverage (your employer or your spouse's) has 20 or more employees, you can delay signing up for Medicare, thus delaying the start of monthly Medicare premiums. Since your employer's plan likely already includes outpatient and drug benefits, you could choose to delay Parts B and D, which cover similar items.

If the employer has fewer than 20 employees, it's crucial that you sign up for Medicare during your initial enrollment period. A small employer's group plan is a "secondary payer" for Medicare-eligible participants, meaning that it covers only the portion of medical bills that the group plan covers but Medicare does not. If you don't sign up for Medicare, you

---

Danielle K. Roberts, founding partner of Boomer Benefits, a Fort Worth–based insurance agency specializing in Medicare-related coverage. She is a Medicare Supplement Accredited Advisor and author of *10 Costly Medicare Mistakes You Can't Afford to Make.* BoomerBenefits.com

could be stuck with out-of-pocket costs until the next general enrollment period.

Example: If a small employer's group plan covers $850 of a $1,000 medical expense while Medicare ordinarily covers $800 of that expense, the group plan may pay only $50 of the expense for a Medicare-eligible employee. If that employee hasn't enrolled in Medicare, the remaining $950 would have to be paid out of pocket.

Signing up for Medicare any later than the initial enrollment period could trigger higher premiums, too.

Example: The premiums for Part B, which covers outpatient medical services, are permanently increased by 10% for each 12-month delay in enrollment. Those higher premiums don't apply if you're covered by a large employer's group plan, however—as long as you sign up for Medicare during an eight-month "special enrollment period" that begins the month after your access to an employer and/or group plan ends.

More details worth noting…

•**It's usually worth enrolling in Medicare Part A,** which covers hospital expenses, at age 65 even if you are covered by a large employer group plan. Part A has no premiums for the majority of Medicare participants, so enrolling usually has little downside.

Exception: It could be worth postponing Part A if you are satisfied with the hospital coverage provided by your group plan and you wish to contribute to a Health Savings Account (HSA). Enrolling in any part of Medicare, including Part A, makes you ineligible to contribute to an HSA.

•**It's not always obvious whether a company has 20 or more employees.** You can't just count heads—part-time or seasonal employees could complicate the math. Ask your HR rep, "Is our group coverage primary or secondary to Medicare?"

•**Don't delay signing up for Medicare because you have retiree or COBRA coverage from a large employer.** Unlike "active employee" coverage from an employer, these coverage types are secondary to Medicare and don't trigger a special enrollment period when they end.

MISTAKE: **Misunderstanding the Medicare/Social Security connection.** These government programs are linked in some ways but unrelated in others, and this partial overlap can cause confusion.

One key connection: If you start receiving Social Security benefits prior to age 65, possibly because of early retirement or working part-time, you will be automatically enrolled in Medicare Parts A and B when you turn 65, and your Medicare premiums will be deducted from your Social Security checks or direct deposits. But just because you've been automatically enrolled doesn't mean that there aren't ways you can and should take charge of your Medicare enrollment decisions. *Three scenarios…*

SCENARIO #1: **You are receiving Social Security benefits when you turn 65 but have large-employer group coverage and don't wish to be enrolled in Medicare Part B.** Watch your mail for a Medicare welcome package, which should arrive about three months before your 65th birthday. You can delay your coverage by contacting the Social Security Administration (SSA) office as soon as possible.

SCENARIO #2: **The SSA automatically enrolls you in Medicare at age 65, and that is what you want.**

There's a catch: You will be automatically enrolled in only Medicare Parts A and B. It's still up to you to select and enroll in a Medicare Part D plan, which covers prescription medications, and to decide whether you wish to enroll in a Medicare Advantage plan rather than "Original" Medicare…or a Medigap plan in addition to Original Medicare.

SCENARIO #3: **You want to enroll in Medicare but don't want to start Social Security benefits yet.** You'll have to pay Medicare premiums out of pocket rather than have them deducted from your Social Security checks/direct deposits. Social Security will send you a quarterly or monthly invoice, or you may set up automatic payment from a bank account to ensure that you don't miss a

Medicare payment—a missed payment could get you disenrolled from Medicare…and if that happens, it might not be possible to rejoin until the middle of the following year.

MISTAKE: **Believing "free" Medicare Advantage Plans are truly free Medicare.** Medicare Advantage plans are alternatives to "original Medicare" offered by private companies. Marketing materials for these plans often emphasize that they charge no or very low monthly premiums…but frequently fail to clarify what that means exactly. While the Medicare Advantage plan itself might have $0 premiums, enrollees still are required to pay the Medicare Part B premium, which in 2022 was typically $170.10 per person per month. Some Medicare Advantage plans cover part or all of this Part B premium for enrollees, but many do not. So read the fine print carefully or work with a Medicare insurance broker who can walk you through the details of the plan.

Worse, people who sign up for these "free" Medicare Advantage plans sometimes fail to pay Medicare bills because they assume these bills no longer apply…and end up disenrolled from Medicare.

MISTAKE: **Signing up for the Part D plan that your spouse or friend has.** In most areas, there are so many Part D prescription drug plans available that many Medicare enrollees grow frustrated trying to choose among them and simply sign up for the plan that a spouse or friend uses…the plan that has the lowest premiums…or a plan offered by a company they trust. Unfortunately, those all are bad ways to pick a Part D plan.

In fact, there's really only one good way to select a Part D plan—use the plan-finder tool at MyMedicare.gov to identify the plans that offer the lowest out-of-pocket costs for the prescriptions you take regularly. That probably isn't going to be the plan your spouse has because your spouse almost certainly takes different prescription drugs than you.

Some people worry, *What if I start taking an expensive drug in the middle of the year?* If that happens, contact the plan provider and ask how you can submit a request for an exception—Part D plan providers often agree to

provide some coverage when otherwise uncovered drugs are prescribed midyear.

Revisit MyMedicare.gov each year during Medicare's annual October 15 through December 7 open-enrollment period to sort through the available Part D plans again—the best one for you could change frequently.

MISTAKE: **Paying an avoidable premium surcharge.** The Medicare Part B monthly premium is $170.10 in 2022…but not for everyone (2023 premiums will be announced in October 2022). If your Modified Adjusted Gross Income is over $91,000 (over $182,000 if married filing jointly), you'll also be charged an "Income Related Monthly Adjustment," which could push that premium up to as much as $578.30 per month…more than $1,100 per month for a married couple. Your Part D premiums would be increased as well, climbing by $12.40 to $77.90 per month. People who are hit with these higher rates usually assume that they have no choice but to pay up—but there sometimes is another option.

The SSA determines whether to charge you these inflated Medicare premiums based on your income from two years earlier. You can appeal the surcharge if your current income is lower than it was two years ago, though only if your income declined because of one of the SSA's approved "life changing events"—work stoppage…work reduction…marriage…divorce/annulment…death of a spouse…loss of pension income…employer settlement payment…or loss of income-producing property. If so, file Form SSA-44, *Medicare Income-Related Monthly Adjustment Amount—Life-Changing Event*…you could save hundreds of dollars per month in Medicare premiums.

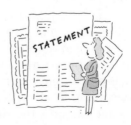

Which Medigap Plan Is Best for You?

Danielle K. Roberts, founding partner of Boomer Benefits, a Fort Worth–based insurance agency specializing in Medicare coverage. She is a Medicare Supplement Accredited Advisor and author of *10 Costly Medicare Mistakes You Can't Afford to Make.* Boomer Benefits.com

Choosing your Medigap plan isn't as daunting as it may seem. Only two of the 10 plans offered in 2022 (and most likely into 2023)—G and N—tend to be worth considering. This supplemental insurance covers many costs that Medicare recipients otherwise would have to pay out of pocket. They are sold by private insurers, but only a limited selection of standardized plans is offered. In most states, those plans are identified by a letter ranging from A to N.

The most popular Medigap plan has long been plan F, which covers all of original Medicare's copays, coinsurance and deductibles. Plan F was discontinued as of January 1, 2020, but remains open to anyone who was Medicare-eligible prior to that date.

What you need to know about Medigap plans (example premiums are for 2022)…

• **Plan F was popular for a reason, but now there's a reason to steer clear.** If you have original Medicare and Medigap plan F, you might never again face an unexpected out-of-pocket medical bill. But now that plan F is discontinued, its enrollees are likely to face large premiums. When the government discontinues a Medigap plan, its premiums tend to shoot up sharply over the years that follow. With no new young retirees allowed to join that plan, those insurers must increase premiums to remain profitable with the enrollees who remain…and if those enrollees have significant health problems, it might be difficult for them to switch Medigap plans. Insurers generally must accept anyone who applies for a Medigap plan during his/her initial six-month Medigap open-enrollment period, but in most states, insurers can reject people who apply after that period. Rejection is likely if the applicant has an expensive medical

condition. So it may be wiser to sign up for a Medigap plan that's nearly as comprehensive as F but not discontinued.

• **Plan G is the new plan F.** The difference is that G doesn't cover the Medicare Part B deductible—$233/year in 2022. It is better to pay that relatively modest deductible than risk higher plan F premiums. Recent plan G quotes included $119/month in Texas or $238 in Florida.*

• **Plan N might save you money depending on your doctors.** Plan N is a lot like plan G, but with lower premiums and a few modest out-of-pocket costs—up to a $20 copay for some office visits and a $50 copay for some ER visits. The other difference is that N doesn't cover part B "excess charges"—if a health-care provider bills more than the Medi-

*All premiums here are for a 65-year-old nonsmoking woman in Fort Worth, Texas, a low health-care cost area…and Miami-Dade, Florida, a high health-care cost area. Men, older applicants and smokers should expect higher premiums. Massachusetts, Minnesota and Wisconsin do not use the Medigap letter codes. If you live in one of these states, tell an insurance broker experienced with Medigap that you are looking for "G-like" or "N-like" coverage.

care-approved amount, plan G will pay the excess, but plan N won't. $88/month in Texas... or $181/month in Florida.

• **High-deductible plan G is a good low-cost option.** If you're looking for a Medigap plan that has low premiums, your best bet may be a "high-deductible" plan G, if it is available in your state. These provide the plan G coverage described above, but with an annual deductible—$2,490 in 2022. $42/month in Texas or $83/month in Florida.

How to Avoid These Affordable Care Act Traps

Maura Carley, MPH, CIC, CEO of Healthcare Navigation, LLC, a patient advocacy and consulting company based in Darien, Connecticut. She is host of Healthcare Navigation's health coverage video series, available on the company's website and YouTube, and previously held senior management positions with Yale New Haven Hospital, Stamford Hospital and Kaiser Permanente.

The Affordable Care Act (ACA) has survived several Supreme Court challenges and has lasted beyond its 12th birthday. Whether that was a happy birthday depends on who you ask. Also known as Obamacare, the ACA makes health insurance more affordable for Americans who lack access to employer health plans and Medicare...but enrollees who don't qualify for the system's subsidies can end up paying steep premiums for coverage with massive out-of-pocket costs—as high as $8,700 for an individual or $17,400 for a family. Insurance can be confusing, whether purchased through this program or from an insurer. *Traps to avoid with ACA health insurance...*

TRAP: Preventive care often is fully covered—but the line between preventive and diagnostic care can be unclear. Insurance sold through ACA marketplaces is required to completely cover the costs of a range of preventive care, such as colonoscopies and mammograms, as long as it is delivered by an in-network provider.

Catch: The same procedure that's covered as "preventive care" could result in treatment that is not preventive care...or the procedure itself might not be considered preventive if, for example, your doctor orders the procedure more frequently than is common because of a preexisting health issue.

Example: A mammogram prescribed more than once a year might be considered diagnostic for a woman who has had a previous diagnosis.

Caution: Some procedures are coded diagnostic rather than preventive simply because someone in the doctor's billing office entered the wrong billing code.

What to do: Before seeing your health-care provider for an exam or test, ask the doctor's office, "Is this a diagnostic procedure or 'well care'?" If the answer is diagnostic and you haven't yet met your plan's deductible, ask about costs. If the procedure is expensive, confirm with your doctor that it is medically necessary...and/or shop around to see if lower rates are available through a local lab or diagnostic center. Confirm that the facility is in-network for your insurance.

If you receive a bill for a procedure that you believed to be preventive, contact your provider's billing department to ask why it wasn't considered preventive and fully covered. If it turns out that the doctor's office simply entered the wrong code, ask for the code to be corrected and the bill to be resubmitted.

TRAP: Not just provider networks are shrinking—hospital networks can be narrow, too. You may know that many ACA plans have limited provider networks—many doctors are "out of network," which means that ACA insurance provides limited or perhaps no coverage for out-of-network services. What many enrollees don't realize is that many plans have narrow hospital networks—and often an area's best hospitals are excluded.

What to do: Before enrolling in any ACA plan, determine if your preferred hospital is in its network. Recheck this during every open-enrollment period.

Reminder: If you have a medical emergency, consider heading to the closest hospital even if it is out-of-network. In emergencies, ACA plans are required to cover out-of-network hospitals as if they were in-network… and under new rules beginning in 2023, an out-of-network hospital typically cannot bill a patient for excess charges if his/her insurance's in-network rates fail to cover the entire emergency care bill.

TRAP: **Your ACA coverage won't follow you if you move to a different state.** The ACA was federal legislation, but individual insurance plans are regulated by state insurance departments and are not portable across state lines—you will become ineligible for your current coverage if you relocate to a new state. That's true even if you relocate only a few miles across a state line and continue seeing the same doctors.

What to do: Visit Healthcare.gov—or your state's marketplace if you enrolled on its exchange—to report your move and sign up for new coverage in your new state. Moving to a new state will qualify you for a midyear special enrollment period.

TRAP: **Your plan might kick you out at year-end.** If you were satisfied with the ACA insurance that you had this year, you might opt to do nothing during the open-enrollment period and let your coverage automatically renew for the next year.

Problem: While taking no action usually results in automatic renewal, insurers occasionally disenroll customers at year-end. This often happens when an insurer isn't offering a similar plan in the coming year.

What to do: Visit Healthcare.gov or your state's marketplace during open enrollment to confirm your coverage for the upcoming year even if you don't plan to make changes. And always read correspondence from your insurance company.

TRAP: **ACA deductibles and out-of-pocket maximums are not prorated for partial years.** ACA out-of-pocket costs can be significant—many plans provide little coverage until you meet a deductible of perhaps $4,000 to $8,000. But as staggeringly steep as those costs might seem, it can get worse—in certain

situations, people must meet two health insurance deductibles in the same year.

If you change insurance plans mid-year—perhaps because you leave an employer, relocate or have another qualifying life event—your deductible will not roll over from one plan to the other…and your new plan's deductible will not be prorated.

What to do: If you or your spouse are leaving an employer and can sign up for COBRA, consider doing so through the end of the calendar year to avoid this partial-year problem. COBRA is a way to continue with your group coverage so that your deductible and out-of-pocket maximum won't reset.

TRAP: **Appointments with specialists might not be covered during the initial months with an ACA plan.** Many ACA plans cover appointments with specialists only if the patient was referred to that specialist by his/her primary care physician (PCP). Many ACA plans also have very narrow provider networks, which forces enrollees to select new PCPs when they join—the doctors they previously saw may not be in network. And PCPs generally won't refer patients to specialists without first examining those patients themselves.

What to do: If you change PCPs when you sign up for an ACA plan that requires referrals to see specialists, make an appointment with this new PCP as early in the coverage period as possible.

Long-Term-Care Insurance Can Pay for In-Home Care

Claude Thau, national brokerage director for USA-BGA, Rancho Santa Fe, California, which provides long-term-care–related support to financial advisers.

Many people would prefer to age at home rather than move into an assisted-living facility or nursing home. But for those who have or who are considering getting long-term-care insurance (LTCI) that raises a question—does this cover in-home care? The answer usually is yes, but there are exceptions. *What you need to know...*

• **Older group policies often don't cover in-home care.** Nearly all LTCI policies issued in this century cover in-home care—including the increasingly popular "linked benefit" life insurance policies that have an LTCI component. But policies issued earlier may have lower maximum benefits for in-home care or don't cover in-home care at all. That's especially likely if the policy was obtained through an employer's group plan.

• **The caregiver choice could determine whether care is covered.** Although most policies pay for a licensed nurse, some cover in-home care only if it is provided by a "licensed home care agency," not an individual caregiver. But if you live in a rural area or expect to retire to one, there might not be any qualifying agencies nearby. If so, look for language in the policy's small print that allows other in-home caregivers if there are no local home-care agencies.

• **Some policies pay loved ones to care for you.** If you see the term "indemnity" or "cash" in your policy's name or description or one of its provisions, it likely pays a fixed cash benefit that you can spend on any form of care—including "informal care" from a family member or friend.

• **Help with household chores could be covered—but the rules can be confusing.** An LTCI policy that covers in-home care likely covers "homemaker services" such as meal preparation and housecleaning—but with some policies, that's true only if these chores are "incidental," meaning that they're provided by a caregiver who also provides covered personal care during the same visit. Avoid potential missteps.

Example: Your caregiver arrives in the morning to help you bathe and dress...then visits a different client before returning to prepare your dinner. The cooking isn't covered.

• **In-home care could increase future nursing home costs.** LTCI policies typically have "elimination periods"—a certain number of days, often 90, during which care must be paid out of pocket before benefits begin. That period usually doesn't begin until paid services are obtained, so if you initially receive uncovered care from a spouse or adult child—not a paid caregiver—then later must move into a nursing home, you might have to pay for a full 90 days of expensive nursing home care out of pocket. Instead, arrange for at least one visit from a paid care provider as soon as you qualify for care under your policy, even if your loved ones initially will provide most of your care. Confirm with the insurer that this paid care is sufficient to start the clock.

Exception: Some policies have "service day" rather than "calendar day" elimination periods—the only days that count are when you receive paid long-term care, so arranging a day of paid in-home care won't help. If a future long-term stay in a nursing home seems likely, consider arranging for a few hours of in-home care on an ongoing basis.

Hybrid Life Insurance/ Long-Term-Care (LTC) Policies Are Gaining Popularity

Traditional LTC insurance is in decline because consumers fear rate increases and don't want to pour money into policies they might never need. Hybrid policies provide a death benefit to heirs if LTC benefits go unused and have guaranteed prices. Providers include Lincoln, Nationwide, OneAmerica, Pacific Life and Securian. If you don't need life insurance, ask your insurer about annuities that include LTC benefits.

Glenn Daily, CFP, ChFC, CLU, a fee-only insurance consultant and cofounder of the LTC policy evaluation service TellUsTheOdds.com.

Don't Miss Out on These Veteran's Benefits

Ryan Guina, a captain in the Illinois Air National Guard and founder of The Military Wallet, a website providing details about military benefits. TheMilitary Wallet.com

Military veterans might be missing out on valuable benefits. Some programs are chronically misunderstood, while others are brand new or have been modified.

•**Whole life insurance for disabled vets.** Life insurance has long been offered to disabled vets through Veterans' Group Life Insurance (VGLI).

But: Veterans had to enroll within 16 months of the end of their service. Starting January 1, 2023, that 16-month deadline has been eliminated, and any disabled vet younger than 81 can obtain a whole life policy with a payout of up to $40,000. VGLI coverage costs more than other insurance, but it is an option for vets whose health is too poor to qualify for coverage elsewhere.

•**Expanded VA Home Loan eligibility for National Guard and Reserve veterans.** VA home loans have been available to National Guard or Reserves veterans only if they had at least six years of service.

New rule: National Guard and Reserves vets must have only 90 days of full-time duty—including at least 30 consecutive days. VA home loans often require no down payment or private mortgage insurance. VA.gov/housing-assistance.

•**VA home loans may be used for rental properties and second homes.** Vets who inquire about VA home loans often are told that these mortgages are available for only primary residences…but there are workarounds.

Example: A VA home loan can be used to buy a rental property with as many as four units as long as the veteran moves into one of the units. And there's no requirement that the property remain the vet's primary residence for the life of the loan.

Information: VeteransUnited.com/valoans/occupancy-requirements-for-va-loans.

•**Property tax breaks.** These breaks often are poorly publicized. Enter "property tax," "veteran" and your state into a search engine.

•**Better burial benefits.** Many vets know they can be buried for free in a national veterans' cemetery…and that they can obtain a free headstone through the VA.

New rules: The names of spouses and/or dependent children can be engraved on VA-issued headstones at no cost, and all family members listed on the headstone can be buried in that grave.

Also: The VA covers the cost of transporting deceased vets' remains to state or tribal veterans' cemeteries as well as to national cemeteries. VA.gov/burials-memorials

•**GI Bill education benefits no longer expire for vets who served in or after 2013—** but only for vets whose service included any date on or after January 1, 2013. The 10- or 15-year expirations still apply for vets whose service ended before then. Benefits.va.gov/gibill

•**New ways to get vet discounts.** Vets now can obtain a Veterans ID card for free through the VA (VA.gov/records).

Also: Most states offer the option of having a veteran's designation included on their driver's licenses. Free online ID-verification services ID.me and SheerID.com are secure ways for vets to verify their service to online merchants.

Note: Vets may get useful guidance from benefits counselors at the Veterans of Foreign Wars (VFW.org)…American Legion (Legion.org)…AMVETS (AMVETS.org)…Disabled American Veterans (DAV.org)…and/or county or state government departments of veterans' affairs.

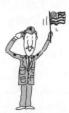

The Auto Insurance Claim Drivers Don't Know to File

J.D. Howard, executive director of the Insurance Consumer Advocate Network, an insurance consumer advocacy organization and diminished-value appraisal provider.

I f your car is in an accident, its resale value could plummet by as much as 35% even if the damage is expertly repaired—but there might be a way to recover that money.

If you were not at fault, you likely can obtain "diminished value" compensation from the at-fault driver's insurer—and in rare cases, you may be able to obtain this from your insurer even if you were at fault.

But you have to take action. The insurer will hope that you don't know to file the claim…or it will offer a fraction of the true diminished value and hope you don't know that you deserve more. *To receive diminished-value compensation…*

• **Check state laws.** In most states, you can make a diminished-value claim only if the other driver was at fault—but there are exceptions…

• You can make a claim even if you were at fault if the vehicle was insured in Georgia and/or the accident occurred in Georgia. You would make this claim under your own policy's collision coverage.

• If the other driver was at fault but uninsured or underinsured, your ability to make a claim depends on whether your policy's uninsured-motorist component covers diminished value.

• You cannot make a diminished-value claim if the accident occurred in Massachusetts or Michigan, regardless of who was at fault, though Michigan does have a comparable "mini-tort" rule that could allow you to recover up to $3,000 if the other driver was at fault.

These and other relevant state law details can be found at ICAN2000-dv.com (choose "Laws" from the "Diminished Value" menu, then select the state).

Helpful: You might be able to file a diminished-value claim even if the accident occurred several years ago and/or you have sold the ve-

hicle. The statute of limitations for claims is between three and five years, though it is one year if the accident was in Louisiana.

• **Put the insurer on notice.** When the at-fault driver's insurer contacts you about the accident, state, "I'm going to explore diminished value."

Warning: If you receive a check to cover diminished value from the insurer, do not sign or cash it until you've taken the steps below to confirm that the amount is reasonable. Some insurers send low-ball payments in hopes that these will be cashed, making it difficult for you to receive additional compensation.

• **Request a free estimate from a diminished-value appraiser.** Reputable appraisers include Collision Claim Associates (Collision Claims.com)…Wreck Check (WreckCheck.com) and my organization, the Insurance Consumer Advocate Network (ICAN2000-dv.com). If you work with a different appraiser, confirm that he/she has been doing diminished-value appraisals for at least five years and has a background as an insurance adjuster or in used-car sales.

Also: If you're asked the approximate pre-accident value of your vehicle, calculate this at NADA.com.

Homeowners Insurance Satisfaction

S cores for customer satisfaction of 10 top homeowners insurance companies, based on a 1,000-point scale: MetLife (904), Auto-Owners Insurance (900), Chubb (896), Nationwide (892), American Family (890), The Hartford (885), Farmers (884), Allstate (882), Liberty Mutual (881) and State Farm (880).

Note: Overall satisfaction with an insurance provider was 19 points higher among customers who used digital tools such as mobile apps to submit their claims…and they tended to receive their payments up to 5.5 days sooner.

Survey of 12,000 customers of homeowners insurance providers reported at JDPower.com.

Buy the Right Flood Insurance

Lisa Sharrard, founder of US Flood Solutions, LLC, a flood insurance consultancy based in Columbia, South Carolina. SimplyFlood.com

Standard homeowner's insurance policies almost never cover flood damage…and that gap can be catastrophic. It takes only a few inches of water to destroy drywall, flooring, furniture and appliances. *What you need to know…*

•**Waterfront homes aren't the only ones at risk.** When people picture flooded homes, they imagine coastal properties slammed by a hurricane storm surge or low-lying homes near major rivers. But the Federal Emergency Management Agency (FEMA) is updating its flood maps, and many seemingly safe properties are being rezoned into "special flood hazard areas" for reasons as innocuous as a nearby creek that might overflow during a rainstorm.

When FEMA estimates that a home has a 1% or higher annual risk of flooding, its owners may be required to obtain flood insurance, assuming that they have a mortgage backed by federal loan guarantees. That insurance could cost thousands of dollars per year, and the flood zone designation could hurt the home's resale value. You may be able to contest FEMA's flood zone designation. On FEMA.gov, select "Change Your Flood Zone Designation" from the Floods & Maps menu for details on how to do it yourself, or contact a surveying or consulting company.

Don't automatically decline flood insurance if your home isn't in a high-risk flood hazard area. About 25% of homes damaged by floods are not in FEMA-designated flood zones. Flood policies for homes in lower-risk areas tend to cost well under $1,000 a year.

•**FEMA's National Flood Insurance program isn't your only option.** Most US flood insurance is obtained through the National Flood Insurance Program (NFIP). This coverage can be purchased through many insurance companies, but its terms are determined by the federal program's rules and will be the same regardless of which insurer you choose.

That doesn't mean you can't shop around for flood insurance—in many areas, non-NFIP–flood coverage is available through the private market. Ask an insurance broker for quotes on NFIP and non-NFIP policies—but don't choose solely on premiums. *NFIP and non-NFIP flood coverage differ in important ways…*

•Long-term availability and pricing. If you choose a non-NFIP or private policy, the insurer can cancel your coverage or increase your rates at its discretion. An NFIP policy can't be cancelled by the provider as long as you pay your premiums…and if the covered property is your primary residence, your rates can't rise by more than 18% per year.

•Lender requirements. If your mortgage lender insists that you obtain flood insurance because FEMA says your home is in a special flood hazard area, that lender might not accept a non-NFIP policy.

• Coverage caps. NFIP coverage is capped at $250,000 for damage to the home and $100,000 for its contents. Non-NFIP policies often provide up to $1 million of coverage or more.

• Basements. Some non-NFIP policies provide extensive coverage for possessions in basements, while NFIP policies provide only very limited coverage there.

Insurance for COVID Travel Emergencies

Meghan Walch, travel insurance expert and product manager at InsureMyTrip.com.

Americans are traveling again. Yet COVID still is very much with us, which is why many people are buying trip insurance. *What you need to know…*

THREE TYPES OF COVERAGE…

• **Comprehensive travel insurance plan covers specific incidents,** such as "unforeseen illness, injury or death." It includes coverage for cancellation and interruption due to named perils as well as emergency medical and medical evacuation benefits. It also includes some travel-delay and baggage-loss/delay benefits. "Cancel For Any Reason" is an option available on some comprehensive plans.

Many plans also offer coverage to cancel your trip if your primary residence or destination is made uninhabitable by a natural disaster. These standard policies lay out specific types of incidents that can trigger a benefit. Read through the policies thoroughly before purchasing so you know what's covered.

For COVID: Most comprehensive policies cover you if you test positive right before your trip and a physician orders you not to travel. A policy also may cover hospitalization while you are abroad and medical evacuation. That means if the attending physician decides that you can't get the necessary care where you're hospitalized, you'll be moved to the nearest appropriate facility, which still could be outside the US. A comprehensive plan also will have travel-delay benefits that could help if you are ordered by a physician to quarantine during your trip. There's usually a per-day limit and a $1,000-to-$2,000 cap. Read the definition of "Quarantine" in your policy—self-quarantine and stay-at-home orders typically are not covered.

• **Cancel for any reason (CFAR).** If you want to be able to cancel because you get cold feet, you need to purchase this option on a comprehensive plan within 10 to 21 days of paying for travel arrangements, insure the full prepaid nonrefundable cost of your trip, and cancel no less than two days before departure. You likely will get back 50% to 75% of the insured prepaid nonrefundable costs.

• **Emergency evacuation memberships may transport you home if you are hospitalized with COVID while abroad.** You pay a membership fee for a single trip or for a full year. If you get sick and are hospitalized more than 100 or 150 miles from home, the evacuation company can arrange to get you stateside on a private medical transport or with a medical escort on a commercial airline.

Mix and match: The above coverage isn't mutually exclusive. You could get a comprehensive travel insurance policy…add cancel-for-any-reason protection…and buy an emergency-evacuation membership. If you had to cancel for a "named peril," you'd be covered for up to 100% of your cost (minus any cap differential). If you wanted to cancel for a reason other than a named peril, you'd recoup 50% to 75%. And if you got sick and are hospitalized, the evacuation membership can help to get you to a hospital at home.

Costs: Comprehensive policy prices vary with the cost of the trip and age of the travelers. The base price of a comprehensive plan could be from 5% to 10% of the trip cost. CFAR could add an additional 40% to 50%. Pricing on an emergency evacuation membership may vary based on whether it's for a single trip or annual travel and the ages and number of the travelers.

What's New in Pet Insurance

Doug Kenney, DVM, general practice veterinarian in Memphis, Tennessee, and founder of the blog "Your Pet Insurance Guide."

Pet adoption skyrocketed during the pandemic. *Result:* Veterinary hospitals are overwhelmed with animals in need of medical attention. And yet the vast majority of pets remain uninsured. That's because pet-insurance policies need to be improved. *Fortunately, insurers are taking baby steps in that direction...*

•**Adding coverage.** Consumers had been reluctant to purchase pet insurance because not enough medical conditions were covered. But today most insurers cover needed services, including wellness, and are offering plans with unlimited payouts. But that has had the unintended effect of driving up costs as more pets need care.

•**Smart restrictions.** Sometimes it's better when insurance covers something only partially.

Example: Medical diets for dogs. It's heartbreaking when a vet prescribes a special diet and the pet owner can't afford the more expensive food.

But: 100% coverage of medical diets makes insurance more expensive for everybody. A smart policy will cover, say, half the cost of a medical diet, putting the price in the same range as that of a normal diet.

Result: The animal gets fed...the owner pays roughly the same amount...and premiums don't spike.

•**Abandoning the reimbursement model.** Possibly the biggest disincentive to pet insurance is that almost all policies require owners to pay the veterinary hospital out of pocket and then file claims to be reimbursed. Most companies still use this reimbursement model, but one company—Trupanion—now provides 24/7 claim approval and direct payment to the hospital. When other companies start providing 24/7 preapproval of claims, those pet owners who can't afford to pay bills up front will be more likely to take out insurance.

11

Tax Talk

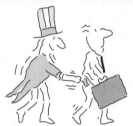

Taxpayer Victories and Defeats—How You Can Benefit from Them

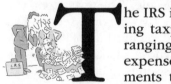The IRS is always challenging taxpayers on matters ranging from business expenses to legal settlements to unusual assets. Thousands of these disputes annually wind up in US Tax Court, an independent judicial authority created by Congress for taxpayers fighting IRS determinations. Whether the result is a taxpayer victory or defeat, court rulings often provide insight into matters that you may be dealing with and that could help reduce what you owe. *Notable cases from 2021...*

DEDUCTING BUSINESS EXPENSES

Ronald Berry and his family, including his son, Andrew, owned Phoenix Construction & Remodeling, Inc., a California real estate de-veloper and builder. The company purchased a 1968 Chevy Camaro racecar body, parts and engine for $121,903 so that Andrew could restore and race the car. Because the Camaro could be a way to advertise the family's business, Berry deducted the car's cost against the company's income.

IRS position: The racecar was a hobby for personal gratification, and the business was not entitled to a deduction. Consequently, Phoenix Construction under-reported its income on its tax returns.

Tax Court ruling: The IRS was correct. The $121,903 was not a legitimate business expense or eligible as a deduction. Section 162(a) of the US Tax Code gives business owners great leeway to deduct expenses paid or incurred in carrying on a trade or business

---

Edward Mendlowitz, CPA, ABV, PFS, partner at WithumSmith+Brown, PC, a national tax and advisory firm, East Brunswick, New Jersey. He is author of 29 books and has tried cases before the US Tax Court and testified before the Congressional House Ways and Means Committee.

as long as the expenses are "ordinary" (ones that commonly or frequently occur in the taxpayer's business) or "necessary" (appropriate and helpful in carrying on the taxpayer's business). But Berry failed to prove there was a proximate relationship between the Camaro expenses and the business operation. No logo or branding was visible in the photograph of the car presented at trial. Nor did Berry produce evidence that contacts at racing events had led to business for Phoenix. Also, the expenses for the car weren't reported as advertising on the company's tax returns but were "buried" among other construction expenses.

Lesson: Business owners often struggle to walk the tightrope between legitimate expenses and quasi-personal purchases. To claim a questionable expense as a deduction, be prepared to quantify to the IRS what value it added to your business…and maintain records to adequately substantiate the nature, amount and purpose of the expense.

Berry vs. Commissioner, TC Memo 2021-42

CASH FROM A SETTLEMENT

When Carol Holliday got divorced in Texas, she retained a lawyer and negotiated an agreement to divide her marital property and assets with her ex-husband. She later had misgivings and sued her lawyer for breaching his fiduciary duties by improperly influencing her to sign the agreement for $74,864 less than she should have gotten and failing to file an appeal for her. The divorce lawyer settled out of court with her for $175,000. After paying her malpractice attorney's fee, Holliday received a check for $101,500. She did not report it as income because she reasoned that property received in a divorce agreement is nontaxable, and the settlement money was compensation that she rightfully should have received from her divorce.

IRS Position: The malpractice settlement of $175,000 should have been reported on her income taxes as taxable income. The $73,500 fee for the malpractice attorney should have been listed as an itemized deduction.

Tax Court ruling: The IRS was correct. A deciding factor was that Holliday "did not allocate any of the settlement proceeds toward any particular claim or type of damages." In other words, her settlement said she was being compensated for legal malpractice. If the settlement said the money was for the return of nontaxable lost capital from her divorce agreement, it's likely that the $101,500 would have been excluded from taxes.

Lesson: Most legal settlements constitute taxable gross income. Even if they do not, the exact wording of the settlement is significant and can trigger taxation. Do not rely on your attorney for tax guidance or expertise before you sign off on a settlement. And consult a tax expert before initiating a lawsuit and before signing the settlement agreement.

Holliday vs. Commissioner, TC Memo 2021-69

WHAT ARE AN ESTATE'S ASSETS WORTH?

Pop singer Michael Jackson died in 2009, at age 50, leaving most of his estate to his mother and three children. On his estate's tax returns, Jackson's executors valued Jackson's image and likeness at $2,105 (a figure they later raised to $3 million). The executors reasoned that Jackson's reputation was in tatters after years of declining record sales, disastrous financial mismanagement, a lurid criminal court case and details about his drug use. When Jackson died, he hadn't made a new album or toured for years and had received almost no revenue related to his image in the previous decade. The executors valued Jackson's other two major assets at $2.2 million—his partial ownership of Sony/ATV Music Publishing whose catalog included the rights to 175 Beatles songs…and the Mijac music catalog which owned the rights to music that Jackson had written. The valuations for the music catalogs were very low, in part because Jackson had taken millions of dollars in loans against them to support his extravagant lifestyle.

IRS Position: The Jackson estate's value was grossly underestimated by nearly a half-billion dollars. At the peak of his career, Michael Jackson was one of the most famous people on Earth, with some of the most popular records ever released. And since his death, he had become one of the world's top-earning celebrities, with his estate taking in tens of millions of dollars annually. The IRS's own expert valued Jackson's image and likeness at $161.3 million and his catalog interests at $320.6 million.

Tax Court ruling: Michael Jackson's estate prevailed over the IRS on several key issues. The court found that the estate overall was worth $111.5 million, four times less than the IRS claimed. It found Jackson's name and likeness were worth $4.15 million, not the IRS figure of $161.3 million. The court noted that the IRS reached its valuations by including the potential revenue from future ventures. While many ventures came to fruition, unforeseeable events cannot be used to value an estate. Only the valuation at the time of death should be considered. In 2009, the Court noted, "Even a rational and undistressed hypothetical seller would have been hardpressed to avoid fire-sale prices."

Lesson: Estate-tax cases can come down to disputes by each party's experts over valuations. If you have high-profile or speculative assets in your estate—say, a piece of artwork, collectibles or a business—consider having valuations done regularly while you are alive to establish a viable track record in case the IRS challenges the item's value after you die. If you fear that a high valuation on an estate asset will saddle your heirs with a large estate-tax bill, strategize ways to lower your estate's value by gifting assets to your heirs and charities while you are still alive.

Estate of Michael Jackson vs. Commissioner, TC Memo 2021-48

When Medicare Premiums Are Tax Deductible

Medicare premiums may be tax-deductible if you are self-employed and make a profit from your business. You can deduct premiums on Schedule 1 of Form 1040 for parts A, B, D, Medigap and Medicare Advantage—the premiums are an above-the-line de-duction, so they reduce your adjusted gross income (AGI). You must be a sole proprietor, partner, LLC member or S corporation shareholder with at least 2% of company stock.

Alternative: You can deduct the premiums by itemizing on Schedule A, although this does not reduce your AGI. You can include Medicare costs in calculating your out-of-pocket medical expenses, which can be deductible to the extent that they exceed 7.5% of your AGI.

Caution: Medicare premium deductions apply to income taxes but do not affect self-employment taxes—which include taxes that fund Medicare. Ask your accountant for details.

MedicareResources.org

TAX SAVINGS...

Medical-Expense Deductions You Might Not Know About

For tax filers who itemize, out-of-pocket expenses that exceed 7.5% of adjusted gross income can be deducted. On the list of allowed deductions are some that many people don't realize they can take, including alternative treatments, such as acupuncture...adaptive equipment, such as wheelchairs, bath chairs and bedside commodes...diabetes costs, including blood strips, batteries and insulin...permanent home improvements to accommodate a disability, such as wheelchair ramps and bathroom handrails...lodging when traveling for medical treatment, up to $50 per night...personal-attendant costs for someone who cannot manage activities of daily living...rehab treatment for alcohol or drug addiction...the initial cost, veterinary bills, food and training expenses for service animals...the amount that exceeds the cost of regular foods for doctor-prescribed special diets...the cost of admission and transportation to a medical conference about a chronic condition from which the taxpayer, spouse or dependent suffers.

Investopedia.com

7 Costly IRA Withdrawal Mistakes to Avoid

Ed Slott, CPA, president of Ed Slott and Company, LLC, a financial consulting firm specializing in IRAs and retirement planning, Rockville Centre, New York. He is author of *The New Retirement Savings Time Bomb*. IRAHelp.com

Economic stimulus legislation enacted in 2020 offers a new opportunity for penalty-free IRA withdrawals—but taking advantage could be costly. And a 2019 law substantially altered IRA-withdrawal rules—but not for everyone, which seems certain to cause confusion.

A single mistake in withdrawing money can derail decades of contributions to an IRA. Taking money out at the wrong time or in the wrong way can trigger tax bills and penalties and also short-circuit future tax-deferred or tax-free investment growth. But IRA-withdrawal rules are complex, and recent changes are likely to complicate matters. Even if you thought you understood the new rules, it's worth reviewing the potential traps. *Seven costly IRA withdrawal mistakes to avoid…*

MISTAKE: **Taking advantage of penalty-free IRA withdrawals.** The Coronavirus Aid, Relief and Economic Security (CARES) Act included a provision allowing people to withdraw up to $100,000 from IRAs without the 10% early-withdrawal penalty that ordinarily applies when money is removed before age 59½. But this rule merely allowed you to raid your own retirement savings before retirement age. Doing so could cost you years of tax-deferred investment growth. (Extensions on this early-withdrawal penalty exclusion ended in 2021.)

This isn't the first time the government has created special opportunities to withdraw money early from IRAs without penalty—another recent rule allows up to $5,000 in penalty-free withdrawals when the account holder has or adopts a child, for example. Ignore all of these early-withdrawal opportunities unless you are desperate for cash and have no other options. Tax-advantaged retirement accounts are the very best long-term savings vehicles

available and should be the last assets preretirees tap when they need cash.

MISTAKE: **Assuming the recent change to required distribution rules applies to you.** Under the Setting Every Community Up for Retirement Enhancement (SECURE) Act, the age at which people must make "required minimum distributions" (RMDs) from retirement accounts has been pushed back from 70½ to 72. What some people don't understand is that this age-72 start year applies to you only if you were born on or after July 1, 1949. If you were born before that day, you still have to begin taking RMDs in the year you turn 70½. Adding to the confusion, no one was required to take RMDs for 2020 because of the pandemic. The penalties for misunderstanding this and missing a withdrawal deadline are steep—a staggering 50% of the amount you were supposed to withdraw.

MISTAKE: **Assuming that the new rules for withdrawing money from inherited IRAs apply to your inheritance.** Prior to the SECURE Act, heirs who inherited IRAs from anyone other than a spouse had the option of removing money from those IRAs slowly, by making annual withdrawals based on their life expectancy. With a few exceptions, the new rules do not require heirs to take annual withdrawals but do require that all of the money be withdrawn from the inherited IRA by the end of the 10th year following the year in which the original account holder died.

On the surface, the changes should help reduce withdrawal mistakes—there's no need to calculate life expectancies or annual withdrawal amounts. But in practice, this is likely to make withdrawal mistakes more common. For one, some heirs will no doubt fail to understand that the new rules don't apply to all inherited IRAs—if you inherited an IRA because of a death that occurred in 2019 or earlier, the old rules still apply. And when the 10-year rule does apply, heirs will have to remember to take the money out by a deadline that's a decade down the road. There are sure to be heirs who lose track of this crucial-but-distant deadline and incur massive penalties as a result. You could add a reminder to yourself in a calendar app or instruct a financial adviser to remind you, but that approach could fail if you're not using the same app or advisor in a decade. Another option is to use multiple reminders, including calendar apps, advisors and asking family members to use their calendar apps, to remind you to do so as well.

MISTAKE: **Failing to follow through after arranging annual early withdrawals from an IRA.** The tax code allows penalty-free withdrawals before age 59½ from an IRA if those withdrawals are made as part of a series of "substantially equal periodic payments." But the rules governing this exception are extremely complex, and if you make a single mistake, the IRS is very likely to spot it and impose harsh penalties. How harsh? To qualify for these penalty-free early withdrawals, you must make a series of withdrawals for at least five years or every year until you turn 59½, whichever is longer—and if you make a mistake with the size or timing of any of these withdrawals, the IRS will impose a retroactive 10% penalty on all the money you have removed from the IRA as part of this series. The rules and calculations required are tremendously challenging, so this is not something to attempt without the assistance of a tax pro.

MISTAKE: **Taking a so-called "60-day IRA loan."** There's actually no such thing as a loan from an IRA, but when you roll over money from one IRA to another, you have 60 days to redeposit it into the new account… so it is possible to give yourself short-term access to your IRA assets without penalty. Don't be tempted—people who attempt this often make missteps that devastate their retirement savings.

The most obvious error is failing to get the money into the new IRA before the 60-day window closes. But that's not the only way "IRA loans" can go horribly wrong. Some account holders misunderstand the rule that limits them to one IRA rollover per year—it's one per taxpayer, not one per IRA. Others fail to understand that the restriction is calculated on a rolling 12-month period, not a calendar year. In other words, you can't do this once in December, then do it again the following January. If you don't get the money into the new account in 60 days or misunderstand the rules and attempt a rollover that you were not allowed, the entire amount transferred will be treated as a withdrawal, potentially resulting in taxes, early-withdrawal penalties and/or the loss of an opportunity for additional tax-deferred or tax-free growth.

The best way to avoid getting rollover rules wrong is to opt for direct IRA-to-IRA rollovers rather than ever taking IRA money you intend to rollover into your possession.

Helpful: The one-per-year rollover rules above apply only to IRA-to-IRA or Roth-to-Roth rollovers, not to 401(k)-to-IRA rollovers or to IRA-to-Roth IRA conversions.

MISTAKE: **Rushing to roll over an IRA inherited from a spouse.** Unlike other beneficiaries, spouses are allowed to roll over inherited IRAs to their own IRAs. But they also are allowed to simply keep the inherited IRA—without the annual withdrawal requirements or 10-year withdrawal deadline faced by other IRA heirs. For widows and widowers who have not yet reached age 59½, initially keeping the money in the deceased spouse's IRA can be the smart move. If the surviving spouse must tap this money before 59½, he/she can do so without penalty—early-withdrawal penalties do not apply to inherited IRAs, but they do when a spouse rolls the IRA into his own IRA. When these widows and widowers reach 59½—or determine that they won't have to tap the account before 59½—they then can roll the money into IRAs in their own names.

MISTAKE: **Assuming an inherited Roth IRA doesn't have RMDs.** Roth IRAs usually do not have RMDs, but there's an exception—if a Roth is inherited by anyone other than the spouse, RMD rules apply just as they do with inherited traditional IRAs. That means if the original owner of the Roth died in or after 2020, the new 10-year deadline applies…or if the death occurred before 2020, the old annual withdrawal rules apply.

You Can Make After-Tax Contributions to Traditional IRAs

Most money put into traditional IRAs is pretax, which is why distributions are fully taxable. But nondeductible contributions also are allowed. There is no adjusted gross income limit on them, and the nondeductible contributed amount cannot be greater than the IRA owner's or spouse's compensation income. Use IRS Form 8606 to report after-tax contributions to traditional IRAs for each year of contribution. The form shows total after-tax dollars contributed since the first such contribution was made.

Important: Be sure to keep the most recent Form 8606, as it is the only record of after-tax contributions. When you take distributions from your IRA, you will need to pay tax on only the earnings for these contributions, not on the basis. It is best to work with a financial or tax adviser.

RetirementWatch.com

Tax-Smart Places to Stash Assets

Larry Swedroe, chief research officer, Buckingham Strategic Wealth, which oversees more than $21 billion in assets, St. Louis. BuckinghamStrategicWealth.com

In the 1990s, tech mogul Peter Thiel invested $2,000 from his Roth IRA in PayPal. Today, his IRA is worth a reported $5 billion—but Thiel won't owe the IRS anything because qualified distributions from a Roth are tax-free. *While tax considerations shouldn't dictate your investment strategy, they do play a role in determining which assets are best held in which accounts...*

• **Taxable accounts.** Retirement savers should max out tax-deferred accounts first because that is the best way to build wealth over long periods. But taxable accounts, such as brokerage accounts, offer the ability to access money penalty-free and harvest capital-gains losses by selling an investment that has fallen in value.

Best for: Volatile stocks and cryptocurrency...tax-efficient funds and ETFs...annuities and municipal bonds, both of which already are tax-favored investments.

• **Traditional 401(k)s and IRAs.** Stash your least tax-efficient investments here, especially those generating interest, income and capital gains, since it can be reinvested and grow tax-deferred.

Best for: Actively managed stock funds with high turnover...dividend stocks/funds/ETFs... REITs...individual bonds/funds/ETFs...CDs and TIPS.

• **Roth 401(k)s and IRAs.** Favor tax-inefficient assets with the relatively highest expected long-term returns and assets that you plan not to touch for as long as possible. Qualified distributions are tax-free, and you don't have to take required minimum distributions (RMDs). Money taken out of a Roth by your heirs is tax-free, and they have 10 years to empty the account after you die.

GOOD TO KNOW...

Another Way Your IRA Can Lower Your Taxes

Contributions made to a traditional IRA can be deducted from income when you file. But not everyone knows about the Saver's Credit, which can be worth 10% to 50% of your contribution, depending on your income.

2022 thresholds for claiming the credit: Adjusted gross income of $68,000 or less for married couples filing jointly...$51,000 for head of household...and $34,000 for any other tax-filing status.

Roth IRAs: While Roth IRA contributions aren't deductible, you still can claim the Saver's Credit if your income makes you eligible.

MoneyTalksNews.com

Best for: High-yield bonds...tech, small-cap and emerging-market stocks, funds and ETFs.

When Filing Taxes, Don't Forget Gambling Winnings

Gambling winnings must be reported separately on Form 1040, Schedule 1, as "other income." The rules are complex. You will receive from the casino an IRS Form W-2G for wins of $600 or more and a payout at least 300 times the wager. For wins of more than $5,000 and a payout at least 300 times the wager, 24% generally is withheld for taxes. Bingo, slot machines, keno and poker each have their own thresholds. Gambling losses up to the amount of winnings can be deducted but only by professional gamblers reporting business expenses on Schedule C or filers who itemize.

Reminder: You also may owe state and local taxes.

Kiplinger.com

Forgiven Student Loans Are Not Taxable

Cancelled student-loan debt is not taxable for loans forgiven as a result of the American Rescue Plan Act (ARPA) passed in March 2021. Borrowers should not put down as income on their tax returns the forgiven amounts of loans discharged from 2021 through 2025. That includes forgiveness of loans for post-secondary educational expenses made, insured or guaranteed by the US, the states or an eligible educational institution. Some forgiven loans made by educational organizations and private lenders also are not taxable.

JournalOfAccountancy.com

Investing Through "Mobile App Brokers" Could Increase Your Taxes

Stock-trading apps such as Robinhood, Webull and Public make it difficult or impossible to specify which shares of a given stock you wish to sell when you sell only a portion of your holdings. Thus you might be unable to minimize capital gains taxes by selling your least-appreciated shares...or offset other profits by selling shares that have declined.

Better: Buy shares through Schwab or Fidelity, which offer specificity and commission-free trades.

Kevin Kleinman, a financial advisor with Blue Haven Capital, Geneva, Illinois. BlueHavenCapital.com

Annuity That Works Like a CD

A multiyear guaranteed annuity (MYGA) provides a fixed interest rate—determined when you buy it—and guaranteed protection of principal. Unlike CD interest, which is taxed every year, interest on a MYGA is not taxed until the funds are withdrawn. Until then, the money grows tax-deferred. A MYGA may allow regular withdrawals of interest during the annuity term—but if it does and you take the interest out, it becomes taxable in the year you receive it. (You also may owe an early withdrawal penalty.) Ask your tax adviser for details.

Money.USNews.com

Alternative Ways with a Roth IRA

Contribute to a Roth IRA if you don't have a conventional job. Roth IRA contributions must be made from "earned income." In most cases, if you pay taxes on any type of income from working, you can make Roth IRA contributions. But earned income doesn't have to come from a conventional job.

Stock options—if you exercise nonqualified options, the difference between the grant price and exercise price is treated as taxable compensation on which you can base a Roth IRA contribution. *Taxable scholarship or fellowship*—stipends or payments for room and board, teaching or research usually are taxable, and the income can be used for Roth IRA contributions. *Spousal income*—if your spouse earns Roth-eligible income but you do not, you can set up your own Roth IRA and use money from your spouse's income to fund it.

Caution: Rules are complex, including income limits for Roth eligibility. It's best to consult a tax adviser.

Investopedia.com

Careful Where You Store Your Precious Metal Assets

Storing IRA assets as gold or silver coins at home is illegal. Contrary to what you may hear in Internet and radio ads, buying gold and silver using IRA assets and then storing them at home or in a safe-deposit box is not legal. It is legal to invest IRA funds in gold and silver coins, but the law does not allow "unfettered access" to these assets. Instead, they must reside in the custody of a third-party fiduciary.

Ed Slott, CPA, president of Ed Slott and Company, LLC, Rockville Centre, New York. IRAHelp.com

12

Retirement Report

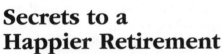

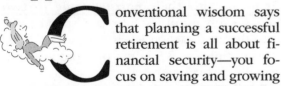

Secrets to a Happier Retirement

Conventional wisdom says that planning a successful retirement is all about financial security—you focus on saving and growing a nest egg and creating a financial plan so that you never have to worry about running out of money in old age.

But financial advisor Wes Moss, CFP, noticed a paradox—many wealthy retirees did not seem significantly happier than retirees who had just a few hundred thousand dollars.

His conclusion: Big retirement accounts let people sleep well—but may not give them enough reason to get up in the morning.

Moss wanted to see if he could reverse engineer what makes for a great retirement, so he launched multiple studies of more than 2,000 older folks to find out what happy retirees were doing right.

Among his surprising findings: Having more money in retirement makes you happier up to a point, then plateaus. Having hobbies to fill up your time isn't enough—you need activities that you are passionate about. You want to live close to your kids—but not too close. And having a busy social life isn't as important as having a few meaningful friendships.

The desire for a realistic vision of retirement has been stoked by the pandemic. Many people working remotely got a trial run at what staying home every day looks and feels like. We asked Moss to highlight the data from his study and explain how to use it to plan a richer, fuller life once your working days are over.

WHAT HAPPY RETIREES KNOW

In my "Retirement Happiness" study, participants answered dozens of questions about their lives and rated their overall satisfaction

Wes Moss, CFP, managing partner and chief investment strategist at Capital Investment Advisors, Atlanta, which oversees more than $3 billion in assets. He is author of *What the Happiest Retirees Know.* WesMoss.com

on a scale of one to five (five being the best). I divided the respondents into two groups—happy retirees and unhappy retirees—and looked for meaningful patterns in the data.

Social data…

•**Happy retirees had an average of 3.6 "core pursuits"…unhappy retirees, fewer than two.** A core pursuit is an activity that brings you an ongoing sense of excitement and fulfillment. The top four core pursuits among the participants were travel…activities with kids and grandkids…playing tennis or golf…and, by far number one, volunteering.

For interesting ideas about where to volunteer: Contact AmeriCorps Seniors (Americorps.gov/serve/americorps-seniors), a federal program with more than 200,000 members that engages volunteers ages 55 and older to serve their communities.

•**Happy retirees maintained at least three close connections beyond their spouses.** The study defined "close" as people you would confide in about good or bad news. Unhappy retirees averaged just 2.6 close connections.

Also: Retirees who took at least one trip a year with a close connection were twice as likely to be happy as the average retiree. And the more close connections retirees had, the greater their levels of satisfaction.

•**Retirees who visited or attended one large "social epicenter" a week were twice as likely to report being happy over the average retiree.** Social epicenters include places of worship, an exercise or golf group, senior centers and/or a charitable or neighborhood group.

Relationship data…

•**Happy retirees stayed married.** Those who were not married were 4.5 times more likely to be unhappy than the average retiree. Being single in retirement didn't doom retirees to unhappiness, but those who were single needed to be very intentional about their support networks and realistic about making lifestyle changes to match their expected income.

•**Happy retirees had sex at least once a month.** If you had sex at least once a week, you were twice as likely as the average retiree

to report being happy. Less than once a month, you were twice as likely to be unhappy.

Personal financial data…

•**Retirees who had paid off their mortgage—or who were within five years of paying it off—were four times more likely to report being happy.** While there can be solid tax and investment advantages to keeping a home mortgage, my study found that older folks got a sense of security from owning their homes debt-free. I typically recommend to my retiring clients the one-third rule—pay off a mortgage only if they can use no more than one-third of their nonretirement savings.

•**Happy retirees had at least $500,000 in liquid net worth.** This included easily accessible investments such as stocks and bonds but not their home and illiquid possessions. Millionaire retirees did report higher happiness levels than others overall. But a half-million dollars was the trigger point for diminishing returns. Happiness levels increased dramatically for retirees who had $500,000 in retirement savings compared with those who had $100,000. But retirees who had more than $500,000 in retirement savings reported far less of a happiness boost.

•**Happy retirees talked about personal finances with their partners one to two hours each month.** Once you spend more than that, satisfaction levels plateau. And discussing finances 3.5 hours or more a month actually was counterproductive.

Family data…

•**Retirees whose adult children were financially dependent on them were 1.5 times less likely to be happy as the average retiree.** The unhappiest retirees often had adult children still living in their homes.

Also: More than 40% of respondents still provided their adult children with some financial support, but happy retirees gave their adult children an average of less than $500 a month…unhappy ones, more than $700.

•**Retirees who live close to at least half of their adult children were five times more likely to report being happy than the average retiree.**

HOW TO IMPROVE
YOUR OWN RETIREMENT

While every retiree's circumstances are different, by emulating and incorporating some of what we learned above, you can reduce the traumatic adjustment that you might experience when you retire. *To implement these ideas...*

● **Write up a nonfinancial plan.** The unhappiest retirees had vague and superficial notions of what retirement would look like, which often led to isolation and boredom.

Better: Set social and lifestyle goals for yourself. The list doesn't have to be comprehensive, but you need to plan enough to create a vision and structure for how you will spend your weeks. This is especially important for men who retire and don't maintain the social support system of their "work families."

● **Practice a faux retirement.** Consider taking an extended vacation without leaving home to experiment with retirement routines and test out what feels meaningful. What you think you need when you stop working may have to be redefined or rethought.

● **Don't count on your to-do lists and bucket list to keep you occupied.** Many people expect to fill up their days with time-intensive tasks and activities that they had been putting off for years, ranging from taking vacations to renovating the kitchen to organizing all the photos on their computers.

Reality: You will get through those lists quickly and need to find ongoing ways to stay busy and maintain a sense of purpose.

● **Get on the same page as your spouse.** Start small. Talk about what your first month of retirement will look like. Be sure to address how your financial situation supports and affects your lifestyle.

Example: If the stock market takes a beating and your finances are tight, what cutbacks are you prepared to make? How long would each of you like to stay in your current home, and what alternatives would you consider?

Don't Let These 5 Surprises Derail Your Retirement

Bob Carlson, editor of the monthly newsletter *Bob Carlson's Retirement Watch*. He is a managing member of Carlson Wealth Advisors and chairman of the board of trustees of the Fairfax County (Virginia) Employees' Retirement System. RetirementWatch.com

My daily expenses will fall when I retire. I'll reap a windfall by downsizing to a smaller home. Medicare will cover all my medical bills. These assumptions play a central role in many retirement plans—but they're often wrong. *Here's a look at five retirement financial surprises that can derail your retirement plans...*

SURPRISE: **Daily expenses often go up in retirement.** Conventional wisdom holds that day-to-day spending drops to 70% to 80% of its prior level when people retire. But many retirees discover that their daily budget increases, particularly during the early retirement years because they have time to do things they've always dreamed of doing. A 2017 study by the Investment Company Institute found that more than half of taxpayers saw spending rise during the first three years after they initially claimed Social Security.

Whether your daily spending goes up or down generally boils down to how you fill those hours that you used to spend working. If you mostly stay home working in your garden or volunteering, your expenses likely will fall. But if you try to fulfill your travel dreams, eat out more often and/or splurge on entertainment, they're likely to rise.

What to do: Be realistic about what you enjoy doing on your free days—are you happy at home or usually out and about? And what are your average day-off expenses when you do go out? Use this info to construct a realistic estimate of daily retirement expenses. If the estimate is more than you can afford, search for low-cost alternatives.

Examples: You might want to combine a movie night out with a special dinner at home that costs far less than a restaurant meal. And a day spent in a park—strolling, reading and picnicking—may be just as enjoyable as a day at a pricey inn or fancy spa.

SURPRISE: Medicare leaves retirees with hefty out-of-pocket costs. If you ask someone who isn't yet retired about Medicare, he/she usually will say that it covers health-care costs for people age 65 and up. But people already on Medicare know the truth—Medicare covers only a portion of health-care costs. Its coverage gaps, deductibles and premiums leave the typical Medicare recipient with more than $5,500 in health-care costs each year.

What to do: Sign up for a Medigap plan when you enroll in original Medicare…or sign up for a Medicare Advantage plan instead of original Medicare. Medicare Advantage plans, offered by private companies, provide an alternative to original Medicare that usually has lower out-of-pocket costs as long as you stay within the plan's provider network. The average premium for Medicare Advantage enrollees was about $20 in 2022 but varies from state to state. But if you don't want to be constrained by a limited provider network, Medigap could be a better option. The plans, which are sold by private companies, supplement original Medicare, covering some health-care costs that otherwise would not be covered. Medigap requires payment of an additional monthly premium, but it's easier to build these predictable recurring premiums into a budget than cope with unexpected out-of-pocket medical bills.

Note: Retiring prior to age 65, the usual age of Medicare eligibility, can trigger an even greater health-care cost surprise. People often don't realize how expensive it is to buy health insurance on the open market—and how limited this coverage can be. Before retiring, ask your employer's benefits department whether you would be eligible to pay to remain on the employer's health insurance for up to 18 months after retiring through COBRA, and if so, how much this would cost. As of 2022, the average cost was more than $7,000 for an individual, perhaps twice that for a couple and more than $20,000 for a family. Also investigate obtaining health insurance through the Affordable Care Act exchanges.

SURPRISE: Your tax bill might rise in retirement. You're no longer earning wages, so your taxes are certain to fall, right? Not necessarily. Money withdrawn from tax-deferred accounts such as traditional IRAs and 401(k)s is taxed as ordinary income. You'll probably have to pay income taxes on your Social Security benefits, too—if your income is $25,000 or more ($32,000 or more if married and filing jointly), up to half of your benefits will be taxed. If it's above $34,000 ($44,000 married filing jointly), up to 85% of your income will be taxed. And once you're fully retired and no longer receiving earned income, you'll no longer be able to lower your tax bill by making contributions to a tax-deferred IRA or 401(k). Add all this up, and your tax bill might not be going down.

What to do: Each year during retirement, try to get a sense of whether your tax bracket will be higher or lower than usual that year. Has the government raised or lowered tax rates? Have your investments risen or fallen in value, causing capital gains or losses? High-bracket years are a good time to make tax-free withdrawals from Roth IRAs or Roth 401(k)s. Low-bracket years are the time to make withdrawals from tax-deferred accounts. Make these withdrawals before the calendar year ends, not as tax-filing day approaches. Roth withdrawals apply to the year in which they are made.

SURPRISE: Downsizing doesn't always generate a financial windfall. Selling one property and buying another is pricier than most people realize—real estate agent commissions, mortgage closing costs, mover's fees and other expenses related to these transactions can consume as much as 10% of the value of the home being sold.

What's more, when people downsize, they often move into properties that are smaller but in more desirable areas. A one-bedroom condo might not cost much less than a three-bedroom house if the house was in a standard suburb but the condo is near the beach or in a vibrant city. Desirable condos often come with steep condo fees, too—sometimes $500 to $1,000 per month.

What to do: Be clear about the reason you are downsizing before you begin shopping for a new home. If "adding to my retirement savings" is at or near the top of your priorities, set your housing budget accordingly. Otherwise it's easy to fall in love with a small-but-pricey residence that undermines the reason you were downsizing in the first place.

SURPRISE: "Gray divorce" is on the rise, so the nest egg might have to fund two nests. The divorce rate among Americans over age 50 has more than doubled since 1990, to around one couple in every 100 per year, even as the overall divorce rate has declined. The cost of divorcing during retirement, including hefty lawyer fees, takes a greater financial toll than splitting earlier. Once someone is retired, it's too late to increase savings to make up for the setback. One 2019 study found that divorcing after age 50 reduces women's subsequent standard of living by 45%…men's by 21%.

What to do: Be honest about the health of your relationship and don't let problems fester. If you divorce during retirement, or appear to be heading toward divorce, immediately reassess your spending—you might have to make significant cuts.

Have Some Fun with Your Portfolio

Allan S. Roth, CFP, CPA, president of Wealth Logic, LLC, a financial advisory firm in Colorado Springs overseeing more than $1 billion in assets. He is author of *How a Second Grader Beats Wall Street.* DareToBeDull.com

Saving for retirement requires careful planning, but that doesn't mean you can't have a little fun along the way. When I started saving for retirement, I dutifully stashed my money in boring, well-diversified Vanguard index funds. It made sense to me as a financial advisor because data showed that by matching the performance of the broad stock market year after year, I could beat nearly 90% of actively managed mutual funds over long periods. Still, it was psychologically hard to accept "average" market returns when picking the right investment could mean far higher returns and early retirement. So I took a tiny portion of my portfolio—called it my "gambling money"—and over the years, I bet on a few dozen of the most volatile and risky long shots. I scored the occasional jackpot, such as a 5,000% gain in my shares of Booking Holdings (formerly known as The Priceline Group). I also picked numerous duds ranging from Eastman Kodak and United Airlines and even a public utility—all went bankrupt. But it's not really about gains and losses. The real benefit of my gambling portfolio is that it satisfied the piece of my brain that wanted to have fun, providing an outlet for my greed and fears of missing out, and allowing me the discipline and wisdom to be, well, boring in the rest of my investment life. *To create your gambling portfolio…*

1. Tap only a tiny portion of retirement assets—5% or less. Keep it in a separate brokerage account.

2. Use any personal investing strategy you want to choose what you invest in—as long as it's fun. Profits can be reinvested or withdrawn, but you never add new money.

3. Maintain an honest and accurate tab of your winners and losers. That way, you won't mistake success for actual genius.

Avoid These Social Security Traps

Martha Shedden, CRPC, RSSA, president of the National Association of Registered Social Security Analysts and founder of Shedden Social Security & Retirement Planning, Capitola, California. She is host of the podcast *Social Security: Answers from the Experts with Martha Shedden.* SheddenSocialSecurity.com

How wise are your Social Security decisions? Social Security benefits account for approximately one of every three dollars received by US retirees, yet many Americans remain unclear about its nuances and unaware of the degree to which their claiming decisions affect the amounts they receive. Most simply start their benefits as soon as they become eligible at age 62...or at a traditional full retirement age between 66 and 67.

But: A 2019 study by investment firm Capital One found that only 4% of retirees make financially optimal decisions about when to claim their Social Security benefits. The other 96% cost themselves an average of $111,000 per household.

Here's what you need to know about the benefits available to you and how to decide when to claim them...

• **Waiting to start taking benefits usually is the smart strategy.** You probably already know that you can start your Social Security benefits as early as age 62 or as late as age 70—or even later, though there's no financial upside to waiting past 70. And you probably understand the basic trade-off involved in that decision—the earlier you start these monthly benefits, the more benefit payments you receive...but the later you start them, the larger each payment will be.

Example: A retiree might receive a $1,050 monthly benefit if he/she starts receiving benefits at age 62...or $1,860 if he waits to age 70. (The amounts you personally receive will vary based on factors including your earnings history and year of birth.)

Problem: There's no way to know for certain whether claiming early, late or somewhere in between will result in the largest total Social Security benefits for you because there's no way to know how long you're going to live. People who live long lives come out way ahead if they claim later...but those who die before approximately age 81 would have been better off claiming sooner. Most retirees will receive more from the Social Security system if they wait until they approach or reach 70 to claim. There are several reasons for this, among them that lifespans are increasing. The rules for how much extra retirees receive if they wait to claim haven't been updated since 1983, when the expectation was that the typical 65-year-old would live an additional 17 years—but today, the average 65-year-old has more than 20 years of life remaining.

Waiting until 70 to claim has other advantages as well. It serves as a sort of longevity insurance—your Social Security benefits are guaranteed to continue as long as you're alive, so maximizing the amount you receive each month reduces the odds that you won't have enough to pay your bills late in a long retirement. It provides a measure of inflation insurance—Social Security benefits include an annual cost-of-living adjustment.

Waiting until age 70 also can have tax advantages if you remain in the workforce well into your 60s—Social Security benefits are partially subject to income taxes above certain income thresholds, so not claiming until you're retired reduces the odds that you'll have to pay a significant share of your benefits to the IRS.

Exceptions: Claiming before age 70 could make sense if you desperately need the money...or if you have serious health problems or a family history that suggests a long retirement isn't likely. It also can make sense for a widow/widower or one partner in a married couple to claim before 70—more on these possibilities below.

• **Married people who earned significantly less than their partners usually should claim years before they reach 70.** The ideal claiming ages for these spouses often is their full retirement age, which is between 66 and 67 depending on year of birth. Married people typically are eligible to receive the larger of their own monthly retirement Social Security benefit or a "spousal benefit" equal to as much as 50% of the spouse's "primary insurance amount" (PIA)—that's the monthly benefit the spouse would receive at his/her full retirement age. If that spousal benefit is the larger of the two, there's no advantage to delay claiming beyond full retirement age—but your retirement benefit, based on your own earnings history, will continue to grow larger for each month you wait to claim from age 62 until 70. Your spousal benefit increases for each month you wait from 62 only until your full retirement age. Some couples overlook this detail and miss out on years of benefits.

One twist: You cannot claim spousal benefits until your spouse also begins collecting his/her own retirement benefit. If your spouse has not yet claimed when you reach your full retirement age, you could initially claim your own benefit, then switch to spousal benefits when your spouse eventually does claim his/her retirement benefits.

Warning: A married couple's claiming decisions can get especially complex. It could be worth asking a Social Security analyst or financial planner to crunch the numbers and work out the claiming dates that make most sense for you and your partner.

•**Widows and widowers often can claim their late spouse's benefits.** If your spouse dies and had been receiving benefits, you likely will be entitled to a "survivor benefit" equal to the amount that your late spouse had been getting from Social Security. If your late spouse died before starting his/her benefits, your survivor benefit will be calculated on factors including the late spouse's earnings record and age at death. Unfortunately, survivor benefits often go unclaimed, especially when the spouse who handled the couple's financial affairs dies first.

Widows and widowers can claim survivor benefits as early as age 60—or age 50 if legally disabled—but claiming before full retirement age reduces the amount received each month.

But: There is no upside to waiting until age 70 to claim survivor benefits—like spousal benefits, these benefits do not continue to increase after the widow/widower reaches full retirement age. People who are widowed before they reach full retirement age often can maximize their total Social Security benefits by either starting their own benefit as early as age 62, then switching to the survivor benefit upon reaching full retirement age...or starting their survivor benefit as early as age 60, then switching to their own benefit at 70.

Worth noting about survivor benefits: Widows/widowers are likely to be entitled to survivor benefits as long as the marriage lasted at least nine months before the late spouse's death.

But: They cannot receive survivor benefits if they currently are remarried unless the remarriage occurred after the surviving spouse's 60th birthday. And they cannot receive both a survivor benefit and their own retirement benefit at the same time—as with spousal benefits, when entitled to multiple benefits, they receive only the larger amount of the two. Survivor benefits could be available even if the late spouse died young, before establishing the extensive earnings history usually required for Social Security benefits.

•**If you're divorced, you might be able to claim benefits based on your ex's earnings.** These benefits are similar to the spousal benefits available to married people—but they're more likely to be overlooked because they could be based on the earnings history of someone you haven't been with in decades. To qualify, the marriage must have lasted at least 10 consecutive years and you must not currently be remarried. You can claim these benefits even if your former spouse has not yet begun receiving his/her own benefits, as long as it has been at least two years since the divorce was finalized.

When your ex dies, you also could be entitled to a survivor benefit based on his/her earnings—again, only if the marriage lasted at least 10 consecutive years.

But: You are not entitled to survivor benefits based on your late ex's earnings if you currently are remarried.

As with other survivor benefits, you can claim as early as age 60—50 if disabled—but the monthly amount you receive will be reduced if you claim before full retirement age. And as with other survivor benefits, there's no reason to delay claiming until after your full retirement age. Claiming benefits based on an ex's earnings has no effect on the benefits received by that ex or his/her new spouse. There's no need to communicate with your ex to claim these benefits.

•**Do-overs are allowed...sometimes.** If you've already started your benefits, you're not necessarily stuck with that decision. *Two options that might be open to you...*

•If less than 12 months have passed since your benefits began, you can "withdraw your Social Security application." You'll be required to repay the benefits that you've received, but once you do that, it will be as if you never claimed at all.

Warning: You can do this only once in your life.

• If you've reached your full retirement age, you can "suspend" your benefits. There's no 12-month time limit with suspending and no need to repay benefits already received. Once you do this, your future monthly benefit will increase by two-thirds of 1% for each month the suspension remains in force up to age 70—that's 8% per year.

These benefit-claiming do-overs are particularly useful at the moment—lots of people claimed Social Security benefits when they lost their jobs during the pandemic but are considering re-entering the workforce now that the labor market is booming.

Self-Employed? Consider a Solo 401(k)

Barbara Weltman, Esq., president, Big Ideas for Small Business, Inc., Vero Beach, Florida. BigIdeas ForSmallBusiness.com

You qualify for a solo 401(k) retirement plan if you are a business owner with no employees. Unlike typical 401(k) plans with employers, you can set up a solo 401(k) at whatever brokerage firm you prefer and invest as you wish. However, since you don't get a salary, your contributions are "effectively" limited to 20% of net earnings from self-employment (up to $20,500 in 2022) plus 20% of your business profits (up to $61,000 in 2022). If you are 50 or older, you can make a catch-up contribution of $6,500, for a total 2022 maximum of $67,500. A solo 401(k) can be set up either to take tax-deductible contributions, like a traditional IRA...or after-tax contributions, like a Roth IRA (within limits). Talk to your tax adviser about whether a solo 401(k) is best for you, compared with other self-employed plans, such as the SEP IRA.

Note: Self-employed retirement plans were formerly known as "Keough plans." Since the law no longer distinguishes between corporate and other plans, the term is no longer used.

When One Spouse Retires Before the Other

Dana Anspach, CFP, retirement management analyst (RMA), founder of Sensible Money, an investment advisory firm that specializes in couples preparing for retirement, Scottsdale, Arizona. She is author of *Control Your Retirement Destiny.* SensibleMoney.com

Many two-income couples assume that they'll retire at the same time and then transition to a new chapter in their lives.

Reality: Only 20% of partners retire within one year of each other, according to a Fidelity Investments study.

Some "staggered retirements" happen when one spouse retires earlier than expected due to health problems or job loss...or one partner extends his/her working years because he wants to qualify for a full pension or enjoys his career.

Retirement expert Dana Anspach, CFP, RMA, says staggered retirement can produce unexpected financial benefits. *Here's how she has helped scores of dual-career couples navigate the financial aspects of retiring at different times...*

WHAT TO CONSIDER

When one spouse continues to work after the other stops working, it often sets into motion three powerful factors...

• **Waiting longer to start taking Social Security increases benefits.** If one or both spouses put off taking Social Security benefits until full retirement age (age 66 to 67 if you were born in 1943 or afterward) or longer, it not only boosts lifetime guaranteed income but increases potential spousal and survivor benefits.

The working spouse can continue to save and invest aggressively for retirement—as much as $27,000 in a 401(k) and $7,000 in an IRA annually (if age 50 or over). He also can contribute up to $7,000 annually to an IRA or Roth IRA on behalf of a nonworking spouse and continue to fund health savings accounts (HSAs)—as long as the working spouse is not enrolled in any portion of Medicare—if the couple has a high-deductible health insurance policy.

Details: IRS Publication 590-A, *Contributions to Individual Retirement Arrangements* (IRAs) available at IRS.gov/publications/p590a.

The nonworking spouse can avoid or limit tapping retirement assets. Assets can continue to accrue, and the couple will need to draw on them for fewer years. This also protects against "sequence-of-returns" risk, which occurs when the first few years of retirement coincide with a bear market, a time when drawing on your portfolio can be damaging to your long-term returns and wealth.

Here's a checklist for couples considering staggered retirement...

#1. Decide how long your staggered retirement will last. Knowing the age at which you both will be retired and drawing on your retirement income allows you to revise your original retirement plan to reach your new goals. You will have to recalculate how much you'll have accumulated by then and the income that you're likely to need in both the staggered and joint retirement phases to cover basic monthly bills, housing, discretionary costs and inflation. For help with these calculations, see the free calculator and tools at NewRetirement.com.

#2. Make sure the nonworking spouse has health-care coverage until eligible for Medicare. The best option typically is for the nonworking spouse to join the working spouse's employer-subsidized plan until age 65. If that's not possible, shop your state's health-care exchange through the Affordable Care Act (ACA) at HealthCare.gov. Your household income may be lower after one spouse retires, so you could qualify for tax credits to offset premiums. The Health Insurance Marketplace Calculator at KFF.org/interactive/subsidy-calculator lets you estimate premiums and subsidies in your state under various ACA plans.

#3. Adjust your monthly budget during the staggered period. Whether your goal is to minimize the financial problems caused by a spouse retiring early or maximize the advantages of a spouse working longer than expected, it's important to make changes during the years when your household has only one income. *Strategies I recommend...*

●Try living on only the working spouse's salary. This may be feasible because expenses associated with working can be eliminated and taxes will be lower. Use the staggered period to see what you can live without when you are both retired and living on a fixed income in the future. If it turns out that you need to supplement your budget, your first step would be to stop contributing to savings, including 401(k) and other retirement plans, and see if you can live on the increased take-home pay. Beyond that, evaluate the tax consequences to determine which assets to tap into next.

●Avoid big splurges until you are both retired. Often the retiring spouse feels that he deserves an immediate reward after decades of labor—perhaps an expensive new car or a kitchen renovation. Not only can this compromise your immediate budget and goals, it can lead to resentment from the working spouse.

●The nonworking spouse should consider part-time work. It's often the most effective solution if one salary is insufficient. *Important:* Run the part-time job past your accountant to find out if the additional income will push you into a higher tax bracket or affect any Social Security benefits you are receiving.

#4. Take advantage of a lower income tax bracket. Many staggered-retirement couples are in a lower tax bracket than before the spouse retired, especially if it is the main breadwinner who stops working. *What to do...*

●Take profits on investments in taxable accounts, especially if you've been reluctant to sell stocks or funds with large, embedded capital gains. For 2022, if you are married, filing jointly and your joint taxable income from all sources after applicable deductions is $83,350 or less, your capital gains tax rate is 0%.

●Consider Roth conversions. It may make sense to pay taxes on the income in IRAs now in order to avoid taxes on withdrawals later if your taxable income at age 72+, when you have added income from required distributions and Social Security, will put you in a higher tax rate than your current rate.

#5. Time Social Security right. If one spouse works longer, a couple can earn tens of thousands of extra dollars over their lifetimes by coordinating when each spouse takes Social Security.

Rule of thumb: If the spouses are close in age, the higher-earning spouse should delay Social Security benefits until age 70. If the age difference is greater than four years, then run your situation through software to maximize your lifetime benefits.

Helpful resources: OpenSocialSecurity.com offers a free calculator that allows you to run Social Security–claiming scenarios. Maximize MySocialSecurity.com is a more powerful calculator developed by Boston University economics professor Laurence Kotlikoff, PhD, which allows you to input a wide range of factors to determine the best claiming strategy.

Cost: $40 for an annual household license.

For unmarried couples: Much of the same advice applies, but you may face additional hurdles and should seek advice from a financial planner.

Example: The retiring partner may not be eligible for coverage under his/her working partner's health-care plan unless he has domestic partnership rights, which vary from state to state. And each spouse will not be eligible for Social Security spousal and survivor benefits if the couple is not married. Also, income tax bills for married couples filing jointly or separately tend to be lower than for unmarried couples filing separately.

Little-Known Tools for Retirement and Estate Planning

Robert Carlson, editor of the monthly newsletter *Retirement Watch*. He is a managing member of Carlson Wealth Advisors and chairman of the board of trustees of the Fairfax County (Virginia) Employees' Retirement System. RetirementWatch.com

The upsides of IRAs and living trusts for retirement and estate-planning are widely known, but even savvy savers might not be aware that there's a type of sav-

ings account that offers more tax advantages than any IRA can offer...and even prudent planners might never have heard of a few tremendously useful types of trusts.

Here are five very useful—and very underused—tools and trusts for retirement and estate planning.

Reminder: For the options below, speak to a qualified financial adviser.

•**Health Savings Accounts (HSAs)**—for retirement savings. You might already know about the advantages of HSAs when it comes to paying medical bills—these accounts let people pay health-related costs using pretax dollars. But the incredible upside of an HSA as a retirement savings tool receives much less attention. These accounts are "triple tax-free"—you contribute pretax dollars...investment profits earned inside the HSA are tax-free... and money isn't taxed when it is withdrawn as long as it is used to pay for qualified medical expenses. No IRA or 401(k) can match that triple tax savings—you can either contribute pretax dollars with a traditional IRA/401(k)... or earn tax-free investment profits and take tax-free withdrawals with a Roth—never both.

Unfortunately, an HSA's unparalleled tax advantages are largely wasted if, like most HSA owners, you simply put your contributions in a low interest rate savings account and then use the money to pay your medical expenses.

To maximize an HSA's upside: Invest contributions in long-term investments such as equity mutual funds, and leave the money there as long as possible. Use other assets to pay near-term expenses.

If your HSA provider doesn't offer appealing investment options, transfer to one that does. Unlike Flexible Spending Accounts (FSAs), with which HSAs are sometimes confused, money in an HSA can be kept there as long as you like—it doesn't disappear early the following year. And unlike traditional IRAs and 401(k)s, HSAs have no required lifetime distributions.

Limitations of HSAs as retirement-planning tools: Most notably, you cannot contribute to an HSA if you have any health coverage beyond a high-deductible health plan—so if you're enrolled in any part of Medicare, you won't qualify.

Important: This high-deductible health plan requirement applies only to making HSA contributions—you can withdraw money from an HSA in a future year even if you have more comprehensive coverage, such as Medicare.

And even if you do qualify for an HSA, your contributions will be capped—as of 2022, the limits are $3,650 per year for an individual or $7,300 for family coverage...though you can make an additional $1,000 "catch-up contribution" if you're 55 or older by year-end.

Also: You will face taxes and penalties if you withdraw money from an HSA for non–health-related expenses (although no penalties once you're age 65 or older), but this causes fewer issues than people tend to imagine. If you don't have sufficient out-of-pocket medical bills to use up your HSA savings when you finally decide to tap this account, you can make withdrawals to reimburse yourself for earlier medical bills, even bills that were incurred many years before.

Helpful: IRS rules don't officially cap how long in the past these reimbursed medical expenses can be, but as a rule of thumb they shouldn't raise IRS eyebrows as long as the medical expense didn't occur before you had an HSA.

• **529 plans—for estate planning.** If you have kids or grandkids, you might have made contributions to 529 plans, a tax-advantaged way to save for educational expenses. But the potential of 529s as estate-planning tools is less well-known—these could be a way to get a large amount of money out of your estate fast without it counting against your lifetime estate and gift-tax exemption. Ordinarily the most one person can give another in a year without incurring tax consequences is $16,000, but with 529s there's a special "five-year election" rule—you can give someone up to five times that $16,000 annual limit and, for tax purposes, treat it as if the gift was spread over five years. That's $80,000 out of your estate in a single year per recipient with no tax consequences—if you have five grandkids,

you could "superfund" five 529s for a total estate reduction of $400,000.

Unlike with most gifts, you don't lose total control of your money when you fund a 529—you still can control how this money is invested...you can shift the money to a different beneficiary if, for example, the original beneficiary doesn't go to college...and you even can withdraw the money for non-educational purposes, though that's likely to trigger income taxes and a 10% penalty.

• **Qualified charitable distributions.** Planning to make a charitable donation this year? If you're older than 70½ and have money in a traditional IRA, whether you claim the standard deduction or itemize your taxes, giving this gift through something called a "qualified charitable distribution" (QCD) could make more financial sense than simply writing a check to the charity. With a QCD, the money you donate counts toward your required minimum distributions and is excluded from your taxable income. Ordinarily charitable donations are excluded from taxable income only for people who itemize their taxes, which is relatively uncommon under the current tax law.

To make a QCD: Instruct your IRA custodian to distribute money directly to the charity of your choice—the custodian might ask you to complete a form. Annual QCDs are capped at $100,000...and the recipients must be 501(c)(3) organizations.

• **Inheritor's trusts.** This underused type of irrevocable trust could be the solution if you have faith in your descendants' financial savvy and want to give them control over the assets they inherit...but also want to protect those assets from creditors and other outside threats. With an inheritor's trust, the adult child—not the parent—sets up the trust and has broad powers over its management and the distribution of its assets. That adult child can access the assets as needed...or leave the assets in the trust to shield them from creditors and divorcing spouses...or let assets pass to their children in a way that avoids future estate taxes. They get all of the benefits of outright asset ownership plus many of the protections of a trust. An inheritor's trust does nothing to protect assets against misuse by its beneficiary, however, so they're not appropriate for irresponsible heirs.

Details can vary, but generally with inheritor's trusts, the adult child is named both the primary beneficiary and a trustee—if you're leaving assets to multiple children, each will need his/her own inheritor's trust. The adult child's children or other relatives might be named secondary beneficiaries, but the adult child has broad power to alter those secondary beneficiaries.

As a trustee, the adult child also has sole control over the investment decisions within the trust. A co-trustee—either a trusted friend of the adult child or a corporate trustee—might be given sole power to make distributions from the trust, but the adult child has broad power to remove or replace that co-trustee, so the adult child truly is in control of the inheritance.

•**Charitable remainder trusts.** This type of irrevocable trust offers a way to convert a highly appreciated asset into both a donation to your favorite charity and an income stream for you—without having the value of that asset diminished by capital gains taxes.

How it works: A highly appreciated asset, such as a piece of real estate, a small business or shares of stock, is transferred to the trust, which typically then sells the asset and reinvests the proceeds. The trust then makes payments to you, either for the remainder of your life or for a set number of years—IRS rules cap the size of these payments based on a number of factors. The remaining assets eventually pass to the charity, but you don't have to wait until that happens to claim a tax deduction—you can take the deduction in the year the trust is funded based on the present value of the amount the charity is expected to eventually receive. This deduction might have to be spread over multiple years if it's more than 50% of your adjusted gross income. A large charity even might be willing to handle the creation and administration of a charitable remainder trust, saving you the legal costs and hassles.

Best Ways to Estimate Life Expectancy

David M. Blanchett, PhD, CFA, CFP, director of retirement research for Morningstar Investment Management, Chicago. Morningstar.com

There are lots of reasons you should estimate how long you are likely to live. It may affect when you retire…whether you buy an annuity or long-term-care insurance…and how big a nest egg you should build.

Your estimate will be more accurate if you go beyond the life spans of your parents or the overly simplistic Social Security calculator. *Instead, use life-expectancy calculators that analyze personal factors and draw on a database of deceased individuals with similar factors…*

•**Living to 100 Life Expectancy Calculator,** created by the medical director of the New England Centenarian Study. It asks dozens of questions about your lifestyle, education, medical and family history, even the air quality where you live and whether you floss daily. LivingTo100.com

•**Actuaries Longevity Illustrator calculator,** developed by the American Academy of Actuaries and the Society of Actuaries, compares your answers for various questions—such as when do you plan to retire and what's your health status—to databases used by insurers setting premiums for annuity products to provide probabilities of how long you will live.

Example: Depending on how he answers certain questions, a 57-year-old man in good health might have a 78% chance of living to 80…a 60% chance of living to 85…a 38% chance of living until 90…and an 18% chance of living until 95. LongevityIllustrator.org

Once you decide on a life-expectancy number you feel comfortable with, take these additional steps…

•**Couples within 10 years of each other's age** typically should use the life-expectancy number of the spouse expected to live longest.

•**When financial planning, singles should add an extra five years to the life-expectancy** estimate...and couples an extra five to 10 years. That provides a cushion in case you live longer than average.

• **Have an extreme-age contingency plan.** Think now about what you might do if you hit your life-expectancy age and are still in good health but running low on financial assets.

Negotiate Your Best Early-Retirement Package

Kimberly Foss, CFP, CPWA (certified private wealth advisor), president of Empyrion Wealth Management, Inc. in Roseville, California. EmpyrionWealth.com

Your company offers you an early retirement or other buyout package with a big lump sum of cash. It's tempting, especially if you've been unhappy with your job...considering a change in careers...or thinking that early retirement might not be so bad. During the pandemic, thousands of employees have received such offers. If offered a package, you typically have just a few weeks to decide what to do. Use the time to put the offer in the context of your overall financial situation including the amount of savings you have, your health-care needs and future sources of income.

Focus on three major provisions in the package...

• **Severance.** This may be paid in a lump sum or annual installments and typically amounts to one to four weeks of salary for every year of service. Calculate whether it's enough to support a smooth transition financially to your next job or to the age at which you would be able to retire without having to depend on an ongoing salary. If not, ask for an additional cash bonus since this portion of the offer has the most room for negotiation.

• **Health-care insurance.** Under the federal law known as COBRA, if your company has a group health insurance plan and at least 20 employees, it must grant you the right to continue group health insurance coverage after a job loss for up to 18 months. Some states have laws that allow employees who do not qualify for COBRA to obtain similar coverage. Your employer may be willing to cover a portion of your COBRA costs.

• **Pension.** If your company offers one, your monthly benefit will depend on how long you have been at the company. Less time may mean reduced payments. There is little you can do to negotiate better terms because pension plans are subject to strict IRS regulations.

Use these strategies to negotiate...

• **Ask whether components of the package that you don't need can be exchanged for cash or other benefits.**

Example: If you can get medical coverage through your spouse's plan, agree to cover your own health insurance in return for higher severance.

• **Request a large severance payment be spread over several years to reduce the tax hit of a lump-sum payment.**

• **Consider what would happen if you turn down the offer and stay.** This could be your best choice if you really enjoy your job... will find it hard to get a comparable one... and/or don't have a big enough nest egg to retire right away. However, keep in mind that you may not get as attractive a buyout offer in the future and even may get laid off.

Workers Overestimate Their Social Security Benefits

Workers overestimate their expected Social Security benefits by an average of $307 a month.

One possible reason: They are unclear how much their benefits would be reduced if claimed before full retirement age. Women were more prone than men to expect too much, overestimating benefits by nearly $4,000 annually. Find personalized estimates

WORKING DURING "RETIREMENT"...

Retirement Business Ideas to Consider

Become a financial adviser if you meet the educational and licensing requirements and have done well with your own money. *Be a consultant* if you are an expert in your field and well-connected with a network of companies. *Help startup companies with administrative tasks* if you have expertise in marketing, accounting, finance or other skills. *Become a landlord* if you can afford to buy properties and enjoy the idea of managing them. *Buy an existing business* if you find one in a field that you like that currently has clients. *Become a franchisee* for a company such as 7-Eleven, The UPS Store, Sonic Drive-in Restaurants or Great Clips. *Become an angel investor* if you want to help someone make a company successful and potentially receive a substantial payoff.

NewRetirement.com

Side Gigs for Easy Money After Retirement

Pet sitting and dog walking: Retirees' flexible daytime schedules make it easier to help pet owners who work long hours. *House sitting:* Again, flexible schedules make it easy to watch homes and water plants when owners travel. *Renting out your car or becoming a driver:* If you are using the car less often, websites such as Turo can help you rent it to others, while Uber and Lyft are always recruiting drivers. *Running errands:* Services such as Postmates and Shipt help connect you with busy people who need small everyday tasks done. *Doing landscaping or gardening:* If you enjoy these activities, you can help neighborhood people who are too busy to do them. *Teaching English:* Instructors are always in demand at websites such as Lingoda and iTutorGroup.

MoneyTalksNews.com

Where to Find Work After Retirement

Retired Brains (RetiredBrains.com) offers employment assistance, résumé-writing help, a list of part-time and temporary jobs in your area, information about seasonal and work-from-home jobs and information on starting your own business. AARP (AARP.org) provides similar information and has a Back to Work 50+ program that helps with job training, networking and career counseling.

MoneyTalksNews.com

depending on the age you start drawing benefits at SSA.gov/myaccount.

Maria Prados, PhD, economist at University of Southern California's Dornsife Center for Economic and Social Research, Los Angeles, and coauthor of a study from University of Michigan Retirement and Disability Research Center.

Pros and Cons of Today's Most Popular Retirement Locations

Dave Hughes, founder of RetireFabulously.com and author of several books about retirement, including *Design Your Dream Retirement* and *The Quest for Retirement Utopia.*

D eciding where to spend your retirement can be both exhilarating and nerve-racking, depending on which aspects you're focusing on.

The fact that a place is prone to wildfires or hurricanes doesn't mean you should scratch it off your list entirely. It just means that you should factor that risk in as you make your decision.

Following is a list of today's popular retirement destinations and some of the primary risks to consider. No place is perfect—or perfectly safe. But it's a smart exercise to ask yourself how you would handle certain contingencies…and not just how you'd handle them today, but 10, 20 or 30 years from now when you may be in much less robust health.

•**The Villages, Florida.** *Heat, storms and sinkholes.* According to the new US Census data, this retirement Shangri-La now qualifies as America's fastest-growing metro area. It's easy to see why—The Villages is its own little world, offering every imaginable activity. But the heat and humidity can be extreme. From May to October, expect temperatures

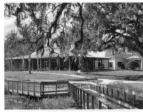

in the 90s, with heat indices often reaching "extreme danger" levels over 100—and climate change will only make matters worse.

Despite its inland setting, The Villages is not immune to storms. It usually is spared the worst of Florida's hurricanes, but it's not uncommon for The Villages to see high winds and heavy rains.

The Villages, together with the surrounding area of Central Florida, is prone to sinkholes. Over the past two decades, The Villages has experienced dozens of sinkholes that have caused significant damage and even evacuations.

●**San Antonio, Texas.** *Fragile infrastructure.* This historic city has become increasingly popular with retirees in recent years. Its housing prices are reasonable...there's lots

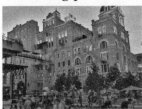

to do...and it retains a small-town feel. But like much of the state, it was hit hard by last year's power crisis caused by devastating winter storms, which revealed dangerous shortcomings in the systems and structures meant to keep Texans safe and comfortable. The outages that left people—many of them elderly—literally freezing to death in their homes or using trash cans to collect water from the San Antonio River were the direct result of poor statewide energy policy choices.

●**Fort Myers, Florida.** *Flooding, rising sea levels and hurricanes.* Not long ago, *US News & World Report* named this southwest coastal city the number-one best place to retire. It boasts numerous parks, galler-

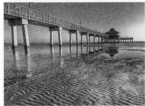

ies and museums, not to mention great beaches. But at just seven to 10 feet above sea level—and with climate-change predictions coming true before our eyes—the chances of serious flooding are increasing. One model predicts that

by 2050, there's a 53% chance that the Fort Myers area will see four-foot flooding likely during a hurricane.

●**Sun City, Arizona.** *Drought and wildfires.* Sun City is a suburb of Phoenix, the fifth-largest (and fastest-growing) major city in the US. The "Valley of the Sun" has been called

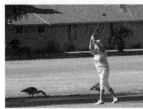

the "least sustainable city on earth"—not surprising given that it sits in the Sonoran Desert. The Southwest is entering its third decade of the worst drought in 400 years. Phoenix's population boom is anticipated to continue indefinitely, but its water supply is finite and shrinking.

Dry conditions contributed to the wildfires that have plagued Arizona in recent years. While the Phoenix metro area proper has not yet been hit, the fires have come too close for comfort. Even if your home is not in the path of a fire, breathing smoky air for months on end—as is becoming the norm through much of the American West—can have serious health consequences.

●**Oklahoma City.** *Tornadoes and earthquakes.* The low cost of living makes OKC one of the country's most affordable cities for retirement. Add to that an average annual temperature of 61°F and sunshine 65% of the days, and the appeal is apparent.

You probably already associate Oklahoma with "tornado alley." And maybe that's okay

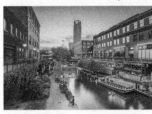

with you, since the chances of your specific dwelling being struck are relatively low. But did you know that Oklahoma has nearly as many earthquakes as California? In fact, earthquakes have become a daily occurrence in the state. Geologists say it's a manmade problem caused by injecting wastewater, a by-product of fossil fuel extraction, deep underground, triggering seismic activity. Most of the tremors are small, but it doesn't take much to make an elderly person fall in the shower—

and chances are, given a long enough timeline, those tremors won't all be mild.

• **Kennebunk, Maine.** *Lack of senior services.* Be sure any area you are considering in this state has a good senior center...transportation vans for people with mobility challenges... 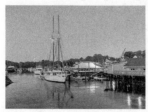 Meals on Wheels... and home health-care providers. Right now, Maine and areas like Kennebunk have a severe shortage of home-care providers. The state has the oldest average population, with many young people having migrated elsewhere for better jobs. Most people don't think about this stuff as they approach retirement or even in the earlier stages of retirement. But by the time it becomes important, it may be too difficult to relocate to somewhere with better services.

• **"That cabin up in the mountains."** *Lack of medical access.* After decades of grinding away at the rat race, fighting our way through commuter traffic and just having too many humans around, many of us fantasize about finally being able to escape to a remote mountain or lake for some blissful solitude. But isolation can entail risk. 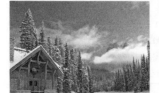 During your earlier retirement years, you'll probably have little need for medical services beyond routine doctor visits. But later, the availability of good doctors, quality hospitals and decent, affordable assisted-living facilities and nursing homes will become crucial. By then, it will be more difficult to relocate to another area to find good health-care options. It makes sense to investigate the services that are available in any area you're considering, and think twice about long-term plans that involve a place with an hour-long drive to the hospital.

• **Your hometown.** *Economic decline.* Surprisingly, most people—53%—don't move when they retire. If you've been fortunate enough to find a place you love...if your house is paid off...if you're surrounded by friends and family...why leave?

But you should apply the same kind of risk assessment to your current location that you would if you were looking into other destinations. Maybe you're fine with the various risks you've been living with. But beware of another risk—a faltering local economy. Is your city on the upswing? Does its future look good? Will home values continue to rise? Will crime rates stay down?

There are several signs you can look for. If the local economy is strong and most employers are in industries with a promising future, such as technology and medical research, that bodes well for a city's outlook. Many people forget that a thriving job market should be an important criterion for retirees—well-employed neighbors make for stability and tax revenues. On the other hand, a heavy concentration of aging manufacturing plants is less promising. And as an area declines, crime is likely to go up. State capitals and university towns are more likely to remain stable over time.

Thinking of Moving to a Senior-Living Community?

Positives: The monthly fee you pay to your homeowner association (HA) most likely will cover outside maintenance such as lawn care and may include utilities, TV and Internet, even meals. Some communities have security gates or walls. You may no longer need to maintain and insure a car, since food, activities and entertainment all may be available within a short walk.

Negatives: The average cost in a community is about $1,000 per month more than the overall average cost of housing expenses for people age 65 and older. Residents also can be hit with special assessments if the community's finances are not in order and well-managed. Rules about visitors may limit your time with friends and relatives.

GoBankingRates.com

13

Consumer Concerns

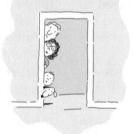

Massive Medical Bills? How to Pay Much Less

Even though Congress passed legislation, which took effect at the start of 2022, to address surprise out-of-network medical expenses at in-network hospitals, there still are many ways that seemingly well-insured patients can be subjected to burdensome health-care costs.

Examples: Out-of-network doctor visits...ambulance rides, which are excluded from the legislation (though air ambulances are included)...and treatments the insurance company or Medicare deems not medically necessary or when patients are uninsured.

Here's a six-step plan for what to do if you receive a massive medical bill—it's often possible to pay much less...

1. Check the "Explanation of Benefits" (EOB) statement before paying. This document details how much your coverage will pay and how much you must pay. It will be mailed to you by your insurer or Medicare and typically is marked "This Is Not a Bill." When you receive it, compare the amount listed under "patient responsibility" or "you owe" with the amount the provider is billing you. These figures should match. If they don't, call both the health-care provider's billing office and the insurer/Medicare until you get an explanation for the discrepancy.

Among the potential explanations: The care provider might have mailed your bill before your insurance/Medicare paid its share... the provider might have submitted its claim incorrectly to your insurance/Medicare...or it might have failed to submit an insurance/Medicare claim at all. If necessary, make sure

Caitlin Donovan, senior director of the National Patient Advocate Foundation, a nonprofit organization based in Hampton, Virginia, that provides case management and financial aid to Americans facing chronic, life-threatening and debilitating illnesses. PatientAdvocate.org

your health-care provider refiles the paper-work properly.

Also: Medical billing errors are very common. Read the bill and the EOB in search of procedures that do not seem relevant to your treatment—a coronary angioplasty if you were in the hospital for a hip replacement, for example—and contact the provider to question whether you actually received these services.

2. Ask your insurer/Medicare why a procedure was not well-covered.

Among the explanations your coverage provider might offer: The health-care provider wasn't in network...the procedure wasn't medically necessary...or the provider failed to submit the information required to process the claim. Don't back down if you believe their explanations might be inaccurate—they often are.

Examples: If you're told the provider isn't in network, you might say, "I confirmed that this provider is in network through your website—why is it being coded as out-of-network?" If you're told the procedure wasn't medically necessary, ask, "How does this need to be coded for you to cover it?" and/or ask your doctor to provide a written "letter of medical necessity" explaining why the procedure actually was necessary in your case. If you're told the claim wasn't submitted properly, contact the health-care provider and ask for it to be resubmitted.

Helpful: If you have Medicare, call 1-800-633-4227 to ask these questions...or visit Medicare.gov, click "Claims & Appeals" at the bottom left of the screen, then click "Go" under "Talk to Someone."

3. File formal appeals with your coverage provider. You have a legal right to submit at least two formal written appeals per medical bill with your insurer/Medicare if you believe it is not covering a bill properly. A free template for these appeals is available at my organization's website, PatientAdvocate.org (select "Free PAF Publications" from the "Explore Our Resources" menu, then click "Engaging with Insurers: Appealing a Denial"). When you complete these appeals documents, keep in mind that you are essentially making a le-

gal argument that the insurer/Medicare is failing to provide the coverage to which you are entitled, not an emotional argument that your bill is crushingly large. Approach this as you would any legal contract, using professional language.

4. Request financial assistance with hospital bills. Ask the hospital's billing department if you qualify for any financial assistance. Most hospitals have programs that can reduce or waive bills for people who can't afford to pay. Eligibility rules vary, but even people with incomes above $100,000 may qualify when bills climb into five figures.

5. Negotiate. You can negotiate medical bills—if you can't pay, the provider will have to sell your debt to a collection agency for pennies on the dollar, a result that the provider wants to avoid.

Strategy: Look up the typical cost paid for the procedures you received. Hospitals now are required to list their negotiated rates on their websites, or check HealthcareBlueBook.com (a membership site benefit provided by some employers) or Medicare.gov/procedure-price-lookup. Compare the prices you find to your bill. Even if you're not going through a hospital system, you still can use your local hospital's list to get an idea of a reasonable charge. Generally, a hospital charge will be more than an in-office service at an independent provider.

Next, call the provider's billing office. Explain that you can't afford to pay the amount billed, then use the lowest price you uncovered for the procedures—that's usually the Medicare price—as the starting point for negotiations. If you can afford to pay immediately, ask if the provider offers prompt-payment discounts or cash discounts.

If you can't afford to pay in a lump sum, ask the provider for a payment plan that fits your budget after you have negotiated a price. Whatever terms you negotiate, get the agreement in writing before making any payment. This written agreement should confirm that the amount you are paying will be considered payment in full...and, if possible, that your failure to pay the entire amount originally billed will not be listed as a late or unpaid debt on your credit reports.

6. Enlist outside help. There are nonprofit organizations that help people find financial assistance or other means of support, such as negotiating a lowered rate. Locate organizations that might help you on PatientAdvocate.org (select the "National Financial Resource Directory" button under the "Explore Our Resources" tab). Also ask any religious and fraternal organizations you belong to whether they have programs that could help. Your town or county might have programs that provide assistance to residents facing financial challenges as well.

Helpful: If you have a chronic, life-threatening and/or debilitating disease, the Patient Advocate Foundation might be able to provide access to a case manager who can review your bills for errors, help you locate financial assistance and negotiate bills on your behalf. We've helped patients with cancer, HIV/AIDs, lupus and diabetes. (You must be receiving care or have received care within the US, and we don't handle behavioral/mental health, accidents or pregnancy.) If you don't qualify for this assistance, you can engage a for-profit medical billing advocate who can vet and negotiate bills on your behalf for a fee—potentially $50 to $100 or more an hour...or 25% to 35% of the amount the advocate gets your medical bills reduced.

Also contact area newspaper and TV reporters who cover consumer advocacy and/or health-care issues. If a reporter starts poking into your case, there's a good chance that the provider or insurer may back down and offer better terms to avoid negative publicity. Reporters can't cover everyone who has huge medical bills, however, so when you reach out to them, stress the ways in which your bills are especially egregious and/or your situation especially heart-wrenching.

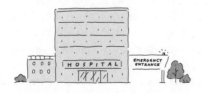

Medical Tourism

Lydia Gan, PhD, professor of economics, University of North Carolina at Pembroke.

Patients from developing nations have long traveled to the United States to access care they couldn't get at home, but the high cost of US care is now sending some Americans in the opposite direction.

COST SAVINGS

For Americans, saving money is the top motivator to travel for health care. Consider heart bypass surgery. In the United States, a patient without health insurance can expect to receive a dizzying array of opaque and confusing bills that add up to between $70,000 and $133,000. But the identical procedure can be performed by Western-trained surgeons in a high-tech hospital in Singapore for about $16,000 or India for less than $9,000-including medical costs, airfare, and hotel. Americans regularly cross the border to Los Algodones, Mexico, also known as Molar City, to save 70% to 80% on dental services such as crowns ($180 vs. $1,250), and dentures ($250 vs. $1,850).

THE HOSPITAL EXPERIENCE

Saving money isn't the only benefit of medical tourism. In many cases, hospitals that cater to medical tourists also offer a more luxurious experience, from private rooms and more personalized attention to dedicated centers that offer assistance with scheduling, interpretation, sightseeing, travel arrangements, and accommodations.

Further, instead of recovering at home, you can combine recovery with a vacation (as long as you stay within doctor-approved activities).

The best hospitals provide Western-trained health-care providers, but not every hospital in every country meets American standards. To ensure safety, seek care only from hospitals that are accredited by Joint Commission International (JCI), which is related to the Joint Commission that accredits hospitals in the United States. Any JCI-accredited hospital meets the same standards as those in America. In addition, seek hospitals that are affiliated with reputable American brands such as

Johns Hopkins, Harvard Medical Center, and Mayo Clinic.

CONSIDER A MEDICAL MIDDLEMAN

While you can arrange for international medical care on your own, it can be helpful to work with a domestic medical tourism facilitator (DMTF), which is essentially a medical travel agency. These companies match you with a doctor or hospital, make your travel plans, pick you up at the airport, offer translation services, secure your medical visa, and may arrange excursions. Look for a DMTF that is based in the United States, is certified by the Better Business Bureau, and works only with JCI-accredited hospitals. A trustworthy DMTF should have physicians on staff or be managed by someone who has an extensive career in health care.

TIPS FOR SUCCESS

Careful preparation can make medical tourism safer and more successful.

•**Plan ahead.** Before you travel, meet with your health-care provider to discuss your health status, the procedure, and travel restrictions before and after the procedure.

•**Make sure you can get any needed follow-up care in the United States.** Call your insurance company, if applicable, to discuss your coverage.

•**Identify where you will be staying immediately after the procedure,** and make sure you have a long enough recovery period. If you have chest or abdominal surgery, cosmetic procedures of the face, eyelids, or nose, or laser treatments, do not fly for at least 10 days to avoid risks associated with changes in atmospheric pressure.

•**Find out what activities are not permitted after the procedure.** Sunbathing, drinking alcohol, swimming, or engaging in strenuous activities may be prohibited.

•**Make sure you're up to date on all vaccinations for your home and destination countries.** Consider adding a hepatitis B vaccine.

•**Buy travel health insurance that covers medical evacuation home.**

•**Take copies of your medical records to your destination,** and bring any new records home with you.

•**Pack enough medications to last your whole trip, plus a little extra in case of delays.** Keep your medication in your carry-on bag.

•**Be aware of antibiotic resistance risks.** The risk of antibiotic resistance varies by location. For example, India has the highest rates of antibiotic resistance in the world.

•**If you are traveling to have a procedure that is not available in the United States,** understand that you may have difficulty getting insurance to cover any post-procedure complications.

Save Money on Medicines with Five Popular Apps

Good*Rx* has a network of 70,000+ pharmacies. *ScripSave WellRx* has more than 65,000. Both *SingleCare* and *Blink Health* have 35,000+ participating pharmacies. *RxSaver* does not say how large its pharmacy network is but says it works at major chains including Costco, CVS, Kroger, Walgreens and Walmart. If you use any medicine regularly, check several apps as well as your regular insurance coverage.

Clark.com

Exercise Bonus—Pay Less for Health Care

Older adults who were moderately active starting in adolescence and throughout adulthood spent $1,200 less on health care per year, on average, than inactive seniors. Older adults who maintained long-term high activity levels saved even more—$1,350 per year. And older adults who did not increase their activity levels until middle age even saved money on health care compared with inactive older adults—$824/year.

Analysis from the National Institutes of Health-American Association of Retired Persons Diet and Health Study, published in *BMJ Open Sport & Exercise Medicine.*

How to Save on Expensive Dental Work

Jim Miller, editor of the nationally syndicated column "The Savvy Senior." SavvySenior.org

Since 1996, average annual dental expenditures have nearly doubled. So unless you've got great insurance, you might need to get creative to avoid serious hits to your wallet if you need dental work.

BEFORE YOU NEED DENTAL WORK

•**Consider a Medicare Advantage plan during open enrollment if you're on Medicare's basic plan.**

Reason: The basic plan does not cover dental work.

•**Consider a Dental Savings Plan.** You pay an annual fee ($80 to $200) and save up to 60% on root canals, crowns, implants and more from participating dentists. You can sign up before an expensive procedure—you won't be denied because of preexisting conditions. To find a savings plan, go to DentalPlans.com.

•**Help for low-income people.** You may get free or discounted treatment at a community clinic. Search at FreeDentalCare.us. Donated Dental Services, a program of the Dental Lifeline Network, provides care to people with disabilities, the elderly and others. Check out your state's program on DentalLifeline.org.

•**Consider private insurance.** Buying dental insurance usually isn't worthwhile—but paying $15 to $50 per month may be worth it if you're shelling out thousands because of chronic dental problems.

TAKE NOTE...

Watch Out for Added Fees to Restaurant Bills

Extra fees—usually 2% or 3% and called "fair wage fees," "kitchen appreciation fees," "equity charges," "COVID surcharges," "wellness fees" or something similar—are being slipped onto restaurant bills. A 15% to 20% "service" or "hospitality" fee also might be added.

Bottom line: Always scan restaurant bills for fees before paying. If a service charge was added, you need to know so you don't double tip. Carefully review menus online for mention of fees before making reservations.

Rafi Mohammed, PhD, author of *The Art of Pricing* and founder of the Cambridge, Massachusetts, pricing strategy consulting company Culture of Profit. PricingForProfit.com

---

WHEN YOU NEED DENTAL WORK

•**Be proactive.** Find out the price tag from your dentist or oral surgeon in advance. Don't agree to a procedure, have it done and only then start looking for ways to bring down the cost.

•**Shop around.** Call other providers to see what they'd charge for the procedure. You'd be surprised at the cost differences between local dentists. For costs of procedures in neighboring zip codes, try HealthcareBlueBook.com or FairHealthConsumer.org.

•**Ask for a discount.** At the least, request a discount for paying in cash, if that's an option. Tell the practice that you're interested in any programs to make the procedure more affordable.

If you really cannot pay: Simply plead poverty—"I just don't have $6,000"—and see what the dentist comes back with.

•**Buy now, pay later.** Some practices have in-house payment programs that charge low or no interest. Others access third-party "buy now pay later" (BNPL) providers that let you pay for procedures at 0% interest over three to 24 months (Sunbit is a market leader). While BNPL solutions won't reduce the procedure's price, they will keep its overall cost down if you must resort to credit.

•**Try a dental or dental hygiene school.** Visit TeethWisdom.org to find schools in your area. All university dental schools and college dental hygiene programs offer dental care and cleanings, often for less than half the cost of what you would pay at a dentist's office. Students are supervised by their professors.

Once Your Gums Are Gone…

"Gum restore" and "gum repair" toothpastes won't bring back receded gums. These products usually contain the antibacterial agent *stannous fluoride* plus amino acid stabilizers, which kill gingivitis-causing bacteria and help to prevent further gum loss. But they don't regrow lost gum tissue—only regenerative periodontal procedures such as gum grafts do that—or address the cause of gingivitis.

Kami Hoss, DDS, is CEO of The Super Dentists, a San Diego–area dental practice and a member of UCLA School of Dentistry's board of counselors. The SuperDentists.com

Frustrating Car Features: How to Live with Them …or Get Rid of Them

Karl Brauer, executive analyst at automotive research firm iSeeCars. An automotive journalist for more than 25 years, he is also a juror and board member for the North American Car, Utility and Truck of the Year Award. iSeeCars.com

Is your car's tech driving you crazy? You're not alone. Modern vehicles are full of features intended to make cars safer, more pleasant or more fuel-efficient—but that actually cause frustration. *Among the most angst-inducing automotive technology today—and what to do about it…*

•**Automatic start/stop systems.** In many modern vehicles, the engine automatically shuts off when the car stops, such as at a red light, then restarts when the driver shifts from the brake to the gas. This boosts fuel economy—but by only about one mile per gallon. Many car owners don't consider that modest savings worth the drawbacks, which include slower acceleration from a stop…loss of power steering when stopped, making it difficult to position the car for a quick lane change when the light turns green…and increased wear on the battery, starter motor and engine.

What to do: Temporarily disabling this start/stop system is simple—look for a button on the dash or steering wheel marked with a letter "A" surrounded by an arrow or read the vehicle's owner's manual for details. But these systems typically turn back on each time the vehicle is restarted, so you'll have to hit this button for every trip.

Caution: Adding aftermarket products designed to shut off the start/stop feature permanently, including Autostop Eliminator and Smart Stop Start, can sometimes cause problems for the vehicle's electronics systems.

•**Warning lights on the dashboard.** A rectangle with wavy arrows? A cartoon image of two cars with a star between them? Dozens of different warning lights can suddenly appear on the dashboards of modern cars, and few car owners know what they all mean. The result is distracted driving and, sometimes, unnecessary mechanic's bills.

What to do: The color of the dash light provides a gauge of how concerned you should be. A red warning light suggests a pressing issue, such as low oil pressure or high temperature—pull over as soon as possible. A yellow light means one of the car's systems is experiencing a problem—there's no need to pull over right away, but repairs might be needed soon. And a blue or green icon is just letting you know that a system is in use.

The much-feared "check engine light" typically isn't reason to panic if it's yellow—it is likely suggesting that there is an issue with the emissions system. In fact, sometimes it can be corrected just by tightening the gas cap.

If you'd like to know a bit more about what a dash light is trying to tell you before taking the car to a mechanic, you can buy an easy-to-use OBD2 code reader at an auto-parts store or online for as little as $25. While the owner's manual may provide a high-level description of what an indicator light means, the code reader will provide a specific answer. It's the same system dealers use to determine what to address when you bring in your car.

•**Proximity key fobs.** Modern fobs communicate wirelessly with vehicles, saving drivers the hassle of fishing the key from their pocket. But is that minor convenience worth the downsides? It used to cost a dollar or two to make a spare car key, but wireless fobs cost $150 to $650 each. And it used to be impossible to drive away without your car key, but now drivers can do just that and end up stranded.

Reason: A car will continue to run if the person holding the fob gets dropped off and the driver leaves without realizing he doesn't have the fob. The vehicle is supposed to immediately recognize the lack of a key…but often it takes several minutes or longer to issue an alert. Finally, these fobs require batteries, which eventually die.

What to do: When you drop off someone who has his own fob for the car, double-check that you have your fob before driving away. If you're prone to misplacing keys, add a wireless key-tracking device to your key ring to reduce the odds that you'll lose these pricey fobs. Buy spare fob batteries, and stash them in your home and car. Also learn how to use your fob if its battery does die—some fobs have old-fashioned physical keys hidden inside, which fit into concealed ignition key slots in the car. Other fobs can be used wirelessly even with a dead fob battery, perhaps by holding the fob directly against the car's start button while pressing it. Find these details in your car's owner's manual…or enter the vehicle's make, model, year and the words "how to start with a dead key fob battery" into a search engine.

•**On-screen phone-dialing systems.** The on-screen buttons on a car's center console screen can be difficult to use to make a call.

What to do: If your car supports Android Auto, Google Assistant and/or Apple CarPlay, use these systems' voice controls to make calls.

•**Lane-keep assist.** This safety feature prevents cars from straying out of their lanes. Unfortunately, many of these systems take control too aggressively, ping-ponging drivers back and forth in their lanes…pulling cars the wrong direction when confronted by complicated situations such as construction-zone lane modifications…and they often can't be counted on to take control when actually needed. When AAA tested five lane-keep assist systems, they experienced one problem per eight miles traveled, a dangerously high error rate.

What to do: If a car's lane-keep assist system frustrates you, turn it off. There's usually a deactivation button on the dash or steering wheel—in some cars, you'll have to deactivate before every trip…in others, it will remain off until reactivated. Or look for this system in the vehicle's onscreen menu.

•**Adaptive cruise control.** This system automatically maintains a safe distance from the car ahead. It can be useful in stop-and-go traffic and on relatively open roads—but frustrating when traffic is fast-moving and congested.

Examples: Sometimes these systems leave such a big gap with the car ahead that other drivers cut in front…or they become confused when the road curves, mistaking a car in a neighboring lane as one that's dead ahead.

What to do: Reduce your adaptive cruise control's following distance…and turn off this system if it frustrates you. Your owner's manual will explain how to do both of these things.

•**One-touch automatic windows.** Pressing the driver's door window control sometimes makes the window go all the way up or down—even if the control is pressed only for a moment. This feature can be annoying when drivers want only to crack the window slightly.

What to do: Use a light touch with one-touch window control. In virtually all vehicles, the window won't automatically open or close all the way if the button is pushed very gently.

Your Car-Towing Plan May Leave You Stranded

Ron Montoya, senior consumer advice editor at Edmunds.com, a leading provider of automotive information.

A re you confident that your car-towing program will provide the emergency help you need when you need it? Don't be so sure.

Roadside-assistance programs are available from many auto manufacturers, auto insurance providers, credit card issuers, cellular-service providers and membership organizations such as AAA and Better World Club. But these programs inevitably have important limits and caveats that many drivers don't know about until it's too late. *Among the details in fine print...*

•**Towing distance caps.** AAA's Classic/Basic membership ($49 to $77 per year, depending on your location) often caps free tows at a mere three, five or seven miles, depending on which regional AAA club you join. Pricier AAA Plus ($60 to $124) and Premier memberships ($77 to $164) generally provide tows up to 100 or 200 miles. Roadside-assistance plans offered by Verizon and certain American Express cards cap towing at 10 miles. Roadside-assistance plans that are included with many auto insurance policies—or available to policyholders for just a few dollars per month—similarly provide free tows but typically only to the nearest repair shop, which often won't be the shop you trust to work on your car. (Auto insurance programs can vary by state, policy and other factors, and they typically include a range of roadside-assistance services, not just towing.)

Exceptions: Progressive offers up to 15 miles of towing or towing to the nearest repair facility, even if that's more than 15 miles away.

Travelers and Nationwide offer tiers of roadside assistance—customers can opt for basic roadside assistance, which provides up to 15 miles of towing, or Premier (in the case of Travelers) or Plus (in the case of Nationwide), which provide up to 100 miles. The higher tiers cost more than the basic tier but still are a fraction of what a membership organization such as AAA charges.

•**Some coverage expires unexpectedly.** Automakers' roadside-assistance programs tend to be available only up to certain vehicle age and mileage limits—similar to auto warranties—so the protection they provide can end suddenly. That could be a problem for drivers who are not paying attention to when their vehicles will reach the age or mileage limit.

Examples: ToyotaCare lasts two years from date of purchase or lease. Honda Roadside Assistance typically expires as soon as the vehicle's three-year/36,000-mile limited warranty ends. Ford's plan lasts five years or 60,000 miles, whichever comes first. Hyundai's plan lasts five years with no mileage limit.

•**Caps on other coverages.** Most towing programs are components of larger roadside-assistance programs that include features such as lockout services, lost-key replacement and jump-starts as well...but details vary.

Examples: If your key is lost or broken or locked in your car, AAA Plus and Premier will compensate you for $100 to $150 in locksmith services, while basic AAA caps this at $50. AT&T Roadside Assistance has a maximum benefit of $75 per incident—though at $2.99 a month, its premiums are relatively low. The roadside assistance provided for free by certain Chase credit cards, including Chase Sapphire Reserve, is capped at $50 per incident.

•**Which drivers, cars and incidents are covered.** Auto-manufacturer programs typically provide assistance no matter who is driving the vehicle, but they don't cover the household's other vehicles. In contrast, Good Sam roadside-assistance plans automatically include spouses, domestic partners and dependent children under age 25 at no additional cost. Good Sam is best known for its RV roadside-assistance plans, but people who don't drive RVs can opt for its Platinum Auto plan, which generally costs $99.95/year but recently was available for $49.95/year. Many other programs, including AAA, cover only one driver, although it's relatively easy to pay additional fees to add other members of the household. And many programs cover only cars, SUVs and small trucks. Only a few extend coverage to RVs, motorcycles and even bicycles.

Example: AAA and Better World Club include bicycle roadside assistance. Bicycle coverage is included at no additional charge with many regional AAA plans...but there's an added fee with Better World Club—$17 to add bike coverage to an auto membership...or $39.95 for a stand-alone bike plan.

And some towing programs cover tows stemming from only mechanical breakdowns, not other events.

Example: AT&T Roadside Assistance's towing program does not cover tows following accidents or even following damage from driving over road debris.

Most programs cap their coverage at either three or four service calls per year.

• **Pay per call.** Some programs don't charge an annual membership fee but instead impose a fee each time the program is used. This is especially common with programs provided by credit cards.

Example: Visa Roadside Dispatch, available with many Visa cards, costs $69.95 per eligible service call—with additional costs for tows longer than five miles.

Buy Your Leased Vehicle When Its Lease Ends

If the lease contract was written before 2020, its "buyout price"—the amount the lessee can pay to purchase the vehicle at lease's end—was based on prepandemic used-car values. But values have risen so sharply since then that the average vehicle coming off lease in late 2021 is

worth 31% more than its buyout price. Leased VW Tiguans, Dodge Chargers and Chevy Camaros are worth more than 50% over buyout prices. You can continue driving your formerly leased vehicle or sell it for a profit.

Karl Brauer is executive analyst at automotive research firm iSeeCars.com.

It Pays to Negotiate with Your Service Providers

Customers who ask often get their Internet, cable and/or cell-phone bills lowered. In a recent survey, 80% of customers who requested reductions succeeded with SiriusXM, Suddenlink, CenturyLink and Dish Network...70% to 79% succeeded with Optimum, Sprint Wireless, ADT Security and DirecTV...60% to 69% succeeded with AT&T, Cox Communications and Verizon Wireless...and 50% to 59% with Frontier, Charter Spectrum and RCN. Savings averaged 10% to 29%—and 40% for SiriusXM customers.

Analysis of data from personal finance app Truebill, reported at MoneyTalksNews.com.

Beware "Buy Now, Pay Later" Plans

Matt Schulz, chief credit analyst with the online loan comparison website LendingTree. LendingTree.com

Make a purchase online these days, and you might be offered the option of splitting the bill into four payments at no additional cost. It's not a scam—"buy now, pay later" programs do allow shoppers to delay all or part of the payment often without incurring interest or fees. Online retailers and the third-party companies that they team with to offer these plans, such as Afterpay, Klarna and Quadpay, extend this no-cost short-term credit because it encourages customers to spend more. They charge a fee to merchants offering their services and assess late fees to customers who don't pay as agreed. *Overspending is the main potential downside of these programs, but there are a few more details worth knowing...*

•**Four payments doesn't mean four months.** These programs trumpet that bills can be spread out over four payments, but they're unclear about the timing of those payments, which generally occur every two weeks, not once a month. Since the first of the four payments occurs immediately, the entire purchase price will be charged to the credit or debit card that you link to the "buy now, pay later" account in just six weeks.

Helpful: Klarna offers the option of deferring the entire purchase price 30 days without interest rather than splitting the bill into four pieces. Klarna can be used at any online US retailer by downloading the Klarna iOS or Android app.

•**Fee structures can be unclear.** Credit cards are required to present terms in an easy-to-understand box. "Buy now, pay later" offers face no such regulations, so you have to read the small print to discover details such as missed-payment penalties. These programs' fees tend not to be exorbitant—often $7 to $10 per missed payment—but you should be aware before taking the offer. Terms vary from program to program and could change with little warning.

•**You might miss out on credit card consumer protections.** If you make an online purchase with a credit card, you can get your money back through the card issuer if the item doesn't arrive or arrives broken and the retailer won't issue a refund. "Buy now, pay later" programs don't offer those safeguards.

Helpful: Link "buy now, pay later" accounts to credit cards rather than debit cards, so that consumer protections still apply.

•**Not all "buy now, pay later" offers are interest-free.** A "buy now, pay later" provider called Affirm lets consumers spread payments over one to 48 months—but while Affirm offers 0% interest on some purchases, it imposes rates as high as 30% on others. Terms vary depending on the retailer and the custom-

er's creditworthiness. Klarna offers an interest-bearing six-to-36-month finance option as well...and American Express's "Pay It Plan It" program, which often gets grouped in with "buy now, pay later" programs, adds fees to the purchase price.

Buy a Mattress That Meets Your Needs

Michael J. Breus, PhD, clinical psychologist in Los Angeles, a Diplomate of the American Board of Sleep Medicine. His latest book is *Energize! Go from Dragging Ass to Kicking It in 30 Days.* TheSleepDoctor.com

Y ou and your bed partner should start by asking yourselves what you need from the mattress beyond restful sleep.

•**If you sleep warm,** which often happens to women after menopause, look for materials that help regulate temperature. A hybrid mattress does a better job of keeping you cool than one that's all memory foam. Latex is naturally cooling, so it's a good pick for hot sleepers.

•**If you need extra cushioning,** consider a pillow-top mattress. Often the body's subcutaneous fat layer (which also helps you regulate temperature) gets thinner with age, meaning that you have less natural cushioning of your own.

•**If you're older and/or have mobility issues,** look for ones with springs or a hybrid mattress but not one that's only memory foam, which may be hard to get in and out of and to turn while sleeping. If you need to sit on the edge of a mattress before standing, you need one that has edge support, a reinforcement you can grab onto so you don't slide off.

•**If you have low back pain and need better support,** an innerspring mattress with coils at its core offers more firmness. Coil technology has advanced—these aren't your parents' innersprings. Plus, you can look for designs that feature comfortable materials in the top layer such as a mix of foam and latex.

Top Mattress Picks from The Sleep Doctor

Avocado Green: This is a certified organic hybrid with a latex, wool and cotton top over support coils arranged in five zones. The company also makes a PETA-approved vegan mattress and a vegan latex mattress. Starts at $1,699.* AvocadoGreenMattress.com

Luma All Latex Slumber System: A great three-layer latex mattress with a latex core, a transition layer and a pillow-top. Luma also makes a variety of hybrids with combinations of base foam, coils and latex tops in natural or synthetic latex. Starts at $2,595. LumaSleep.com

Helix Midnight Luxe: This mattress features a coil core layer for support and even weight distribution and a gel-infused memory foam layer for comfort plus a pillow-top that cushions joints and wicks away heat. Starts at $2,049. HelixSleep.com

Purple Hybrid Premier 3: The most technically innovative product currently on the market, the Purple mattress's proprietary "grid" top layer is like nothing I've seen—an open-channel gel-based material offering support and cushioning in one, set over wrapped stainless steel coils. *Full disclosure:* I was so impressed that I recently became the company's chief sleep advisor. Starts at $2,999. Purple.com

—Dr. Michael J. Breus

*All prices are for queen size

• **If you snore...or your partner snores... or one of you has GERD**—or if you enjoy sitting up in bed to read before sleep—an adjustable base under the mattress can form a slight incline to raise the bed. Look for a mattress specifically designed to work with this kind of base. The Purple Ascent Adjustable Base is a great one and works with mattresses other than its own, such as the Nectar.

• **If you want to have better sex,** an innerspring or hybrid will be better than memory foam, which is less effective in supporting your body during sex.

MAKING IT TO TRYOUTS

There's no substitute for in-person mattress shopping. This often is possible even with offerings from online companies—some have brick-and-mortar stores or sell their mattresses through furniture stores.

Example: Raymour & Flanigan stocks Casper, Nectar, Purple and more.

Some companies allow you to try out a bed in your home for a certain period of time. One of the biggest mistakes people make is giving up on a new mattress too soon. It can take three weeks before you'll know if a mattress is a good fit. Some companies even insist that you keep their mattress for at least 30 days.

Reason: The return rate goes down the longer a mattress is in your home. But regardless of timing, if you determine that a mattress is not a comfortable fit for you, do not hesitate to return it.

WHAT ABOUT BOX SPRINGS?

Before the popularity of the platform bed and its cousin, the futon, innerspring mattresses came with a box spring—a separate base with coils that supported the mattress and gave it more lift. Many mattresses today go directly on what's called a "foundation," or a "base," some of which might be made of attractive wood or covered in upholstery. Many companies still term it a "box spring," but there are no springs.

WHAT ABOUT PRICE?

It is hard to get a great mattress for $600 to $800—these beds-in-a-box are fine for a guest room or limited use. But expect to pay closer to $2,500 (or more) for a great queen-size mattress, topper and base.

DO YOU REALLY NEED A NEW MATTRESS?

Beyond sagging and wear-and-tear, if you wake up more than three days a week with body-wide stiffness that lasts 20 minutes, then goes away, you likely need a new mattress.

Alternative: A latex topper for your existing bed. It can help with heat regulation and offer extra comfort.

"Energy Vampires" Wasting Your Money?

Some appliances continue to use electricity even when turned off if they're plugged into electrical outlets.

Worst offenders: Phone chargers that are not in use…computers left in "sleep" or "hibernate" mode…televisions—a red power light means the TV is pulling electricity…game consoles left on so you can pick up where you left off (even turned off they use power for software updates)…printers left in standby mode (wireless ones use even more energy to maintain an active Wi-Fi signal).

What to do: When it is practical, unplug devices…use outlet timers to turn off devices…plug multiple devices into a single surge-protector power strip so it's easier to turn them all off with one switch.

Komando.com

Trader Joe's Trivia

The store has a no-questions-asked return policy, even if you opened the item and tried it. Trader Joe's stores donate unsold food that is still safe for consumption to local food banks and soup kitchens through their Neighborhood Shares Program. The site also has a "Request a TJ's in My City" page where you can ask about getting a store brought to your area. And those ship's bells located near cash registers that are used to signal employees that someone needs help—one ring means another register needs to be opened…two rings mean a customer has questions…three rings call for a manager to help out.

Kiplinger.com

GOOD TO KNOW…

Walmart Allows Return Items from Home

You no longer have to go to a store or post office to return an item that you ordered online and that was shipped and sold by Walmart.com. The company has partnered with FedEx to arrange for a carrier to pick up the item from your home. Just print and affix a label to your packed item, schedule a pickup date via Walmart's website or app, and a FedEx driver will pick up the package. If you don't have a printer, you can drop the item off at a FedEx location.

MarketWatch.com

Home Depot Has Expanded Its Military Discount

Eligibility for The Home Depot Military 10% Discount, which was newly expanded in 2022, includes active members and veterans of the Army, Navy, Air Force, Marine Corps, Coast Guard, Space Force, National Oceanic and Atmospheric Administration (NOAA), US Public Health Service Commissioned Corps (USPHS) and National Guard…and the spouses of eligible members who are currently enrolled in the discount program. Also, it can be used online, not just in stores. Dependents of military members enrolled in the program are not eligible for the discount. To receive the discount, register online at HomeDepot.com/military/discount or through The Home Depot app.

MilitaryTimes.com and HomeDepot.com

"We-Buy-Homes" Signs Often Are Legitimate

These signs may be posted by real estate investors who buy houses—frequently sight unseen—for less than the market value, then fix them up and flip them or turn them into rental units. Prices paid usually are based on the market value of a fully restored home in the same neighborhood, comparable sales, the cost of repairs and the cost of holding the house until the investors resell it. Owners who need to sell quickly may be able to get a cash sale in a week, compared with the 30-to-45-day time frame for standard closings. But these fast-cash sales never deliver top dollar—and inexpensive repairs, such as fresh paint and an upgraded backyard, can add thousands of dollars to a home's selling price.

Beware: There also are scammers operating in the cash-sales area—so if you are considering such a sale, check out the group's website, trace the phone number listed on signs and ask your local real estate agent for an opinion.

Money.com

Don't Spend More Than $500 on Your Next Cell Phone

Because of trickle-down technology from flagship phones of a few years ago, today's basic low- or mid-range cell phones are among the market's most attractive and affordable phones. Previously, such phones were stripped-down versions of flagship models, but they now have great displays, biometric security such as fingerprint sensor, good cameras, and reliable and timely updates.

ReviewGeek.com

How to Find the Cheapest Gas

Gas prices can be volatile, varying as much as 20% within one city. If you're looking to save some money when gassing up, the website GasBuddy.com can help. Enter your zip code, and select what kind of fuel you need—regular, midgrade, premium or diesel—to get a list of gas stations near you with up-to-the-minute pricing.

Komando.com

Great Buys at Yard Sales

Le Creuset cookware and *Pyrex glassware* can be resold or used in your own kitchen. *Specialty appliances* often can be found for very low prices—much better than buying a new gadget. *Legos* often are available as mixed or partial sets. *Baskets* are inexpensive and great for gift packaging. *Exercise equipment* often is available virtually new...as is *sports gear* for a kid trying out a new sport. *Musical instruments* can be great buys, and ideal for kids just starting out. *Halloween costumes* can be found in both child and adult sizes. *Fancy clothing,* such as wedding dresses and prom outfits, may show up as well.

MoneyTalksNews.com

Cha-Ching!! Yard Sale Success Secrets

Cindy Sabulis, author of *The Garage Sale How-To Guide* and *Collector's Guide to Dolls of the 1960s and 1970s.* CindySabulis.com

The pandemic put the brakes on yard sales—but now they're in full swing. Everyone who held off disposing of their accumulated junk now is looking to get

205

rid of it. One rule has stayed the same—the more planning you put in, the more money you're likely to make. *Here's what you should do for yard sale success…*

GETTING READY

● **Logistics.** Your first step is to find out what is permitted in your town…not just whether you can hold a yard sale but also where you can place signs to draw people to your event.

The next step is to pick tentative dates. Spring and fall are excellent choices because the weather isn't too hot or cold. Most sales last from one to three days.

Rule of thumb to get rid of most items: The more stuff you have, the longer the sale.

Also: Get a commitment from at least one friend or family member to help you—he/she also will be another pair of eyes to prevent theft.

● **Prepping your stuff.** Get a few small or medium boxes, and start filling them with items grouped by category, such as books, collectibles and clothes.

Don't stop to evaluate worthiness at this stage. Some things you think are questionable might not sell, and you can toss or donate them after your sale. But there's a buyer for almost anything!

One caveat: Presentation matters, so clean off dust from each item before you put it in a box. You don't have to mend things, but if you do sew the rip in a coat, for instance, you'll probably get a few more dollars for it.

Important: Check everything completely for hidden or forgotten items. I've heard dozens of stories about people finding gift cards, cash, jewelry and all kinds of hidden treasures inside furniture and clothing they purchased at a sale.

● **Pricing.** To find the sweet spot for pricing all types of items, visit an area thrift shop or even someone else's yard sale—what are they selling hardcover books and small appliances for? Many sellers also look at eBay for pricing guidance, but the best you can hope to get at a yard sale is between 50% and 75% of what a comparable item sold for on eBay—eBay asking prices don't count.

Battery Savings

Save Money With a Battery Tester

Most people replace all the batteries in a battery-powered device when it stops working. But batteries do not all drain at the same rate, so you could be throwing out batteries that still have some juice in them.

Solution: Check batteries with a battery tester, and replace only the ones that are dead.

Good testers to consider: Amprobe BAT-250 ($6.25)…WeePro Universal Battery Tester ($5.85)…Gardner Bender GBT-500A ($13)… D-FantiX Digital Battery Tester ($11). All are available on Amazon.

Clark.com

Save Money With Rechargeable Batteries

They've come a long way in recent years and now make good financial and practical sense. Rechargeables can be used hundreds or even thousands of times and are at least as powerful as traditional batteries. And today's rechargeables won't lose power sitting on the shelf— they'll hold their charge for up to five years. Usually one rechargeable AA or AAA costs the same as four or five traditional batteries, but you can reuse it instead of throwing it away.

Best brands: Panasonic Eneloop Pro, Energizer, Amazon Basics and Ikea Ladda. What about the charger? Expect to pay as little as $10 for a four-battery model, $15 to $25 for an eight-battery, or up to $40 for an 18-battery setup. You'll often get a good deal on a charger when it's bundled into a battery purchase.

MoneyTalksNews.com

Or you can just ask yourself how low you're willing to go to make a sale and still be satisfied. Keep in mind that buyers love to haggle, so leave yourself some wiggle room.

To save time later, put a price sticker on each item as it goes into a box.

Important: If you have pristine collectibles or designer clothing, you might do better on eBay or a resale website such as Poshmark or TheRealReal. Yes, it takes more time to photograph and post items, but if raking in money is a priority, take a divide-and-conquer strategy—decide which items will be earmarked for the yard sale and which will be sold through more profitable sites.

GETTING THE WORD OUT

• **Not publicizing your yard sale well enough is a big mistake.** People often put up a few signs and leave it at that...or they take out a single ad, not realizing that there are many places to list yard sales for free. Postings on key websites bring in dealers and collectors, usually at the start of your sale, while strategically placed signs bring in people driving by throughout the day.

• **Online options.** You can post ads online as late as the night before your yard sale if you're unsure about the weather. *Consider these options...*

• Your local Patch online site, both for your town/area and those near you. Patch is a website that has news and events about your local area.

• Facebook groups. Join as many local yard sale or buy-sell groups as you can. When you join one or two, Facebook will suggest other groups to you. Always find out what a group's rules are before posting. Create ads to run at different times in different Facebook groups. I might post 10 different ads on Facebook the night before a sale. Sponsored ads that cost a few dollars may be worth it to target Facebook members who live within a certain distance of your location.

• Free yard-sale listing sites such as Gsalr.com, YardSaleSearch.com and GarageSaleFinder.com.

• Craigslist, not only under the category of yard/garage sales but also under all relevant categories of items you are selling. Place the ads a few days in advance, and give only your street, not your house number, to avoid aggressive people showing up on your doorstep prematurely.

• Church or local town e-newsletters or bulletins. Find out when ads are due and will appear in the bulletins to time these mentions.

Important: Check the weather forecast before you start actively advertising. If the chance of rain is better than 20%, consider postpon-

---

---

ing your sale for a week—rain definitely cuts down on buyers and makes it logistically difficult to hold a sale in your yard or driveway.

• **Craft your postings and ads carefully.** Be specific with a bulleted list of big and expensive items and items you have a lot of or that are unique or interesting. This will entice buyers looking for specific items as well as buyers who figure that you might have other good stuff even if they didn't see anything they wanted on your list.

Reminder: A picture is still worth 1,000 words—include individual photos of big items and group photos of smaller, interesting things in the ads and posts. E-mail your ad to all your local friends and neighbors to let them know about the sale.

•**Signs.** Scout out where you'll put signs as far in advance as you'd like, but don't actually place them until the day before or even the morning of your yard sale. If you live in a very rural area, you might put your first sign a few miles away. You'll need one at every turn along the most highly trafficked routes to your house.

Signs should be least 14 x 18 inches (but bigger is better). Stores such as The Home Depot, Lowe's and Staples sell corrugated plastic yard sale signs that hold up to rain and moisture better than cardboard and often come with a stake.

Make eye-catching signs by stapling fluorescent poster board onto them and writing with thick, waterproof markers. Use red for "YARD SALE" at the top, and draw a big red arrow to indicate the direction to your sale near the bottom. In between, use black (easier to read) to write your address on one line and the dates and times on another.

Early-bird buyers, especially dealers, often will show up 30 to 60 minutes before a sale starts. Keep that in mind so that you leave yourself enough time to stake signs and organize your tables well before the sale starts.

ON THE DAY OF YOUR SALE

•**Make your displays enticing.** Most items look best set out on tables. Cover your tables with cloths or plain fabric. Lightweight plastic shelves placed on tables increase your display area. Clothes look best (and will stay neater) when hung on rolling racks.

•**Refresh your displays as the day goes on.** Sometimes people gravitate to a certain area, making it a hot spot for sales—if so, move items to that area every time some get sold. Fill in any big empty spots as needed so

people won't assume that all the good stuff is gone. Move unneeded tables off to the side.

•**Know how to haggle.** Many buyers will try to negotiate the price. Don't take it personally if someone offers $3 for something you think is worth $10. You might accept $3 if you want to get rid of the item…suggest meeting in the middle at $6 or $7…or say, "I just dropped the price" or "I priced it low for quick sale and can't go any lower." Whatever decision you make, do it with a smile—people respond better when you're nice about it.

Avoid these money pitfalls…

•**Have $50 to $100 in small bills,** including plenty of singles, in advance. Invariably your first buyer will hand you a $20 for a $1 item!

•**Keep the doors to your home locked,** even if you have helpers, so that no one can sneak in when you're distracted.

•**Don't leave cash from your sales within anyone's reach,** and don't use a cash box. Instead, wear a fanny pack or a money pouch. Empty it inside your house periodically.

•**Get the money in hand before you help a "buyer" load up his car**—thieves will distract you and take off before you know what's happening.

The Newest Collectibles: Old iPhones, Boomboxes and More

Eric Bradley, vice president of editorial content at WorthPoint.com, the largest resource worldwide of antiques and collectibles pricing…and Valarie McLeckie, spokesperson and video-games consignment director for Heritage Auctions (HA.com), the largest collectibles auction house in the US. Bradley is author of a dozen books on collectibles, including *Picker's Pocket Guide: Toys.*

There are plenty of gadgets gathering dust in American attics that could fetch $50 to a few hundred dollars on eBay or Facebook Marketplace, including…

•**Early Apple computers.** There may not be an Apple 1 in your closet—only a few hundred of those were made. But the Apple II sold well in the late 1970s and early 1980s. And the Macintosh 128K—the original Mac—was popular in the mid-1980s, so you could easily own one. They won't bring life-changing money, but they could be worth enough to buy a brand-new Macintosh computer.

Examples: An Apple II with a low serial number sold for $7,155, and other Apple IIs bring $500 to $1,000.* Macintosh 128Ks often sell for $500 to $2,000, or as much as $5,000 with their original boxes.

•**Early Apple iPhones and iPods.** Apple's early phones and digital music players are collectible even though they're less than 20 years old.

Examples: First-generation iPhones, released in 2007, sell for between $40 and $350 depending on condition. Never-used ones sealed in their original packaging often go for around $8,000. First-generation Apple iPod 5GB music players, originally sold in 2001, can bring $150 to $400.

•**Video-game cartridges.** The value of old video games has skyrocketed in recent years, but generally it's only the games sealed in their original packages that generate big bucks. *Super Mario Bros.*, a 1985 game for the Nintendo Entertainment System, sold for $114,000 in 2020 because it was sealed in its original packaging and in mint condition—that game is worth around $10 if you have just the cartridge. If you have old video games, look them up on PriceCharting.com or GameValueNow.com to see if they're worth selling.

Examples: Donkey Kong Jr. Math for the Nintendo Entertainment System sold for around

---

*All prices in this article are for devices in working condition, unless otherwise noted. Nonworking examples might have some value but usually much less. Prices are from recent sales on eBay, at Heritage Auctions or from other auction sales.

$100 without packaging. *River Patrol* for the Atari 2600 sold for $770 without packaging.

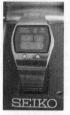 •**Digital wristwatches from the 1970s and 1980s.** Watch-collecting has been red hot lately, and not just classic luxury brands such as Rolex and Patek Philippe—early digital watches from Casio, Pulsar and Seiko are collected as well.

Examples: Hamilton Pulsar LED men's wristwatches, among the earliest digital wristwatches, can bring from $200 to $500 in working condition—potentially more if you have the original box. The Casio 79QS-39 digital watch often sells for $70 to $100...the Casio DBC-630 digital calculator watch, $90 to $130. The Seiko model 0634-5009 LCD sells for $100 to $350.

 •**Sony Walkman.** These famed portable music players might seem unnecessary now when you can choose from millions of digital songs to play on your phone, but collectors are paying hundreds of dollars for some vintage Walkman models.

Examples: The Walkman model TPS-L2, first sold in 1979, often brings $350 to $700 depending on condition—it's the model featured in the 2014 film *Guardians of the Galaxy*. The Walkman model WM-D6C, made from 1984 through 2002, can bring $200 to $600—or over $1,000 if you have one that's unused in its original packaging. Walkman models that play compact discs have begun to be collected as well—the Sony D-5 can bring around $200.

•**Handheld electronic games from the 1970s and early 1980s.** These battery-powered toys don't have video display screens, just LED lights that turn on and off during game play.

Examples: Mattel *Battlestar Galactica Space Alert*, a game that went on sale in 1978, fetches $20 to $60 depending on condition... or $100 or more with its original packaging. Coleco *Electronic Quarterback*, a handheld football game from 1978, brings $30 to $40 but can reach $60 to $130 with original packaging. *Pokédex*, a Pokémon-themed handheld electronic game, often sells for $40 to $60—or $100 to $250 if still sealed in its original packaging—even though it dates back to only 1999.

•**VHS tapes from the 1980s and 1990s.** Get ready for the next big collectible. Vintage VHS tapes are being graded and encapsulated in sealed, Lucite cases as movie buffs pre- serve a bit of nostalgia. These obsolete cassettes represent the first time a film could be watched outside of a theater. A new company called VHSDNA is leading the effort to grade boxes and tapes—sealed tapes are worth more than those that were opened and played—and they are bringing big bucks online. VHS copies of *Star Wars: Episode IV—A New Hope* are selling for more than $1,000...and a tape of *Star Wars: Episode V—The Empire Strikes Back* sold for $280.

•**Wood stereo speakers from the 1950s, 1960s and 1970s.** Buyers snap up old speakers that have stylish wooden cases, then replace the electronics inside with Bluetooth speakers. There also are some old speakers that are prized for their audio quality. Small "bookshelf" speakers made from mahogany, maple or teak are popular...old oversized speakers and oak construction are less desirable.

Examples: A pair of Pioneer CS-99A speakers from the 1970s recently sold for $1,500. A pair of Tandberg 112-7 speakers from the 1960s recently sold for $250.

•**Small kitchen appliances from the 1950s, 1960s and 1970s.** Cooking and baking have been popular hobbies of late. Some 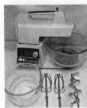 kitchen converts have begun seeking out gadgets from the kitchens of their childhood homes for nostalgic reasons. The devices in demand tend to be those that have distinctive retro styling.

VHS Tape Photo: Copyright © VHSDNA.

Examples: GE Spacemaker 10-Cup Coffeemakers from the 1970s sell for $30 to $80 depending on condition, or $150 to $200 for unused examples in their original packaging. Oster electric mixers and blenders from the 1970s and earlier can bring anywhere from $35 to $300 depending on model and condition.

•**Boomboxes from the late 1970s and early 1980s.** These portable-but-bulky cassette-tape player/radios are not an especially convenient way to listen to music, but they are an 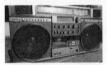 iconic item from their era, and certain models now are collected. Boomboxes that include compact disc players are less likely to be collected. The bigger and showier a boombox, the more likely it is to have value—especially if it's made by a respected manufacturer such as Sharp, Sanyo, Panasonic or Magnavox.

Examples: Panasonic RX-5500, which was first sold in 1979, now sells for $150 to $500. Sharp GF-8989, first sold in 1981, now sells for $150 to $250. Even nonfunctioning boomboxes can be worth around $50 or so—collectors try to fix them or use them for parts.

•**Portable radios and clock radios from the 1960s and 1970s.** Radios made by big-name electronics brands such as GE, Pana- 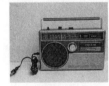 sonic, RCA and Sony tend to be especially desirable—but any radio that has a distinctive retro look might be collected.

Examples: Panasonic model RQ-831 recently sold for $125. GE Superadio model 7-2880B recently sold for $100. Weltron "Radio Ball" Model 2001 AM/FM 8-Track players from the 1970s sell for $200 to $500 depending on condition—collectors love their space-age styling.

14

Emotional Help

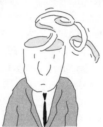

5 Surprising Causes of Hidden Stress...and How to Overcome Them

The way we treat our bodies—from how we move and eat...to the people, objects and energy surrounding us—has a direct impact on our stress response whether or not we realize it, promoting inflammation, accelerating aging and hindering the body's anti-stress efforts.

If we know where stress hides in our lives, then we can combat it. *Headaches and digestive issues are common, but here are five hidden sources of stress—and how to overcome them...*

***HIDDEN STRESSOR #1:* Poor foot biomechanics.** Feet are true taskmasters, keeping us moving while bearing the brunt of our weight. Poor foot biomechanics—the way the toes and feet function as they interact with our muscles and gravity—can reach up the body, making it hard for the other muscles and joints to work properly and leading to hip and back pain, poor balance and more. When feet are under stress, the whole body feels stress!

Ill-fitting shoes are a cause of stress in your feet, as are thick-soled shoes that prevent feet from receiving the stimulation they need to keep them strong and supple.

The fix: Walk barefoot. Feet are built to walk on varied terrain and need the stimulation that comes from that. Walking barefoot engages the bones, joints and dozens of muscles that work together to keep communications flowing through your body and improve your balance and feeling of stability.

Frank Lipman, MD, founder of Eleven Eleven Wellness Center and chief medical officer at The Well, both in New York City. He is author of six books including *The New Rules of Aging Well: A Simple Program for Immune Resilience, Strength, and Vitality.* DrFrankLipman.com

Even better: Walk barefoot outside. The subtle negative electromagnetic charge from grass, moist soil and sand helps balance the positive electromagnetic charge that builds up in the body from the stress of daily living.

Also: Stimulate and massage bare feet by rolling them over a tennis ball for five minutes a day. Strong, flexible feet translate into a strong, flexible body.

HIDDEN STRESSOR #2: **Nighttime eating.** Research shows that late eating puts stress on the brain and the body, both of which interpret the incoming calories as *Food is coming in…time to start producing energizing hormones.* That, in turn, interferes with sleep.

The fix: After consuming a healthful meal balanced with adequate protein, carbs and fat, stop eating by 8 pm. This will help lead your body toward restful sleep.

HIDDEN STRESSOR #3: **Clutter.** In a study in *Personality and Social Psychology Bulletin,* women who described their homes as "cluttered" or "disorganized" (as opposed to "peaceful" or "comforting") experienced cortisol levels that indicated chronic stress. Our brains like structure and order. Piles of paper and overflowing closets can hinder concentration and are linked with procrastination, both of which further contribute to stress.

The fix: Purge, hide and donate. If you have time to tackle only one area: Focus on your bedside table. It often becomes cluttered with books, tissues, beauty products and more. Seeing a big mess right before you go to sleep can cause your stress hormones to spike…precisely when you don't want them elevated.

HIDDEN STRESSOR #4: **Out-of-whack light and dark cycles.** Humans run on an internal 24-hour body clock that naturally syncs with the sun and moon. Morning light signals the brain to stop producing sleep-inducing *melatonin* and increase levels of energizing hormones. As darkness falls, melatonin production ramps up in preparation for sleep.

But modern life makes it easy to ignore these light and dark signals. Smartphone, tablet and TV screens emit a blue light that is similar to the color and wavelength of day-light. Looking at these screens at night tells the brain to stay awake.

The fallout: Poor sleep, which is linked to numerous stressors and impairment of the body's glymphatic system, which cleanses and clears the brain of toxins created throughout the day while you sleep. When these toxins accumulate, they can lead to cognitive decline and even Alzheimer's disease.

The fix: Expose yourself to bright light in the morning. Help reset your body clock by throwing open the curtains as soon as you wake up. Even better, step outside. As your eyes adjust to daylight, your hormones will program your internal clock to help energize you all day.

At night, power off screens by 10 pm and dedicate at least 30 minutes to a relaxing transition activity—take a warm bath, read a book, etc.

HIDDEN STRESSOR #5: **Stressful texts and e-mails.** Junk e-mail…unnecessary texts…robocalls—we've come to accept these intrusions as normal parts of modern life. But anything that makes you feel annoyed, angry or harassed triggers the same fight-or-flight hormonal stress response designed to propel you out of dangerous situations.

Surprising: Even happy texts can create stress if announced with a *Ding!* on your phone—it diverts your attention and creates a sense of anxious anticipation that won't dissipate until you check the text.

The fix: Unsubscribe! Turn off your phone's notifications so that you don't hear that ding every time a message arrives. Limit your time reading or watching upsetting news…or at least try to balance things by purposefully seeking out feel-good news at sites such as GreaterGood.Berkeley.edu

How to De-Stress Your Smile

The high stress of recent years has led to increased dental problems, including tooth grinding, jaw clenching, chipped and cracked teeth, and jaw pain.

Relieve jaw pain/spasms: Lightly hold (but don't bite) a pencil horizontally in your front teeth for about 20 minutes to loosen jaw muscles.

Prevent pain/strengthen jaw muscles: Place a thumb under your chin, and open your mouth, pushing against the thumb for five seconds...then try to close your mouth while pushing your chin down to keep it from closing.

Relax your jaw at bedtime/reduce night-time clenching: Close your eyes, press your tongue against the roof of your mouth, and breathe deeply through your nose for several minutes.

Helpful: An ergonomic desk chair supports your back and encourages good posture, reducing muscle stress in your shoulders, head and neck, which will relieve stress in the jaw.

Real Simple. RealSimple.com

Stress Buster: It's Your Heart—Not Your Brain

Leah Lagos, PsyD, licensed clinical psychologist Board Certified in Biofeedback (BCB) who specializes in health and performance psychology in New York City. She is author of *Heart Breath Mind: Train Your Heart to Conquer Stress and Achieve Success.* DrLeahLagos.com

No matter how much stress you had in your life before 2020, the pandemic has put everyone on edge. If you're like most people, you may have relied on one or more of the go-to approaches to tamping down that stress—mental imagery, journaling, knitting, reading a novel...you name it.

What you may not realize: The most widely used calming activities are based on the belief that stress lives in your brain, and if you can just think your way through it or distract yourself from it, it will improve.

But here's a secret that can revolutionize the way you deal with stress—it actually lives in your body, not in your brain. To tap into your body's hidden calming capacities, one of the

most effective self-regulation approaches is to train your heart rate variability (HRV).

Here's what you need to know about training your heart to ease day-to-day stress...

WHAT IS HEART RATE VARIABILITY?

Most people think that the heart beats with the regularity of a metronome. But the truth is, when you inhale, your heart rate naturally quickens...and when you exhale, it slows down. The result is a slight variation in the time between heartbeats—so slight that it's measured in milliseconds.

The degree to which the heart rate accelerates on inhalation and decelerates on exhalation varies from person to person. The more variation you have in those intervals—your HRV—the better. Too little variation suggests a condition called *sympathetic dominance*, meaning that the nervous system is essentially stuck in fight-or-flight mode. Sympathetic dominance is all too common today.

The goal is to balance the sympathetic nervous system and parasympathetic nervous system—the "rest and digest" or "tend and befriend" branch that handles day-to-day vitals such as digestion, along with helping the body relax and de-stress. When balanced, HRV is high, reflecting a strong ability to tolerate and bounce back from stress.

THE GOOD NEWS ABOUT HRV

Just as HRV responds to everyday life's stressors, it also can be significantly improved by strengthening your parasympathetic nervous system to assist your body in handling stress.

Result: Higher HRV...improved health and longevity...and a happier you.

In addition to mental and emotional resilience, high HRV is linked to a host of health benefits, including reduced blood pressure, improved cardiovascular health, lower rates of depression and more. In fact, research has shown that HRV is a more accurate predictor of future cardiac events in people who don't have heart disease than cholesterol, blood pressure or resting heart rate.

To track your HRV, you can use an HRV sensor, which usually comes as a chest-strap monitor...a fitness tracker, some of which

Exercise Eases Stress and Anxiety

Regular Aerobic Exercise Fights Stress Best

Walking, running, biking and/or swimming at least a few times a week much more effectively strengthens the brain's resilience when stressful events occur than non-aerobic exercise such as weight lifting. And regular workouts are much better than any form of exercise done only when a stressful event occurs—such as doing a 10-mile run the day before something stressful is anticipated. An ongoing exercise regimen leads to an increase in the protein *galanin*, which promotes behavioral resilience after stress occurs. Higher galanin levels do not reduce immediate feelings of stress, but they help the body cope with its impact more effectively.

Study by researchers at Emory University School of Medicine, Atlanta, published in *Journal of Neuroscience*.

Exercise Away Your Anxiety

According to a recent finding, participants in a 12-week exercise program that included a 60-minute training session three times a week, including strength-training and aerobic exercises, had improved anxiety levels. Most participants reported going from a moderate or high level of anxiety to a low level. Those who did moderate exercise were three times as likely to report fewer and less severe symptoms of anxiety…and those who exercised strenuously, nearly five times as likely.

Study by researchers at University of Gothenburg, Sweden, published in *Journal of Affective Disorders*.

have a wristband embedded with a sensor…or a fingerprint-scanning app.

Even though it can be interesting to have an exact measurement, most people can safely assume that they need to improve their HRV. The breath-pacing exercises below are easy and highly effective for most people.

WAYS TO BOOST YOUR HRV

Increasing evidence shows that HRV can help anyone improve his/her physical and mental health—often by practicing for 20 minutes twice a day for four weeks. After 10 weeks of practicing at this frequency, you'll develop a reflex that kicks in during moments of stress to help you reset and recover. *Here's how…*

STEP 1: **Change your breathing.** Instead of breathing at a rate of 12 breaths per minute—as most adults do—slow it down. Breathing at a rate of approximately six breaths per minute triggers a systemwide relaxation response.

Inhale through your nose for four counts, filling your belly with air, and exhale for six counts through pursed lips, as if you're blowing on hot soup. Belly breathing stimulates the parasympathetic nerve receptors found in the lower lungs, helping to spread a sense of calm throughout the body and mind. When you breathe only into your chest, those lower-lung receptors go untouched.

Start with 10 minutes twice a day.

Helpful: Try a free app, such as *Awesome Breathing*. For maximum benefits, work your way up to 20 minutes twice a day. Don't try this while reading, watching TV or listening to music. For best results, forgo other sources of stimulation and enjoy the feeling of your breath.

Fascinating research: Reciting the "Ave Maria" or a mantra can slow breathing to almost precisely six breath cycles per minute, according to a study published in *BMJ*. This may be one reason why people find the recitation of these words to be calming—it improves HRV.

STEP 2: **Don't skimp on cardiovascular exercise.** Cardiovascular fitness and HRV are strongly correlated—the fitter your heart, the higher your HRV. Follow the guidelines for physical activity—150 minutes per week of moderate-intensity aerobic exercise (challenging enough that you can carry on a conversation but not sing) or 75 minutes per week of vigorous-intensity aerobic activity (you can't say more than a few words without having to catch your breath).

Helpful: Try to incorporate some high-intensity interval training (HIIT) workouts, which alternate quick, intense bursts of cardio exercise with periods of low-intensity activity. Research shows that HIIT has even better potential for improving your body's response to stress because alternating the intensity of your workout challenges your nervous system. Start out with a 1:2 ratio—run for one minute then walk for two, and repeat…or go all-out on the elliptical for 30 seconds, then slow down for a minute, and repeat. Most people can aim for a 10- to 20-minute HIIT session.

STEP 3: **Practice "emotional pivoting."** The next time you're feeling stressed—after a difficult conversation with a coworker, for example—try this mind-body strategy. Think back to a time in your life when you felt an incredible amount of love, gratitude, awe and/or safety. Take 10 breaths, focusing on the positive experience as you inhale for four counts through your nose. Really try to connect to the memory, almost as if you're reliving it. Exhale through your mouth for six seconds, releasing any anxiety, stress or fear along with your breath. Do this for about five minutes after a stressful situation. With practice, this can help improve your HRV, allowing you to easily pivot away from negative emotional states.

STEP 4: **Limit those cups of joe.** Getting too much caffeine—for example, three or more cups of coffee a day—can reduce HRV. That's because excess caffeine stimulates the sympathetic nervous system.

Helpful: Consider swapping your coffee for green tea. It has less caffeine than coffee, so it's energizing without feeling overly stimulating. Green tea also contains an active compound called *L-theanine*, which can boost your HRV by increasing production of various calming neurochemicals while lowering levels of stress-producing brain chemicals.

STEP 5: **Try cold therapy.** Exposure to a cold temperature can increase HRV. Though no one knows exactly why, it's often attributed to a physiological survival mechanism called the "diving reflex," which kicks in when a person dives into cold water. The body responds to this sudden underwater immersion by conserving oxygen (via decreased heart rate) and prioritizing blood flow to the heart and brain. Don't worry—you don't need to sign up for a local polar bear plunge. You can trigger the diving reflex by splashing very cold water on your forehead, cheeks and nose. Try this before your breathing practice to jump-start your HRV.

The Dopamine Dilemma: Wanting What We Don't Have

Daniel Z. Lieberman, MD, professor and vice chair for clinical affairs in the Department of Psychiatry and Behavioral Sciences at George Washington University, Washington, D.C. He is the author of *The Molecule of More*.

Anyone who has made a large purchase, fallen in love, or overeaten at a party knows that humans face a perpetual pull between what we want and how we feel once we have it. Dopamine is the brain chemical that induces pleasure when you are *pursuing* things, but it offers no such benefits once you have them. In fact, part of its role is to make you dissatisfied with the present, so you'll be motivated to work harder to improve the future.

Let's take a closer look at this lesser-understood chemical.

DOPAMINE WANTS MORE

The dopamine desire circuit is a system in your brain that constantly scans the environment for new resources that will improve your chances of surviving and keeping your DNA replicating. As such, its primary focus is food, sex, and the ability to win competitions.

When the circuit finds something potentially valuable, dopamine floods the brain and creates feelings of pleasure, desire, and excitement to convey the message, "You desperately need this!" Whether you actually need something in the moment is irrelevant because dopamine is entirely focused on stockpiling resources for the future.

It's like a person at the beginning of the pandemic who stockpiled toilet paper. No one needed or enjoyed having 200 rolls of TP, but dopamine insisted that it was important to have just in case. Dopamine does the same thing with all sorts of resources. It can make your perfectly good house seem inadequate. It can make a new acquaintance seem more interesting and desirable than a current partner. It can make space for a third piece of cake even though you feel uncomfortably full.

The cruelty of the dopamine desire circuit is that as soon as you get what it told you that you wanted, its job is done and dopamine levels plummet—along with those feelings of desire and excitement. Buyer's remorse, the sinking feeling of regret that occurs after making a big purchase, is a perfect example of a dopamine drop.

Wanting and liking are produced by two different systems in the brain, so enjoying things once we have them requires finding balance between dopamine and the here-and-now chemicals. (More on that shortly.)

OVERACTIVE DOPAMINE CIRCUITS

Some people have more active dopaminergic circuits than others, which can make finding that balance more difficult. People with elevated activity in the dopamine desire circuit can become trapped in an endless cycle of chasing the buzz and fall prey to compulsive spending, hypersexuality, gambling, or even becoming addicted to drugs, which provide an intense dopamine rush. (One in six people who take *levodopa* [L-Dopa], a Parkinson's disease drug that replaces missing dopamine, has a similar response.)

Others have too much activity in the dopamine control circuit. The dopamine *desire* circuit gives us urges, while the dopamine *control* circuit, when working properly, gives us the ability to manage those urges and guide them toward profitable ends. The latter lets us imagine the future to see the potential consequences of decisions we might make right now, and it gives us the ability to plan how to make that imaginary future a reality.

But when people have an overactive dopamine control circuit, they can become addicted to achievement. For them, life is about the future, improvement, and innovation—at the expense of being able to experience the joys of the present. This can cause people to neglect their emotions, abandon empathy, and miss out on enjoying the present. If you ignore your emotions, they become less sophisticated

over time and may devolve into anger, greed, and resentment. If you neglect empathy, you lose the ability to make others feel happy. Living for the future can also rob you of the pleasure of the sensory world around you. Instead of enjoying the beauty of a flower, you can imagine only how it would look in a vase.

FINDING HARMONY

Dopamine naturally decreases as we age, so part of successful aging is transitioning to the here-and-now chemicals. Just as too much dopamine is detrimental, too little is problematic as well. Without adequate dopamine, you lose motivation and drive, and no longer experience excitement at the prospect of a brighter future. *There are many ways to balance dopamine with the here-and-now neurotransmitters…*

• **Master a skill.** Mastery is the ability to extract the maximum reward from a particular set of circumstances. That satisfies dopamine and causes it to pause for a little bit and let the here-and-now neurotransmitters shine. You can gain mastery over a game, a sport, an art, a musical instrument, or anything else that you enjoy.

• **Pay attention to what you are doing in the moment.** By spending time in the present, we take in sensory information about the reality we live in, which allows the dopamine system to use that information to develop plans that maximize rewards. That's dopamine and the here-and-now neurotransmitters working together. Further, when something interesting activates the dopamine system, if you shift your focus outward, the increased level of attention makes the sensory experience more intense. Being in nature is particularly beneficial because it's complex, has unexpected patterns, and there is a virtually limitless amount of detail to explore.

• **Download a meditation app.** You can strengthen your ability to be in the present with practice. It's like lifting weights. In fact, brain scans show that parts of the brain are thicker in people who meditate.

• **Create.** Because it is always new, creation is one of the best dopaminergic pleasures. Satisfy both your dopamine and you're here-and-now chemicals with activities like woodworking, knitting, painting, decorating, sewing, and using adult coloring books.

• **Fix things.** Solving problems by fixing things is a dopaminergic activity, but it also leads to a satisfying solution in the present. Plus, learning to fix your own broken appliances or other objects boosts your sense of self-efficacy and saves money.

How to Get Through Any Crisis and Come Out Stronger

Jennifer Love, MD, and Kjell Tore Hovik, PsyD, PhD. Dr. Love is board-certified in psychiatry, addiction psychiatry, and addiction medicine. She is currently in group practice with Amen Clinics. Dr. Hovik, a clinical neuropsychologist, is an associate professor of psychology at the Inland Norway University of Applied Sciences and editor-in-chief of *Nevropsykologi,* the peer-reviewed journal of the Norwegian Neuropsychological Society.

When you're in the throes of a crisis—whether it's a pandemic, the loss of a loved one, or a major life change—you may feel overwhelmed, stressed, and even physically unwell. The crisis may consume your every waking moment, making it hard to see a path forward.

Jennifer Love, MD, and Kjell Hovik, PsyD, PhD, have developed a process that will help you manage any crisis—and emerge even stronger. In their book *When Crisis Strikes: 5 Steps to Heal Your Brain, Body, and Life from Chronic Stress*, they describe five strategies and explore how different people (themselves included) applied the process to deal with a wide variety of intensely stressful situations, from chronic illness, depression, and cognitive decline to cancer chronic pain and addiction. They share stories of people who have overcome abusive parents, mass shootings, bullying, suicide, and sexual abuse.

Here's a look at those five steps…

STEP 1: Get a Grip.

Your brain and body are wired to respond to stress quickly, not to pause and deal with complex threats. Step one is about learning how to override your brain's automatic tendency to freak out. It challenges you to identify what your life crisis is triggering from deep within you and to unearth past experiences that may be amplifying your physical and emotional response to your current situation.

Think of your crisis as a meteor landing in a sandy field. The meteor is the main problem, but it's surrounded and hidden by a cloud of sand and dust made of the multitude of thoughts and threats that swirl around you when you're dealing with a crisis. You have to make your way through the chaos to identify and focus on the core problem before you can begin to solve it.

To do that, you can practice using attentional focus (which is often called mindfulness) to train yourself to deal with the chaos by choosing which thoughts to quiet and which to pay attention to.

It can help to write down key words and descriptions. The physicality of writing and creating something on the outside to mirror a thought or feeling on the inside can help you better "see" a problem. From there, you can begin to examine the thinking behind the emotions generated by the problem.

STEP 2: Pinpoint What You Can Control.

In a crisis, it may feel like nothing is within your control, so it can be easier to do this exercise in reverse. Identify what is *beyond* your control. Let's use illness as an example. If your spouse has been diagnosed with a serious illness, you can't control the diagnosis or how your partner responds to it. So think about how you can manage the things you can't control. This step involves pinpointing options, not committing to acting on them. You are training your brain to step beyond reacting to your crisis. You are designing a measure of control over your circumstances. You may consider attending a support group or researching specialty medical centers.

Once you eliminate what you can't control, you can shift your focus on where your energies are better spent. Think about things you can control, such as what you eat, what time you go to bed, and whether you get out of the house to spend time with friends or to exercise.

STEP 3: Push into Motion.

Next, you need to find your inner motivation to take whatever action you need to move forward. If your crisis is job loss, that action might be moving to another state with more opportunity. If your crisis is depression, it might be seeing a therapist.

If you're finding it difficult to commit to a decision, try this exercise. Divide a piece of paper into four quadrants. Label one "Benefits of Action," one "Consequences of Action," one "Benefits of Inaction," and one "Consequences of Inaction." Fill in the boxes with any and every argument; then highlight the three most important items on the page. This exercise will give you a powerful visual image of what is most important to you.

Next, break down the tasks you need to accomplish into easy and tough actions. The true test of whether you are ready to push into motion and move on to the next steps is whether you can start doing easy actions on a daily basis.

If you're not ready, don't worry. You might need to spend more time on step one, find more easy actions to start with, or reach out to a friend or therapist for help and support. Once you've completed your easy tasks, you'll be better prepared to deal with the tougher challenges.

STEP 4: Pull Back.

Step Four is about finding balance, so that despite our life crisis, our emotional responses can be appropriate for what is going on in the moment. Ruminating on past events and worrying about the future won't solve a medical problem or save you from financial troubles, but stopping the worrying in this moment will offer a much-needed respite from overthinking.

Once you've practiced being in the here and now, reflect on these questions…

• **How am I adding stress to my life?**

• **Which of my daily habits and routines are healthy, and which are too complicated or stressful?**

• **How am I willing to simplify these habits and routines?**

• **What is important in my life, and are my actions aligned with that?**

Be honest in your reflections and kind in how you treat yourself. Shame and self-judgment lead to isolation and depression, but curiosity creates a space where change becomes possible.

STEP 5: Hold On and Let Go.

In this step, you work on cultivating the personality traits, characteristics, relationships, and lifestyle choices that you want in your life moving forward.

Before there was a crisis and before you grew up, there was a time in your life when you were young at heart, with infinite possibilities and few responsibilities. What positive qualities do you think of when you reflect on that time? Humor, curiosity, playfulness, intensity, orderliness, correctness, mischievousness, generosity?

Step Five is also a time to let go of the things that don't support your well-being: unhealthy thinking patterns, grudges, or personality traits that prevent you from being the person you want to be.

Seeking Mental Health Services

Charles B. Inlander, consumer advocate, healthcare consultant and author or coauthor of more than 20 consumer-health books.

In addition to the tragic loss of life caused by COVID-19, the pandemic has taken an enormous toll on our mental health. Few people have ever experienced anything close to the stress, anxiety, and restrictions this dreadful virus has brought to us all. The worry of contracting the disease, the isolation from family and friends, and the fear of being exposed in public settings have changed all our lives in ways we never anticipated.

Studies show the pandemic has caused a major uptick in mental health problems. Doctors report many of their patients are suffering from mild to severe depression and anxiety because of the pandemic. Fear has caused many of us to avoid necessary medical tests, such as mammograms, prostate screenings, and even routine blood work. Many of us feel helpless in these very trying times.

But there is help available. No matter where you may live, mental health services are available to help you get through this (or any) difficult period. These services may be as close as your computer or telephone, located at a nearby hospital or associated with a church or other religious-based organization. Some are free services, others may have fees, and many are covered by Medicare or Medicaid or your private health insurance.

Here's how to find mental health services...

• **Start with your primary care physician.** Your primary care doctor is a good starting point. Frankly discuss what you are feeling. Ask for suggestions or referrals to the best mental health professionals in your area that might be appropriate for your needs. Don't be surprised if the doctor suggests a non-physician such as a licensed social worker, psychologist, guidance counselor, or stress management classes run by county or municipal health departments.

• **Widen your search.** There are many possible sources of counseling and stress manage-

ment you should check out. Many people turn to their pastor, rabbi, or other religious leaders for counseling. You may also find services at locally run senior centers. Check with your local Department of Welfare or Area Agency on Aging (most counties have one) for a list of available services. Go online or have someone search for mental health services in your area.

• **Seeking specialized help.** There are numerous mental health support programs when you may be suffering from severe stress or anxiety. Call 911 if you are feeling suicidal and you'll be connected to a trained professional to help you. There are special services for veterans that can be accessed through the Veterans Administration and/or county government. These services can be found online. Search for "mental health services in your community."

When Depression Drugs Don't Work

Stephen S. Ilardi, PhD, an associate professor of clinical psychology at the University of Kansas, and the author of *The Depression Cure: The Six-Step Program to Beat Depression Without Drugs*.

Since World War II, the rate of clinical depression, also called *major depressive disorder*, has risen tenfold. It's not surprising, then, that about one in eight Americans takes a daily antidepressant.

For many of those people, though, antidepressants just aren't effective enough. In the largest "real-world" study of antidepressants—one that looked at more than 4,000 patients—fewer than 10% of those taking an antidepressant experienced complete remission that lasted longer than a year. Antidepressants can also deliver a slew of common side effects, like headaches, dry mouth, insomnia, digestive upset, sexual problems, weight gain, and fatigue.

Healing depression typically requires combating the disease from several different angles at once—and the following non-drug methods have particularly strong scientific support.

EXERCISE

This is the single most powerful tool we have for overcoming depression, probably because it affects so many systems in the body: It regulates neurotransmitters, improves sleep, and decreases brain inflammation, to name just a few. It's not an exaggeration to say that if all of the benefits of exercise could be packaged in one pill, it would instantly become the most useful overall medication in our psychiatric armamentarium.

Based on the best research, just 30 minutes of brisk, aerobic walking three times a week is usually effective. There is some evidence that boosting the exercise "dose" may carry even greater antidepressant benefits. If your depression makes it hard to exercise, a personal trainer, friend, or loved one who can walk with you regularly can help you start and keep up with this depression-busting habit.

DIET, FISH OIL, AND FIBER

The Mediterranean diet, which emphasizes fish, vegetables, fruits, beans, whole grains, nuts, seeds, and olive oil, fights depression, likely because it controls inflammation. (The inflamed brain is usually a depressed brain.) You can also fight inflammation—and depression—with 1,000 to 2,000 daily milligrams of eicosapentaenoic acid (EPA), a powerful omega-3 molecule derived from fish oil. To

avoid the dreaded "fishy burps," buy pharmaceutical grade, enteric-coated fish oil and store it in the freezer. Take your pill with a meal.

The Mediterranean diet also delivers high levels of plant fiber, which encourages the growth of healthy microbes in the gut, preventing or reversing dysbiosis, an imbalance of good and bad gut bacteria that has been linked to both depression and anxiety. To get even more fiber, take a soluble fiber supplement, such as psyllium husk or chicory root, at a dose of 5 to 7 grams each day. Cutting-edge research suggests we can also boost beneficial, depression-fighting gut microbes with probiotic supplements, especially those that feature lacto and bifido bacterial strains.

Caution: If you have a gastrointestinal problem such as irritable bowel syndrome or ulcerative colitis, talk to a gastroenterologist before taking fiber or a probiotic.

ACETYL-L-CARNITINE (ALC)

This brain-produced nutritional compound supplies energy to brain cells (neurons). ALC levels are often low in people with depression, particularly those over age 40. Several studies show that supplementing the diet with 2,000 mg of ALC can produce anti-depressive results comparable to medication, but with effects that kick in faster (about a week, as compared to four to six weeks for medications) and with minimal adverse side effects.

BRIGHT LIGHT

If your depression starts in the fall or winter, when the days are shorter, you may have seasonal affective disorder, which is best treated with bright light therapy. The eye is an outpost of the brain, and light works like a drug, resetting your body clock and normalizing the natural sleep-wake cycle (the circadian rhythm) for better mood, sleep, and appetite. Research also shows that light boxes are beneficial for anyone with depression, at any time of year.

To get the benefits of light therapy for depression, you need about 30 minutes of exposure to 10,000 lux, a unit of illumination, within an hour of waking up. It's important to read the manufacturer's instructions and use a measuring tape to make sure you're sitting at

---

EASY TO DO...

Shedding Light on Therapy Boxes

Researchers who study the benefits of light therapy use devices that emit 10,000 lux, a measurement of how much light falls on a surface, at a distance of about 20 inches. To attain the benefits seen in research, consumers need light therapy devices that are comparable.

Three commercial devices studied were close to the quality used in clinical trials. These larger units are preferred as a first-line approach to bright-light therapy because they provide the most power, the least glare, and give you more freedom to do other things during the session to make it less burdensome.

- **SunRay II** (The SunBox Company, Sunbox.com)
- **NorthStar 10,000** (Alaska Northern Lights, AlaskaNorthernLights.com)
- **Day-Light Classic** (Carex Health Brands, Carex.com)

For people who prefer smaller devices, three met our standards if used closer and with less movement.

- **BOXelite** (Northern Light Technologies, NorthernLightTechnologies.com)
- **Day-Light Sky** (Carex Health Brands)
- **Sun Touch Plus** (Nature Bright Company, NatureBright.com)

We also identified two promising visors that allow users to move around freely.

- **Feel Bright Light** (Physician Engineered Products, PEPonline.com)
- **SolarMax Light Visor** (BioBrite, BioBrite.com)

Paul H. Desan, MD, PhD, is an assistant professor of psychiatry at Yale University.

---

the correct distance to get the full brightness. Sitting too far away can reduce or eliminate the benefits of light therapy. (See the sidebar above for tips on choosing the best box.)

SPEND TIME WITH PEOPLE

Social connection is a key component of overcoming depression, but when you're depressed, your brain tells you to stay away from people. It also says they don't want to be around you, anyway. That's the disease talking: Disregard the message and spend time with friends and family members in shared activities that you enjoy. For the 25% to 30% of depressed people who don't have supportive friends or family, a psychotherapist or therapy group can provide that type of support. You can also build connections by taking classes or participating in organized or informal group activities. Try Meetup.com to find groups of people who are interested in things that you are.

STOP RUMINATING

Nonstop negative, anxious thinking about the past or the future creates a runaway stress response that worsens depression. To stop ruminating, you need to first notice that you are doing it, and then focus your attention elsewhere.

Cognitive-behavioral therapy and mindfulness-based stress reduction are excellent tools in this process.

A rumination log can help, too. Every hour or so, note whether or not you've been ruminating. Over time, you'll develop a spontaneous "mental alarm" that will alert you any time your thoughts take a ruminative turn—and stop them.

Nitrous Oxide May Improve Symptoms of Treatment-Resistant Depression

In a small study, breathing the anesthetic drug, commonly called laughing gas, with oxygen for one hour significantly improved symptoms, and the benefits lasted for several weeks. The most common side effect was nausea. Nitrous oxide binds to N-methyl-D-aspartate glutamate receptors on neurons, as does ketamine, another anesthetic drug that is being widely studied for its antidepressant effects.

Charles R. Conway, MD, professor of psychiatry, Washington University School of Medicine in St. Louis, Missouri.

sponsibly, perhaps tapering is not the wiser strategy. The risks and benefits of ongoing therapy for the individual patient should be regularly evaluated.

If the decision is made to taper, it must be done gradually and with support. An occasional 20-minute office visit with a doctor is not enough. Additional oversight should be provided by psychologists specializing in pain management, social workers and/or other trained caregivers.

Also: The doctors may have to slow or suspend the tapering process if the patient starts experiencing distress.

Also: Family members should ask their loved one's health-care providers to teach them how to identify opioid overdoses and administer naloxone, an effective opioid-overdose treatment.

Beware the Mental Health Risks of Tapering Opioids

Alicia Agnoli, MD, assistant professor of family and community medicine at UC Davis School of Medicine and lead author of the study "Association of Dose Tapering with Overdose or Mental Health Crisis Among Patients Prescribed Long-Term Opioids," published in *Journal of the American Medical Association.* UCDavis.edu

The dangers of long-term opioid use are well-documented—addiction, overdose, bone fractures, heart attacks and more. But new research shows that the seemingly sensible step of gradually reducing opioid doses dramatically increases the odds of a mental health crisis including major depressive and anxiety-related events and suicide attempts. Tapering off opioids also significantly increases overdose risk, perhaps because patients who are struggling with smaller doses sometimes compensate by taking illicitly obtained opioids.

What to do: Patients prescribed long-term opioids—such as *hydrocodone* and *oxycodone* (Percocet)—and their doctors should weigh the risks of continued opioid use against those of tapering. If the patient has used opioids re-

Obsessive Compulsive Disorder Breakthrough

James Greenblatt, MD, chief medical officer at Walden Behavioral Care in Waltham, Massachusetts, and assistant clinical professor of psychiatry at Tufts University School of Medicine and Dartmouth College Geisel School of Medicine. He is the founder of Psychiatry Redefined, as educational platform dedicated to the transformation of psychiatry.

It's human nature to have occasional worried thoughts or to overanalyze important decisions. Normally, these thought patterns dissipate quickly, but in people suffering from obsessive compulsive disorder (OCD), letting go of repetitive thoughts isn't so effortless. Instead, relentless ideas, impulses, or images inundate the brain, mentally imprisoning the individual in recurrent, irrational thought patterns.

These senseless obsessions often drive the individual to ritualistic behaviors or compulsions—like handwashing, hoarding, counting or hairpulling—in an attempt to temporarily relieve their anxiety. A person with OCD staggers through life with a sense of powerlessness—fully aware the behavior is abnormal, but unable to stop.

> ## An Undertreated Ailment
>
> OCD is the fourth most common psychiatric illness in the United States. In fact, it's estimated that OCD is more common than diabetes. But in spite of its prevalence, it is underdiagnosed and undertreated—with more than half of people receiving no treatment at all.

TREATMENTS MISS THE ROOT CAUSE

There are two standard treatment options: selective serotonin reuptake inhibitors (SSRIs) and cognitive behavioral therapy (CBT). But even with these two treatments, only one out of five patients experiences complete recovery from OCD, and relapse is common. The reason for this failure: Conventional treatments don't address the root cause of OCD.

INFLAMMATION AND OCD

Inflammation is a natural feature of the immune system. When there is a virus, bacteria, or other foreign invader, the immune system activates to neutralize the threat, producing the telltale redness, swelling, heat, and pain that are the signs of acute inflammation. But an immune system that is out of balance can generate low-grade, chronic inflammation—including inflammation in the brain (neuroinflammation). In the brain, cytokines produce an enzyme called IDO (indoleamine 2,3 dioxygenase). IDO decreases the level of serotonin, the neurotransmitter that regulates mood and anxiety. (Every medication approved for OCD works by increasing serotonin levels.)

Along with this biochemical understanding, there is a growing body of clinical and scientific evidence that immune dysregulation underlies OCD. Psychiatrists know that autoimmune disease—when the immune system attacks the body as if it were a foreign invader—is rampant among those with OCD. For example, a 2021 study in the *International Journal of Environmental Research and Public Health* showed that people with OCD had triple the risk of developing the autoimmune illness Sjogren's Syndrome than the non-OCD population.

Researchers have identified two other neuroinflammatory disorders that play a role in OCD: pediatric autoimmune neuropsychiatric disorder associated with streptococcus (PANDAS) and pediatric acute-onset neuropsychiatric syndrome (PANS). In PANDAS, children who have had a streptococcal infection go on to rapidly develop OCD, practically overnight, because the immune system attacks the part of the brain (basal ganglia) where OCD is thought to originate. In PANS, other types of infections, such as Lyme disease, mononucleosis, and the flu, are also thought to quickly trigger OCD.

NUTRITIONAL SUPPORT

Along with neuroinflammation, a number of other factors affect serotonin levels, including genes, diet, stress, and neurotoxins. Those factors can be directly affected by nutritional therapy—a key treatment for OCD that is overlooked by conventional psychiatry.

Integrative psychiatrists, on the other hand, are open to both conventional and natural treatments for OCD. (You can find a list of integrative psychiatrists at PsychiatryRedefined. org/directory.)

ANTI-OCD SUPPLEMENTS

An integrative psychiatrist may recommend one or more of the following commonly used supplements. *Always talk to your physician before taking any new supplements...*

- **5HTP.** 5-hydroxtryptophan is a precursor of serotonin that has provided relief for many patients with OCD. The typical dose is 100 to 300 milligrams (mg). In some cases, doses as high as 600 mg may be needed.

- **Vitamin B12.** A deficiency of this serotonin-boosting B vitamin is common in OCD. Although most conventional doctors consider blood levels between 200 to 1,100 picograms per millilitre (pg/mL) normal, any level under 500 pg/mL should be considered low. If a patient is low, a weekly intramuscular B12 injection until the blood level reaches 900 pg/mL can be effective. Some patients experience a dramatic decrease in symptoms with just this treatment.

- **Folate.** This B vitamin is crucial in the manufacture of serotonin, and it can boost the effectiveness of antidepressants. However, some people with OCD can't metabolize folate because of a genetic abnormality. If you have OCD, consider having a methylenetetrahydro-

The Little-Known Neurotoxin That Can Trigger OCD

The toxic gut bacteria *Clostridia* can generate 3-(3-hydroxyphenyl)-3-hydroxypropionic acid (HPHPA), a compound that disrupts normal brain function. High levels of HPHPA are a feature of many psychiatric diseases, including OCD. Your doctor can order a urine test for HPHPA from a laboratory that specializes in digestive disorders, such as the Great Plains Laboratory. If HPHPA is detected, consider high-dose probiotics that supply 50 to 300 billion colony-forming units daily. You might also need to take an antibiotic, such as *vancomycin* (Vancocin).

folate reductase mutations (MTHFR) test to see if you lack the enzymes to process folate. If the test is positive, you may need to take one to 15 grams of folate daily.

•**Zinc.** This mineral is a crucial cofactor in the production of serotonin. A zinc deficiency also can have a number of other negative consequences for health, such as depression, poor metabolism of essential fatty acids, lower melatonin, more vulnerability to stress, and digestive difficulties. Consider a dose of 30 mg daily.

•**Inositol.** In some patients, supplementing with inositol—a vitamin-like compound that affects the serotonin receptors on cells—is the only treatment needed for OCD. Consider taking 5 to 10 grams (g) daily, starting off with 1 g and increasing by 1 g weekly. Taking too much inositol too quickly can cause gastrointestinal discomfort.

•**Omega-3 fatty acids.** The brain is 60% fat, and optimal brain function requires healthy fats such as the omega-3 fatty acids eicosapentaenoic acid (EPA) and *docosahexaenoic acid* (DHA) found in fish oil. Consider a daily supplement containing 3 grams of omega-3 fatty acids with a slightly higher ratio of EPA to DHA.

•**N-acetylcysteine (NAC).** This compound is a derivative of the amino acid cysteine and helps produce glutathione, a powerful anti-inflammatory antioxidant. In a study published in the *Journal of Clinical Psychopharmacology*, 36 women with OCD who didn't respond to serotonin-boosting medication were divided into two groups: One group took NAC daily and one group took a placebo. A total of 53% of the NAC group had significant improvement in OCD symptoms, compared with 15% of the placebo group. Consider taking 2 to 3 g of NAC daily.

•**Glycine.** This compound is a precursor to glutamine and gamma aminobutyric acid (GABA), two calming neurotransmitters that can inhibit obsessive thinking. Consider taking 3 to 6 g of glycine daily.

•**Vitamin D.** This vitamin can lower neuroinflammation. Your doctor can test you for vitamin D deficiency (blood level below 30 nanograms per milliliter [ng/ml]). If you're deficient, take 2,000 to 4,000 international units (IU) of vitamin D daily to bring levels to at least 50 ng/ml.

•**Magnesium.** To cool inflammation, take 400 to 800 mg of magnesium citrate or glycinate daily, divided into two or three doses.

LIFESTYLE SUPPORT

Several lifestyle factors can also affect OCD...

•**Poor sleep.** Treat insomnia with improved sleep hygiene. Go to bed at the same time every night and get up at the same time every morning, giving yourself at least seven hours in bed.

•**Stress.** Stress not only causes inflammation but also worsens the symptoms of OCD. Reduce stress by learning and practicing mindfulness-based stress reduction techniques.

•**Eliminate gluten and casein.** People who are missing the digestive enzyme DPP-4 can't adequately break down certain proteins from dairy (casein) and wheat (gluten), producing morphine-like compounds (*casomorphin, gliadorphin*) that can play a role in OCD. Taking the DPP-4 digestive enzyme, which breaks down gluten, and eliminating dairy and gluten-containing foods (wheat, rye, barley, oats) sometimes significantly or even completely resolves symptoms, particularly in children and adolescents with OCD. The Great Plains Laboratory tests for casomorphin and gliadorphin in the urine (GreatPlainsLaboratory.com).

Adult Attention-Deficit Disorder: Hope Is Here

Richard Gallagher, PhD, director of executive function and organizational skills treatment programs, Institute for Attention Deficit Hyperactivity and Behavior Disorders of the Child Study Center at NYU Langone Health, New York.

Researchers estimate that 4% of American adults meet the diagnostic criteria for attention-deficit hyperactivity disorder (ADHD) .

This chronic condition can make it difficult to focus, to sit still, to be organized, and much more, affecting sufferers' personal and professional lives. It can lead to depression, anxiety, and a higher risk of substance use.

IF YOU SUSPECT YOU HAVE ADHD

The table below lists some common attributes of the two main subtypes of ADHD. (You can have both in what's called combination ADHD.) If these statements ring true for you, particularly if you've had symptoms since childhood, talk to your physician, a mental health professional, or a neurologist with ADHD expertise for a full evaluation. In some cases, ADHD symptoms become apparent only as life and work demands increase in adulthood.

TYPES OF ADHD	
Hyperactive/Impulsive	Inattentive
I feel compelled to move around.	I don't pay close attention to details.
I get bored easily and crave excitement.	I have difficulty sustaining attention.
I generally feel restless.	I often don't listen when people speak.
I have a difficult time waiting in lines.	I don't follow through on instructions.
I finish sentences for other people.	I have difficulty organizing tasks.
I talk excessively.	I am easily distracted.
I fidget whenever I need to sit still.	I lose things that are necessary for tasks.
I have trouble keeping quiet when working or engaging in leisure activities.	I dislike and avoid tasks that require sustained mental effort.

TREATMENT OPTIONS

While ADHD is a lifelong condition, with the proper recognition and diagnosis, treatments can reduce the impact of the symptoms.

●**Medication.** Daily medication can help ADHD sufferers improve their focus and behavior control. The most effective medications stimulate the brain areas responsible for directing and sustaining attention as well as those responsible for selecting and moderating behaviors and choices. These include drugs like *amphetamine* and *dextroamphetamine* (Adderall) and *methylphenidate* (Concerta). These medications come with potential side effects, however, including sleep problems, decreased appetite, weight loss, increased blood pressure, dizziness, headaches, stomachaches, moodiness, and irritability.

●**Psychotherapy.** Whether it's used instead of, or alongside, medication, cognitive-behavioral therapy can help people with ADHD identify and correct thinking errors. For example, many people with ADHD believe that they work best under time pressure, which can lead to procrastination. A therapist can help those patients understand that they are embracing this mistaken belief to avoid completing tasks that are difficult because of a lack of attention control.

Once patients recognize and accept this common pattern, they can start to learn how to use tools and routines to make tasks more manageable. A psychotherapist can help adults with ADHD learn how to slow down to write things down, develop plans for complicated tasks, manage emotional reactions, and build social skills.

Inviting family members into therapy sessions can help adults with ADHD improve relationships, too.

NEXT STEPS

Researchers are developing and testing tools such as mindfulness meditation training and brain stimulation through the use of low-power magnetic fields and low-power infrared light to ease ADHD symptoms. Initial results are promising, but these treatments are not yet widely available.

The Benefits of Regret

Daniel Pink, JD, author of several books including *The Power of Regret: How Looking Backward Moves Us Forward*. He previously was a contributing editor at *Fast Company* and *Wired* magazines and host and co-executive producer of "Crowd Control," a National Geographic Channel series about human behavior. DanPink.com

Regrets are viewed as negative forces in our positivity-promoting society. But the secret to life isn't getting through it without accumulating any regrets. It's keeping regrets in perspective…and learning to shape these powerful negative feelings into positive thoughts and actions.

Research suggests that it's possible to derive powerful benefits from regret…

• **Improved decision making.** A 2021 study of senior business leaders by researchers at Bentley University found that reflecting on their regrets improves business leaders' future decisions. The deeply unpleasant feeling of regret likely reminds them not to rush into decisions and/or to remain wary of past mistakes.

• **Improved performance.** A 2019 study by researchers at Northwestern University's Kellogg School of Management found that scientists who narrowly miss receiving prestigious grants go on to produce more hit research papers than those who are narrowly approved for grants. Missing out on grants triggers regret…but that appears to lead to self-improvement.

• **A more meaningful life.** A 2017 study by another professor at Kellogg School of Management found that when people spend time thinking about what might have been if they'd made different choices, they tend to come away feeling a deeper sense of purpose in the life that they're living, as well as elevated levels of spiritual feelings. Similarly, when researchers involved in a 2010 study at University of California's Haas School of Business asked college students to imagine that they had selected a different school—and consequently were on a different campus with different friends—those students ended up sensing greater meaning in their friendships and college choices. When we regret a path not taken, it reminds us that our lives could have gone in a million different ways—that makes the path we did take seem very special, even miraculous.

What to do with regret to make it work for you…

• **Write it down.** A 2006 study by a psychology professor at University of California, Riverside, found that talking or writing about a negative experience for 15 minutes a day for three consecutive days boosted the writer's psychological well-being in ways that simply thinking about the experience did not. When we think about a regret, we might tell ourselves that we're sorting through what happened, but there's a good chance that we're letting the regret remain a mental abstraction—a big, ill-defined cloud of negativity that we're afraid to examine closely. When we write or speak out loud about the regret, we force ourselves to analyze our thoughts on the subject, and that can help us see our regrets for what they truly are—ordinary missteps, not evidence that we're fools or monsters.

Interestingly, researchers also found that it's best not to talk or write much about life's happy memories. Analyzing these too closely tends to sap the sense of joy they provide, just as analyzing regrets saps their sorrow.

• **Practice self-compassion.** Treat yourself with the same understanding you would offer a friend if he/she made the mistake—this is known as self-compassion. When a regret nags at you, remind yourself that you're not the first person to make this mistake and you won't be the last. Self-compassion doesn't let you off the hook, but it does normalize and neutralize your regrets.

Studies conducted by University of Texas psychologist Kristin Neff, PhD, over the past 15 years found that self-compassion is linked with optimism, happiness, wisdom, initiative and mental toughness…and it's negatively correlated with depression, anxiety and shame.

Wisdom and Loneliness Linked to Microbial Diversity of the Gut

Researchers discovered that people with higher levels of wisdom, compassion, social support, and engagement have more diverse bacteria in their guts than people who report high levels of loneliness. That diversity may increase immunity and decrease systemic inflammation.

UC San Diego School of Medicine.

Verbal Habits to Boost Relationship Health

Count to five before replying to someone to give yourself time to think of the best thing to say. Avoid immediately reacting when something upsetting occurs—wait a day or half a day to get your emotions under control. Ask questions when speaking to people to get them talking more—do not spend your time talking to or at them. Repeat back what another person has told you even if you don't agree—this shows that you are paying attention and trying to understand. Increase the effectiveness of compliments by first saying, "You might not know this, but…"—the phrase gets people tuned into what you say next. Start conversations with specific questions, not throwaway lines—instead of "How are you?," try saying, "How was your weekend trip?"

Inc.com

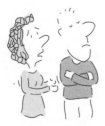

Say "No" to a Drink at Social Gatherings

Ruby Warrington, creator of the term "sober curious" and author of multiple sober-curious books including *The Sober Curious Reset: Change the Way You Drink in 100 Days or Less*. Warrington is host of the "Sober Curious" podcast. RubyWarrington.com

Are you "sober curious"? You're in good company! According to Google Trends, searches for "benefits of quitting drinking" spiked 100% since 2021 in the US…and sales of nonalcoholic beer have increased 86% over the past three years, per Instacart marketplace data. Being sober curious doesn't mean swearing off wine, booze or beer forever. It simply means that you're questioning your personal relationship with drinking and the way society views alcohol.

But a significant portion of the population continues to drink, and that means you may face pressure to imbibe at social gatherings. *Here are some strategies to take a temporary break from alcohol or quit altogether…*

• **Carry a beverage.** Club soda or sparkling water with a citrus wedge looks enough like a cocktail to dissuade most people from asking, "Why aren't you having a drink?" You don't need to hold one all night long, but if it helps prevent unwanted conversations, go for it.

And thanks to a boom in nonalcoholic beverages, many restaurants and bars are stocked with innovative no- or low-alcohol options, from alcohol-free spirits and beer to creative mocktails. These fun drinks replicate the festive feel of social gatherings, taste delicious and won't cause a hangover.

• **Craft your "no" script.** If you're empty-handed at a social gathering, chances are someone is going to offer you a drink. Be prepared with a few possible responses. At a business event, a simple, "No, thanks" or "I can't…I'm driving" should suffice. At a family gathering, respond with what feels comfortable. That might be a quick "I'm not drinking this month—like Dry January, only it is Dry [insert current month]."

GOOD TO KNOW...

Hobbies Are a Form of Self-Care

Try This Relaxing and Fun New Craft

Dot Mandala rock painting...water-based acrylic paint is used to create colorful, symmetrical patterns.

How to do it: Place a large dot of paint in the center of a smooth stone. Place four smaller dots evenly spaced around the center one. Then place four more dots, one between each of the first four dots, evenly spaced. Continue to add dots of different sizes using different colors of paint, spacing the dots evenly to keep the design symmetrical. Let dots dry between additions to keep the paint from flowing together.

Variations: Use a pin, toothpick, crochet hook or similar tool instead of a brush...use a pin or toothpick to drag the edge of still-wet dots in a curve. For inspirational examples and instructions, see RockPainting 101's Dot Mandela tutorial at bit.ly/3fuD2Or.

Miranda Pitrone, rock-painting artist, Lake Erie-Painesville, Ohio. MirandaPitroneArt.com

Hobbies Don't Have to Become Side Hustles

If you've picked up a new hobby during the pandemic, you may want to resist the urge to commercialize it (unless you're truly desperate for money). The happiness and well-being that come from taking time to do something for the pure joy of it can vanish when you pressure yourself to compete in the marketplace.

Self.com

If anyone pressures you, it likely has more to do with their own relationship with alcohol—perhaps they are concerned that they're boring without a few drinks or they're drinking to escape a personal problem.

• **Enlist your friends.** If alcohol usually makes an appearance at your monthly get-togethers with friends, you may want to mention ahead of time that you won't be drinking.

Examples: "I know we normally drink wine, but would you mind if I bring my own soft drinks? I'd love to feel fresh the next morning"...or "I'm trying something new. Instead of meeting for dinner and drinks, why don't we grab coffee and take a long walk?"

• **Remember your why.** Make a list of the reasons why you're reexamining your relationship with alcohol. Shine a light on what you'll be gaining rather than focus on what you'll be missing. Are you seeking better health? Better sleep? To be more productive or more present for your kids? Have you been disappointed with how you act when under the influence? Write your reasons on a piece of paper or in your phone's notes app, and reread it before entering alcohol-related settings.

• **Celebrate your first successes.** You'll have many "sober firsts"—your first sober wedding, dinner party, vacation. Most people get a wonderful confidence boost after each sober first, as you prove to yourself that you don't "need" alcohol. Let yourself feel proud... and congratulate yourself on prioritizing you.

15

Happy Home

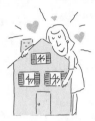

5 Myths About Couples and Sleep

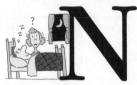Not sleeping well? Your problem might be your partner. Sharing a bed with a loved one often means that his/her sleep problems create problems for you, too. Fatigue might not be the only fallout—poor sleep has been linked to increased risk for health problems ranging from heart disease to Alzheimer's...and when a partner is the cause of poor sleep, relationships often suffer as well.

Some aspects of couples' sleep issues are widely misunderstood. *Here, five myths that cost couples sleep—and what to do about them...*

MYTH: **Never go to bed angry.**

Reality: Conventional wisdom holds that couples should always work through conflicts before retiring for the night. But the evidence suggests otherwise—going to bed angry often is preferable to arguing right before bed, from both a sleep and a relationship perspective.

Research conducted at University of Utah found that anger before bedtime does not disrupt couples' sleep...but conflict before bedtime does. Nighttime conflicts are likely to escalate, potentially to relationship-straining levels. Partners tend to be tired as bedtime nears, so they're not thinking and listening at their best—that may cause arguments to descend into unproductive bickering.

Better: When you and your partner start to get upset at one another late in the evening, put the matter on hold...even if that means going to bed while you are at odds. Say something like, "Let's table this discussion—it's

Wendy M. Troxel, PhD, licensed clinical psychologist, certified behavioral sleep medicine specialist and senior behavioral and social scientist at RAND Corporation, a research and analysis organization, Pittsburgh. She is author of *Sharing the Covers: Every Couple's Guide to Better Sleep.* WendyTroxel.com

too important for us to try to figure out when we're tired and unlikely to listen well."

MYTH: **One partner can tell how well the other slept.**

Reality: Your observations about your partner's sleep are not a fair assessment of how tired he/she is.

Example: Women suffer from insomnia at about twice the rate of men, so researchers at University of Michigan were shocked to discover that women actually sleep 23 more minutes per night than men, on average. While women get more sleep, they tend not to sleep as deeply as men—women's brains remain more active during sleep, perhaps because throughout human history mothers have had to be attentive to their babies' nocturnal needs.

Result: Women can wake fatigued even if they get lots of sleep.

Gender-related sleep misconceptions can work the other way, too.

Example: Some women complain that their husbands fall asleep as soon as their heads hit the pillow, while these wives struggle to rest—and that sometimes is exacerbated because their husbands snore. But snoring could be a sign of sleep apnea or a serious difficulty that's reducing the quality of their partners' sleep.

MYTH: **Sleeping apart leads to lonely, sexless relationships.**

Reality: If you or your partner regularly cost each other sleep by snoring, thrashing or some other issue, sleeping together is more likely to leave you lonely and sex-deprived than sleeping apart. A series of studies conducted at University of California, Berkeley, found that enduring poor sleep increased feelings of loneliness the next day. Researchers also found that when women sleep poorly, they report lower sexual desire and less sexual activity the following day...and men who consistently get insufficient sleep experience a significant drop in testosterone levels, reducing their sex drive. Sleep-deprived couples tend to be more short-tempered with each other as well, which can exacerbate feelings of loneliness and make sex even less likely.

Having separate bedrooms is not the solution for all couples' sleep problems. Sharing a bed has benefits, too—it gives couples time to bond and boosts their levels of *oxytocin*, a hormone that reduces stress and promotes feelings of comfort.

But: Separate bedrooms should not be ruled out when couples struggle to sleep together. Most of the benefits of sharing a bed occur before sleep, so one option is to spend presleep bedroom time in the same bed, talking, cuddling and/or having sex...then one partner can move to a different room.

MYTH: **When one partner's restless leg syndrome is keeping the other partner awake, the only effective solution is a prescription.**

Reality: Iron deficiency is a common cause of restless leg syndrome. Taking iron supplements might prevent you from accidentally kicking your partner awake at night.

Caution: Ask your doctor to test your iron levels to confirm a deficiency before taking iron supplements—too much iron is just as unhealthy as too little.

MYTH: **A compassionate partner should express concern for his/her partner's struggle with insomnia.**

Reality: Loving partners tend to voice their sympathy for their significant others' sleeplessness. Many also suggest that their partners sleep in, nap or head to bed early.

Unfortunately, this concern is counterproductive. Insomnia is, in part, a "thought" disorder—the more the insomniac focuses on it, the more difficult it is to overcome. Partners' concerned questions and sympathy encourage rumination on the subject. And while sleeping in, going to bed early and napping might seem like obvious solutions to offer an insomniac, spending more time in bed struggling to sleep only worsens insomnia. Instead, it is better for him/her to stick to a regular daily sleep schedule and restrict his hours in bed to the hours when he/she is most likely to achieve sleep, probably at night.

Keep a Crush from Ruining Your Marriage

Raffi Bilek, LCSW-C, director of the Baltimore Therapy Center, where he specializes in marriage counseling. BaltimoreTherapyCenter.com

Even people in good relationships can find themselves attracted to people other than their partners. And a crush is powerful—you feel giddy or melty when you're with the person, and that's a feeling you like.

Crushes and affairs are invariably more exciting than marriages. They are new and secretive and don't come with any of the challenges of a marriage. But in terms of your own feelings, the fact that you use the word "crush" is telling. A crush is just, well, a crush. You don't love this person. Remember in junior high when you had a huge crush on that cute girl or boy who sat next to you in class? Odds are that a few months later, you were over it. You won't have these feelings forever…but you may be prolonging them by keeping yourself in close proximity to the object of your crush.

There is no quick trick you can use to make a crush disappear. If you are committed to your marriage and want it to continue to flourish, you need to take deliberate precautions to avoid taking your crush too far.

Ask yourself how much time you really need to spend with this other person. The less time you spend together, the easier it'll be to shake off that crush.

Example: If it's a workmate, you don't have to have lunch together.

If you suspect that the other person shares your feelings, and thus this crush is an imminent threat to your marriage, the best course of action is to change the circumstances entirely. See whether you can be assigned to another work project. Or if this crush comes from a social or volunteer environment, spend less time with the associated group.

Have a Happy, Successful Remarriage

Terry Gaspard, MSW, LICSW, therapist in private practice in Rhode Island and author of *The Remarriage Manual: How to Make Everything Work Better the Second Time Around.* MovingPastDivorce.com

"Love is better the second time around." That's what the song says, but remarriage is far from easy.

Fact: Although more than 40% of first marriages end in divorce, the divorce rate for second, third and fourth marriages is 60% or higher.

After interviewing more than 100 remarried couples, I've found that it's common for one or both partners to assume that a second union will automatically be better than the first because they think they've learned from past mistakes. In reality, many people haven't taken the time to examine their prior relationships for clues to why they failed, potentially dooming them to repeat self-sabotaging relationship patterns.

Second marriages also come with complicated relationships when kids are involved. Children can be a big factor in second-marriage failures if you and your spouse are not communicating well.

Whether you are newly remarried or you've been remarried for a while, here is advice for ditching unresolved baggage and putting your remarriage on the right path…

RULES FOR A HAPPY REMARRIAGE

•**Cultivate realistic expectations.** In second marriages, couples typically get to know each other more quickly than first-time couples, have more baggage and have more complicated lives—especially if they have children from prior marriages.

•**Don't make assumptions about how your remarriage should work.** That can lead only to misunderstandings and disappointment. No matter how much you love someone, you are going to have different ways of doing things when it comes to managing conflict around money, parenting, dealing with in-laws and ex-partners, and other issues. In

231

many cases, new partners haven't yet learned successful ways to manage conflict. It usually takes a few years for family members to adjust to a remarriage or living in a stepfamily.

●**Abandon the power struggle.** The need to be right is prominent in second marriages because partners have typically lived on their own for some time and figured out what they think is the best way to do things.

Example: Samantha and John, both of whom were left by their previous spouses, bicker a lot as they try to get the other to do things his/her way. They have trouble finding the middle ground without feeling as if one of them is losing.

Better: They need to learn to trust that they can be open with each other about what they really want in a given situation without feeling rejected or weak.

Many couples have hidden issues with control, and this usually means that they need to feel cared for and loved. Rather than digging their heels in and getting into a power struggle, they can ask for what they need in a positive way. Partners who learn to say "Yes" more often and see things from their partner's point of view are happier. And they need to learn how to compromise so that both feel like they are satisfied with the outcome. Those who can accept each other's influence are open to their partner's point view even when they disagree. You can learn to do this by being more self-aware of your control issues and listening with curiosity to your partner's perspective.

KNOW YOUR TRIGGERS

We all have basic needs and desires for acceptance, attention, safety, love, respect, being in control and being needed. In remarriages, each partner's unmet needs and desires may come to the surface and bump into the other spouse's vulnerabilities. Some of us may have trust issues or a fear of abandonment, while others have anxiety about being stifled or controlled.

To gain self-awareness about your triggers when interacting with your new spouse, notice situations when your muscles tense up… your heart rate increases…you have hot or cold flushes or tingling…and/or you are hav-

ing repetitive or intense thoughts such as *I can never win* or *This is so unfair.* Notice what is going on when you have these physical responses or thoughts. Is your partner speaking very loudly? Are your children arguing? Did you have a stressful day at work?

Important: The more intense your reaction to your partner's behavior or words, the more likely it is your own issue that is causing the problem.

Remarriages often take more effort than first marriages because you are dealing with more baggage and more family members. But they also can be stronger and more resilient because both partners typically have some experience with marriage. Critical to success is that both partners need to be open and vulnerable when communicating with each other, as well as kind and forgiving when misunderstandings occur.

Friend or Foe? Getting Along with Your Son- or Daughter-in-Law

Ruth Nemzoff, EdD, resident scholar at Brandeis University's Women's Studies Research Center and author of *Don't Roll Your Eyes: Make In-Laws into Family* and *Don't Bite Your Tongue: How to Foster Rewarding Relationships with Your Adult Children.* RuthNemzoff.com

---

In-law relationships can be thorny. Virtual strangers are suddenly family. When your child marries, you may be dreaming of gaining the son or daughter you never had.

But your new child-in-law may not share the same enthusiasm for being part of your family as you do. Worse yet, you may not like or approve of your child's new partner, and this judging gets you off to a bad start—no one wants to be seen as unworthy. Or you may feel competitive with your in-law child and fear that you might lose the affection of your own flesh and blood.

It takes time to build a relationship, particularly because so many adult children live far away from their parents so there often are fewer opportunities to talk and bond today than in the past.

Example: As landlines have disappeared and individual cell phones have proliferated, spontaneous conversations and check-ins between parents and in-law children have become less common since calls typically go directly to the child.

Here's how to build a great relationship with your child-in-law in today's world...

• **Deal with real life, not your hopes and dreams.** Examine the hidden expectations you are bringing to your in-law relationship... and discard them. Except in rare instances, they can create only friction and disappointment. *Questions to ask yourself...*

What expectations do I have for this relationship? Does everyone have the same expectations, or might others see my wishes in a different light?

What worked well in my relationship with my in-laws, and what could have gone better?

Does my partner have a different relationship with the in-law child that works better than mine? If so, can I adopt a similar relationship?

• **Stay open.** Don't take offense at behaviors that you don't understand. Different families have different expectations of family members, which affects their expectations of in-laws.

Example: Carl's mother never let guests lift a finger to help in the kitchen—it was her domain—so Carl never offered to help his mother-in-law in the kitchen. Carl thought he was being respectful, while his mother-in-law thought he was being lazy.

• **Don't expect to be a parent.** Many in-law children already have their own parents and aren't looking for more. They may be close to their own parents, or they may be suspicious of their in-laws if they have a poor or complicated relationship with their own family.

Example: Elaine and Don had hoped to be close with their daughter-in-law, Ashley, whose parents had divorced and remarried. Ashley was exhausted by the thought of finding a way to accommodate a third family at Christmastime, so she retreated from every-

one. Elaine and Don, feeling terribly disappointed, ask their son if they have offended Ashley, and he explains her history. Elaine and Don decide to back off to give Ashley some time. Eventually, Ashley begins to figure things out, and she and her husband make a tradition of coming to Elaine and Don's house on Christmas Eve.

• **Don't compete with your in-law child's parents.** You may feel resentful that your child-in-law's family spends more time with the children than you do. But if you make a fuss, you will place excess pressure on the couple and may lose out on seeing them at all.

Better: Rather than waste your energy comparing the types of activities your family does versus your child-in-law's family, do what your family enjoys. Invite the couple to come along. If they decline, accept their choice but don't stop trying.

• **Don't expect your daughter-in-law to be responsible for your relationship with your son.** In years past, women took care of the family relationships. In today's world, if your son isn't calling you, it's usually his doing...or not doing.

• **Listen without judging, criticizing, confronting or giving unwanted advice.** Being critical is the fastest way to sink a newly forming relationship.

Example: When I had my first child, my own mother was ill and couldn't help me. My mother-in-law came to visit and saw that I was holding my baby by his neck like a chicken. She said, "That's so interesting how you're holding your baby. Did they teach you that at the hospital?" She asked this question with love and curiosity, not judgment. I was feeling very insecure and unknowledgeable about babies, and I would have gotten defensive if she had told me I was doing it wrong. Instead, I said, "Oh no, how should I hold the baby?" She set me straight and I was grateful instead of resentful.

If you cannot change a situation or if your child and his spouse don't want your advice, find a way to understand and accept it. Continuing to push will only drive a wedge in your relationship, and maybe even force your child into choosing between spouse and parent—a battle that you're likely to lose.

- **Take the long view.** Relationships grow. Young couples often don't need or want to see their parents often, but later in life—when they have kids of their own or become ill or injured—they may need your help.

Example: Marlene was cordial to her in-laws as a newlywed but often turned down invitations from her mother-in-law, Andrea, to meet for lunch or shopping. Andrea was hurt, so she took a step back. Years later, she was thrilled when Marlene welcomed her help as a grandmother to her children. Marlene never disliked Andrea—she just didn't need to be as close to her as her mother-in-law had hoped.

- **Maintain your relationship even if the couple splits.** If you want to see your grandchildren, stay cordial and neutral with your in-law child.

Example: Charlene and Phil, Jake's parents, tried to stay close to their grandchildren after Jake and his wife Irma went through an acrimonious divorce when Jake cheated on his wife. Irma blamed her in-laws for Jake's behavior. Charlene and Phil never took sides—although Jake wanted them to—and continued to call their daughter-in-law offering to help with the children, sent presents and invited the children and their mother to holiday gatherings. Eventually, Irma came around and saw that Charlene and Phil were good people and she allowed her in-laws to see the children.

6 Strategies to Help Your Child Buy a Home

Keith Gumbinger, vice president of New Jersey–based HSH Associates, which publishes mortgage and consumer loan information. HSH.com

Young adults aren't just borrowing from banks to buy their first homes—many are asking for help from mom and dad. The median US home price surged above $400,000 in 2021. And a 2019 survey found that 43% of homeowners younger than age 35

received financial help from their parents, and more than half of would-be homebuyers in this age bracket expected to get such support.

But there's a dark side to this assistance: Many parents put their own retirements at risk when they help kids buy homes, and, counterintuitively, this aid sometimes damages parent-child relationships. *Here are strategies to help your kids without blowing your retirement…*

STRATEGY #1: Gift money to help with the down payment. A 20% down payment on a $400,000 home is $80,000. A cash gift from a parent can be a big help, and no-strings-attached gifts are less likely to have unforeseen financial consequences than most of the alternative strategies that follow. *Still, there are details to consider…*

- **If you have more than one child, gifting a large amount of money to one could create family disharmony.** Potential solutions include gifting money to the other kids, too, if you can afford to do so…or adjusting your estate plan so that your kids receive equal amounts in the end.

- **Your child's lender likely will insist that you sign a "gift letter."** This letter should state that you gave the money free of any encumbrance. In other words—that it is not a loan you expect the child to repay.

- **Large gifts occasionally have tax consequences—but the limits aren't as strict as many people think.** You might have read that as of 2022, the maximum amount one person can give another without potential tax consequences is $16,000—but there are ways around this.

Examples: If you're married, you and your spouse each can give $16,000 to your child…and if your child has a partner, you and your spouse could each give your child and his/her partner $16,000, boosting the total no-tax gift cap to $64,000. And even if you do exceed the annual cap, it won't necessarily result in a tax bill—the excess will count against your lifetime gift-tax exemption, which is $12.06 million. This exemption changes over the years, but unless your estate is well into the millions, federal gift taxes are unlikely to affect you. Speak with your financial or estate planner for details.

Is this strategy right for you? Cash gifts are the most straightforward and often the best—assuming that you have the means to give a sum of money without risking your own retirement. Choose an amount that fits into your financial plans even if it's only a fraction of what your child needs—it's better for your child to save a little longer before buying a home than for you to outlive your savings.

STRATEGY #2: **Loan money to the adult child.** A loan might seem like the sensible solution if you have sufficient savings to help your child with his/her down payment but you eventually need that money back for your retirement. *Two big drawbacks…*

• **You might not get the money back.** Many intrafamily loans are never repaid—a 2019 survey reported that 37% of these loans resulted in financial losses for the giver. Moreover, tensions triggered by intrafamily loans damaged 21% of giver-recipient relationships.

• **An intrafamily loan could make it harder for your child to get a mortgage.** Your child's "debt to income ratio" is among the key stats that lenders will evaluate when deciding whether and at what rates to offer a loan. The money you lent your child will increase his debt.

Is this strategy right for you? Only if you cannot afford to make this money a gift… and you have confidence that your child will repay you…and this loan would not inflate your child's debt-to-income ratio to levels that lenders might consider problematic. An online mortgage calculator such as HSH.com's "Home Affordability Calculator" can help determine whether this might be a problem, or ask a mortgage lender or broker.

If you do lend money to your adult child: Put the loan terms in writing, and charge sufficient interest so that the IRS accepts it is a loan and not a gift. As of February 2022, rates as low as 0.59% were acceptable for loans up to three years…higher minimums applied to longer-term loans. Enter "Index of Applicable Federal Rates" into a search engine to find the minimum rates for the month when the loan is made.

STRATEGY #3: **Let your child live in your home rent-free while he saves for a down payment.** If you have more free space than free cash, inviting your child to temporarily move in could help. If this saves the child $2,000 per month in rent and utilities, that's the equivalent of a $24,000 gift each year.

The downsides here are relationship related—not every parent and adult child could live under the same roof without getting on each other's nerves.

Is this strategy right for you? It could be if you have the space and everyone enjoys living together. Discuss the details before it begins to reduce the odds of problems. *What house rules would you request? How would household chores and expenses be divided? Is there an end date by which you would expect the adult child to move out?*

STRATEGY #4: **Co-sign the adult child's mortgage.** Adding your name to a child's mortgage application could help him qualify for a loan—lenders will take your credit score, assets and income into account as well as your child's. When co-signing goes well, it's a way for parents to help their kids buy homes without handing over any cash—but it doesn't always go well for the following reasons…

• **Co-signers have a legal obligation to make mortgage payments if the primary borrower fails to do so.** You could end up saddled with a long-term financial obligation for a home you don't own.

• **Co-signing could damage your credit score, particularly if mortgage payments are late or missed.** That could make it more expensive for you to borrow if, for example, you later wish to refinance your own mortgage or obtain a car loan.

Is this strategy right for you? Only if your credit score is significantly higher than your child's—otherwise adding your name to mortgage applications won't sway lenders—and only if you are very confident that your adult child will make his mortgage payments on time.

STRATEGY #5: Be a "co-borrower" on the adult child's mortgage. As with co-signing, this means lenders will consider your credit score and financial picture along with your child's. But as a co-borrower, you're not just required to step in if the child misses mortgage payments—you share the primary obligation to make these payments and share ownership of the home. And as with co-signing, your credit score could suffer if your child fails to make his mortgage payments on time—even if you paid your share.

Is this strategy right for you? Only if you're able to pay part of the mortgage each month and you're confident that your child will pay his share. This also makes sense if the plan is for you to eventually move in with this adult child.

STRATEGY #6: Buy a home, and rent it to the child. This avoids the financial entanglements of co-signing or co-borrowing—the property belongs to the parent. It's like buying an investment property. *But there's still plenty of room for this to go wrong...*

• **Adding a landlord/tenant component to the parent/child relationship can create family strife.** It could undercut your investment, too. Just think—would you evict your child if he didn't pay the rent?

• **Investment property mortgages have higher rates and down-payment requirements than those for primary residences.**

Is this strategy right for you? Only if you're looking for an investment property in the area anyway and your child would be a reliable tenant and doesn't have his heart set on becoming a homeowner. You and your child should discuss how property maintenance will be handled—is this a traditional landlord/tenant relationship where the tenant calls the landlord whenever something breaks...or do you expect your child to handle such things, perhaps in exchange for a below-market rental rate?

Avoid These Common Etiquette Mistakes

*D*rinking to your own toast—when you're being honored, the other guests are drinking to you, so hold off on quaffing your own beverage. *Replying to a "thank you" with "no problem"*—the thanker was expressing gratitude, not suggesting that you should have viewed the act as a problem. Instead, say, "You're welcome." *Setting your phone on the table*—it signals that you have more important things on your mind than your fellow diners. *Starting "fun" conversations about politics*—stick with safe topics such as friends, family, hobbies and so on. *Oversharing on social media*—it's just as off-putting as when you do it in real life. *Sitting while being introduced to someone*—show they're important enough for you to stand for a moment. *Leaving in your earbuds when someone is talking to you*—take them out to give the person your full attention.

Lisa Grotts, etiquette expert and author of *A Traveler's Passport to Etiquette*, quoted at RD.com.

How You Can Spot Heart Trouble...In Your Parents

Bobbi Bogaev, MD, board-certified specialist in cardiovascular diseases, advanced heart failure and internal medicine. She is medical director, heart failure, at Abiomed, maker of Impella, a heart pump for patients with severe coronary artery disease.

Thanks to the far-reaching effects of the COVID-19 pandemic, the American Heart Association predicts that rates of heart disease, already the number-one cause of death in the US, will rise. This has to do with pandemic-related delays in seeking care...weight gain, inactivity and poor eating habits that developed while staying at home for extended periods...excess stress...the psychological toll of isolation...and heart damage from COVID-related cardiovascular complications. These risks increase with age, leaving the elderly most vulnerable.

Many of us may be unaware of our older loved ones' new heart-related symptoms. Now that more people are vaccinated, it's an ideal time to take a closer look and see if parents or other older relatives may be showing signs of heart disease.

EASY-TO-MISS WARNING SIGNS

When most people hear the words "heart disease," they think of chest pain, labored breathing, high blood pressure and rapid heartbeat. And those certainly are indicators of heart disease, a heart attack or heart failure. (Contrary to how it sounds, heart failure doesn't mean that the heart has stopped but rather that it can't pump enough blood to keep up with the body's demands.)

But did you know that your 80-year-old father quitting his golf game…your 90-year-old mother no longer wearing her trademark lipstick…extra pillows on your parents' bed…or a switch from them cooking to eating frozen meals all could be signs of failing heart health?

HEART DISEASE SIGNS

Recognizing often-disguised heart-health warning signs could mean the difference between life and death for your aging loved ones. *The next time you see them, ask yourself…*

•**Are they no longer doing the things they used to love?** Fatigue is one of the most common symptoms of heart failure, a symptom of heart disease and the leading cause of hospitalization in people over age 65. If your parent used to love playing golf several times a week but has stopped…or no longer gardens even though it gave him/her great joy, that could be a tip-off that heart failure–related fatigue is keeping them from their usual passions.

Depression also can cause people to disengage from formerly enjoyable activities, and depression and heart disease often go hand in hand. Depression can increase risk for heart attack and/or heart disease by increasing inflammation or causing platelets—cells that help with blood clotting—to become too sticky, clogging arteries in the process…or heart disease can fuel depression when one

feels too tired to engage in favorite pastimes and begins to feel hopeless or worthless. At least one in five people with heart failure develops depression.

•**Are they cooking meals…or stocking premade and frozen foods?** Cooking requires a surprising amount of mental and physical energy, from recipe planning to grocery shopping to meal preparation. That's a lot of effort for someone who feels exhausted. Check your parents' kitchen for evidence of cooking. Is the olive oil bottle full? Is the fridge produce drawer full of fresh vegetables—or worse, produce past its prime? Or is it relatively bare and the freezer full of frozen dinners? Complicating matters, premade, frozen and shelf-stable meals are notoriously high in sodium, which can aggravate existing heart issues.

•**Do you notice puffy weight gain?** Heart failure can cause people to accumulate fluid around the liver and the ankles. It may appear to have developed out of nowhere and is more likely to happen if high-sodium foods are being consumed. A parent may report that it's suddenly hard to button his pants.

Don't mistake excess body fat for fluid—25% of adults over age 76 reported weight gain as a result of the pandemic, according to a 2021 Harris Poll conducted for the American Psychological Association. This type of weight gain tends to be all over the body, while fluid accumulation due to heart failure is localized around the middle and in the legs and ankles. It also feels different—when a physician thumps the belly of a patient with fluid buildup, it has a dull sound, like tapping a watermelon.

Other signs: Swollen ankles…a visibly pulsing jugular vein in the neck…and tenderness under the right ribcage (from fluid accumulating in the liver).

•**How many pillows are they using?** Heart failure can cause fluid to accumulate in the lungs, leading to shortness of breath, especially when lying flat. Patients often say that it feels like they're suffocating when they lie down, so they prop themselves up to avoid that feeling. Some people take to sleeping in a recliner. Patients also may awaken from sleep with shortness of breath and have to sit bolt upright to breathe easily.

•**Does Mom pass "The Lipstick Test"?** It's always reassuring when an older patient reports to a doctor's appointment wearing lipstick. It shows that she has the energy to keep up her normal routine. This is the type of clue you may not have noticed if you haven't seen your parents in person in several months. Is mom still putting on lipstick? Is dad still shaving? Are they showering regularly? Do their clothes look wrinkled? If parents seem to be letting themselves go, it can be a tip-off to start asking more questions.

Other signs: Is mail piling up that didn't used to? Did they not decorate for the holidays even though they've been hanging Christmas lights for decades? These are similar red flags of low energy.

•**Are there bottles of antacid everywhere?** If you spot antacids in the medicine cabinet, on the kitchen island and on their bedside table, ask about episodes of heartburn. Chest pain (angina) often masquerades as heartburn, especially chest pain that worsens with exertion, such as during a brisk walk. It even can be a symptom of a heart attack. The acid indigestion–like feeling can be accompanied by shortness of breath or fatigue. Although this "angina equivalent" can feel like heartburn caused by reflux, it has everything to do with the heart. Women are especially likely to experience atypical heart attack symptoms such as heartburn-like pain, fatigue and shortness of breath, as opposed to classic symptoms such as crushing chest pain.

•**Can they walk for six minutes straight… or sit and stand five times in a row?** If your loved one gets winded from navigating stairs or struggles to get up from a chair, suggest taking a walk together. If he can't walk for six minutes without stopping, he may have heart disease. Pay attention to whether he tries to make excuses to stop during the walk, such as chatting or tying his shoes.

You also can suggest they try the "5 Times Sit-to-Stand Test." This is a simple way to look for a heart disease symptom called frailty.

Frailty is an age-related syndrome involving deteriorations in several body systems, including stamina, strength, weight and fitness.

How to do it: Have your loved one sit in a standard-height chair with his back against the back of the chair. Using a timer, ask him to stand up straight as quickly as he safely can, five times in a row without stopping, his arms remaining folded across his chest. Stop timing him when he stands for the fifth time. Someone age 70 to 79 ideally will finish in 12.6 seconds or less…someone age 80 to 89, 14.8 seconds or less.

Recent finding: A 2021 BMC Geriatrics meta-analysis concluded that frailty is an increasingly common heart disease symptom in older adults, affecting nearly one-fifth of heart disease patients.

NEXT STEPS

If you recognize any of these symptoms, encourage your parent to schedule a visit with his primary care physician. If you can't attend the visit, help make a list of concerns to show the doctor. (This is especially helpful for adults with memory issues.) With a little investigative work, you can help get Mom or Dad back to playing golf, gardening and feeling engaged with life.

Protect Your Loved Ones from Nursing Home Neglect

Annette Ticoras, MD, founder and patient advocate, Guided Patient Services, Inc., Columbus, Ohio. GPS Columbus.com

The five-star rating system for nursing-home quality is far from perfect. Even high-ranking facilities had appalling instances of neglect and abuse, according to a recent exposé in *The New York Times*. The pandemic has made things worse, exacerbating existing staffing problems and, thanks to social-distancing rules, making oversight nearly impossible. *When choosing a home for a loved one...*

Talk to residents and their families about their experiences and, to the extent allowed, conduct a "secret-shopper"–style investigation. Are there opportunities for fresh air, socializing, and exercising mind and body? Unpleasant smells? If your loved one has any special needs, such as dementia, ask if the staff has specialized training. *Once you've chosen a home...*

• **Visit frequently, sometimes unannounced and during off hours.**

If in-person is impossible: Make generous use of video calling, keeping an eye on the background and listening to how the staff speaks to your loved one.

• **Ask staff members how you can ease their burden.** Approach them with openness and cooperation. In-the-trenches nursing home work is demanding yet poorly compensated. Lots of positive communication goes a long way toward making sure your loved one gets the attention he/she needs.

• **Get to know the director of nursing.** He/she is supposed to notify you when there is a change in your loved one's treatment, including medications, and when there is a need for evaluation.

• **Create a care plan for your loved one.** Each resident should have a personalized care plan, with goals and preferences—even things as simple as, "Don't park Mom in front of *Jeopardy!*—she hates that show." The plan should be updated periodically.

If you spot true abuse or neglect: Gather as much information about the incident as you can, and contact the facility's long-term-care ombudsman or your nearest Area Agency on Aging to file a detailed complaint. The name and contact information for the ombudsman, an unbiased third party who does not work for the facility, must be provided to loved ones as well as publicly posted at the facility.

Nursing-Home Patients Are Being Misdiagnosed ...Deliberately

Michael Wasserman, MD, chair, Public Policy Committee, California Association of Long-Term-Care Medicine, Santa Clarita, California.

Alzheimer's and other forms of dementia can cause nursing home residents to be agitated and challenging to work with. An appealing proposition for some short-staffed nursing homes facilities is to give such patients antipsychotic medications to render them more docile.

But: Antipsychotics are associated with negative outcomes, including increasing risk for death for elderly patients with dementia. These drugs are so concerning that nursing homes must report their use to the federal government, and a high rate of antipsychotic-drug use can negatively affect a facility's quality rating on the Centers for Medicare and Medicaid Services' nursing home comparison website (Medicare.gov/care-compare).

But nursing homes have found a loophole: They aren't required to report prescriptions for schizophrenia patients, so it is possible to simply diagnose residents with schizophrenia so that they can be prescribed antipsychotic medications.

A *New York Times* investigation found that more than one in five nursing home residents take antipsychotics, even though schizophrenia affects only one in 150 people, most of whom are diagnosed before age 40. With more nursing homes coming under scrutiny, many have shifted away from antipsychotics in favor of antiseizure medications such as *gabapentin* (Gralise) and *divalproex sodium* (Depakote). But these, too, are being prescribed for their side effects—lethargy and quiescence.

To protect your loved ones: When you're choosing a facility, ask what training the doctors and other caregivers have when it comes to dementia. Once your loved one is living in a nursing home, insist on an up-to-date list of all prescriptions. Ask the doctor the reason for every drug on the list. If you see an inappropriate prescription, take it up with the facility's ombudsman.

Preparing for the Stages of Alzheimer's

Monica Moreno, senior director for care and support at the Alzheimer's Association in Chicago, where she works with families after an Alzheimer's disease diagnosis. Alz.org

---

Alzheimer's disease is life-altering and frightening not just for the person receiving the diagnosis but also for his/her family. When you or a loved one hear this diagnosis, you likely will think of the end—or final—stages of this disease. However, diagnosed individuals can continue to live meaningful and productive lives in the early stages.

The first step is to understand and accept the diagnosis. That starts with getting educated about the stages...how the disease will progress...and what treatments and services are available today and in the future so that you can be prepared. There is a lot of information available...in fact, so much that it can be overwhelming. Take your time and go at your own pace. Alzheimer's is a journey, not a sprint.

Most important: You do not have to go through this alone. Once you reach out and get support, you will feel some relief and less isolated.

Each person's progression is different, but there are changes that characterize each stage and things you can do to prepare for the next stage...

EARLY-STAGE OR MILD ALZHEIMER'S

What to expect: In the early stage, people often still are independent and able to drive and can continue to enjoy being social, though they might have a hard time planning and organizing tasks.

Symptoms: Mild memory issues, including struggling to find the right word when speaking...forgetting words or something you just read or heard, perhaps the name of someone you just met. You may start to lose things.

Loved ones may notice these problems, but they might not be obvious to the outside world.

Steps to take...

•**Take care of yourself.** Many people who are newly diagnosed take the opportunity to look at their lifestyle and make changes that will enable them to live their healthiest life. Adopting lifestyle changes, including controlling blood pressure, healthy eating, exercising and staying socially and intellectually engaged, may help slow cognitive decline and preserve existing cognitive function longer.

•**Discuss medications.** Early detection gives you the chance to start taking medications that might help now. It also provides an opportunity to enroll in a clinical trial exploring new medications and treatments. Talk to your doctor.

•**Prioritize what matters to you.** In the wake of a diagnosis, many people choose to spend time doing meaningful activities and spending more time with the most important people in their lives.

•**Build your support team.** This is a good time to start building the right support team so that you'll have people to rely on as the disease progresses. This also is important for the spouse or care partner, whose support needs will grow as well.

One option: Connect with others who are living with Alzheimer's or other caregivers by joining an Alzheimer's Association support group (see the next page for suggestions). Being able to share your experiences with others living your journey can be helpful.

•**Take practical steps to prepare.** Put legal and financial documents and end-of-life plans in place. Doing so now allows the person with Alzheimer's to be part of the conversation and share his/her wishes with family and friends. Later on, family members will have peace of mind knowing that they're following their loved one's wishes.

•**Put safety measures in place.** Most people want to stay in their home as long as possible, so creating a safe environment is critical. Remove tripping hazards such as throw rugs, and secure bookshelves and other heavy furniture to prevent them from tipping over.

Other steps become more important when Alzheimer's worsens and affects judgment—securing hazardous items, such as medication, liquor, sharp objects and cleaning products, from easy access...putting stickers on glass doors to prevent walking into them...and securing exterior doors or installing motion detectors to prevent wandering from the home. Remove locks on bathrooms and bedrooms so the person cannot lock himself in accidently. When to take these actions will depend on Alzheimer's progression.

•**Consider when to stop driving.** This is a very difficult and complicated decision. The Alzheimer's Association offers online tools to help families discuss this sensitive topic, including signs of unsafe driving and transportation alternatives.

MIDDLE-STAGE OR MODERATE ALZHEIMER'S

What to expect: This often is the longest stage—it can last for many years, and the person living with dementia can require more and more care as damage to nerve cells in the brain increases. Dementia symptoms become more pronounced, and loved ones may see clear personality and behavior changes.

Symptoms: Worsening language and cognitive problems, forgetting basic personal information and not knowing what day it is...difficulty doing—or even refusing to do—everyday activities such as bathing or needing help with those tasks...and emotional issues that manifest as anger and frustration and refusal to participate in social situations. Wandering and getting lost—either on foot, by car or on public transportation—may become a problem and pose a threat to safety.

Also: The person may become increasingly suspicious, have delusions or engage in repetitive compulsive behaviors. Physical changes can include sleep problems, such as nighttime restlessness and daytime sleepiness, and difficulty with continence.

Steps to take...

•**Consider additional help.** As care needs increase, families may consider adult-day-care centers, aides and other outside support. These resources not only provide additional

assistance but also offer caregivers a break to attend to their personal care and well-being.

•**Adapt your communication.** As the disease progresses, and communication becomes more challenging, adapt your communication. This may include slowing down and making eye contact with the person as you speak... and using short, simple sentences. Ask one question at a time, rather than overwhelming the patient with a series of questions. Give him time to process and respond before continuing the conversation.

LATE-STAGE OR SEVERE ALZHEIMER'S

What to expect: This is the most difficult stage, with profound changes, such as loss of speech and movement and the inability to walk and swallow. General health worsens with an increased risk for infection, especially pneumonia. Significant personality changes may take place, and there may be little awareness of recent experiences or one's surround-

---

More from Monica Moreno...

Help When You Need It

General help: The Alzheimer's Association has a 24/7 helpline at 800-272-3900 with masters-level counselors available to guide you. There also are chat boxes throughout the website. Alz.org

Online community: The website AlzConnected.org connects you to people who have walked in your shoes and will provide support by sharing their experiences, tips and strategies.

Action plans: At AlzheimersNavigator.org, you can create your own action plan for any of 10 of the most common concerns facing caregivers, such as care options and legal planning. For each topic, you'll answer a group of questions and, based on your answers, receive back an action plan along with resources to help you apply it. Over time as your needs change, you can go back and answer the questions again.

E-learning: At the Alzheimer's Association Education Center, you'll find many Alzheimer's and dementia learning programs available online. Alz.org/education

ings. But the person living with Alzheimer's still can benefit from some types of interaction and may be soothed by relaxing music or a gentle touch.

Steps to take: Around-the-clock assistance for daily personal care usually is needed. Families may consider nursing homes or other long-term-care options. Hospice care may be available for individuals nearing the end of life. See the box on page 241 for resources that can provide help.

Help for a Depressed Family Member

Mark Pollack, MD, a board-certified psychiatrist and chief medical officer for Myriad Mental Health.

Caring for family members with depression is often challenging, but your support can make all the difference.

1. Keep trying to talk. It can be awkward to ask about someone else's mental health but initiating the conversation can reduce the sense of isolation for someone who may be suffering in silence. Patience, compassion, and active listening can help. For some, talking about feeling "stressed" as opposed to "depressed" may be less likely to engender defensiveness or denial. Talking to someone about sleep disturbance, loss of appetite, or low energy (all symptoms of depression) may be a more acceptable way to start the conversation.

2. Help your loved one get help. For older people taught to "keep a stiff upper lip," stigma about addressing mental health issues may be ingrained. A nationwide poll found that nearly two-thirds (61%) of Americans ages 65 or older who have concerns about having depression will not seek treatment. Nearly one in three seniors believe they can "snap out" of it on their own. Yet depression is not a moral failing but rather an illness, like heart disease. It can and should be treated.

3. Take care of yourself. You cannot be an effective caregiver if you don't address your own needs. Make sure that you are doing

what you can to keep yourself as physically and emotionally resilient as possible.

Gens X and Y Are in Poorer Health

Generations X and Y are in poorer health than their parents and grandparents were at similar ages. These generations also show higher levels of behaviors that endanger health—such as alcohol use and smoking—and have more depression and anxiety. Generation X, born 1965 to 1980, and Generation Y (aka Millennials), born 1981 to 1996, are more likely to have decreases in life expectancy than prior generations—and to have more disability and morbidity as they age.

Analysis of National Center for Health Statistics data by researchers at The Ohio State University, Columbus, published in *American Journal of Epidemiology.*

Sugary Beverages and Brain-Health Link

Drinking sugar-sweetened beverages in youth may affect cognition in adulthood. Researchers discovered that rodents who drank a sugary beverage every day in their adolescence showed impaired performance on a specific learning and memory task when they reached adulthood. They believe that changes in gut bacteria may be to blame. Early life sugar consumption elevated levels of the bacteria *Parabacteroides*, which is associated with memory deficits.

University of Georgia.

Dangerous Concussions

More than one-third of kids with concussions experience mental health problems.

Recent finding: 37% of children who had concussions developed problems with anxiety, depression, withdrawal or PTSD, and 20% developed problems with aggression, hyperactivity or attention—and some problems persisted for years. While a history of mental health issues raises risk for more after a concussion, 26% of the children with such issues had no history of them.

Vicki Anderson, PhD, pediatric neuropsychologist at Murdoch Children's Research Institute, Parkville, Australia, and leader of a study of 90,000 concussion cases, published in *British Journal of Sports Medicine.*

Marching Bands Should Have Athletic Trainers

When researchers monitored core body temperatures and other physiological measurements during practices and games, they found that band members often were overheated and underhydrated. Wearing heavy uniforms and performing on blacktop or artificial turf make matters worse. Although such conditions put musicians at a level of risk similar to that of athletes, most bands lack access to trainers familiar with how to properly schedule hydration breaks and deal with heat injuries.

Study led by researchers at University of Kansas, Lawrence, Kansas, published in *Journal of Athletic Training.*

How to Make Sure Your Kids Graduate College

Mark Kantrowitz, financial-aid and college-savings expert who has testified before Congress on student debt issues. He is author of *Who Graduates from College? Who Doesn't?* Kantrowitz.com

The cost of a college education can be staggeringly steep—and for many students, that investment will be wasted. Only 41% of students who enroll in bachelor's programs earn degrees in four years, and only 60% do so in five years. The rest will be saddled with debt for decades but without the en-hanced earnings potential that a degree might have provided.

It is possible to predict which college students are unlikely to earn degrees and identify strategies that could improve their odds of graduating.

IN HIGH SCHOOL

Parents should encourage students to do these things in high school to improve their odds of graduating from college…

•**Take challenging classes.** High school students face a strategic choice—should they take easy classes to boost their grade point averages (GPAs) or more difficult classes that will push them academically? Higher GPAs are correlated with better college-graduation rates, but the data strongly suggests that kids who take tough high school classes are especially likely to earn bachelor's degrees.

Example: Students who take at least one advanced placement (AP) class or class that provides college credit are nearly twice as likely to earn bachelor's degrees as those who don't take advanced classes. This is in part because the smartest high school students are most likely to take AP and college courses—but it also is because students who are academically challenged in high school tend to be better prepared for the educational rigors of college.

•**Push particularly hard in math**—even if the student doesn't intend to major in math. Every additional math course a student takes in high school significantly improves that student's odds of earning a bachelor's degree in any major. If the most advanced math class a student takes in high school is algebra 1, the odds of earning a bachelor's are just 7%…taking high school geometry ups that to 21%… algebra 2 to 39%…trigonometry to 63%…precalculus to 73%…and calculus to 83%. This data is in part simply showing that good students tend to get further in math than weak students—but, again, the differences in college outcomes are so dramatic that this seems unlikely to be the only explanation.

Two possibilities: There is something about high school math that identifies the students destined to succeed in college…and/or that helps students succeed in college.

243

One theory: Kids who study advanced math develop their ability to think rationally, which is valuable in any academic field.

• **Take on the right extracurricular activities.** Should high school students who wish to graduate from college focus on academics or join teams, clubs and groups? The answer is… it depends. There's strong evidence that joining high school math clubs and science clubs increases the odds of later earning a bachelor's degree. Joining student government, the student newspaper or yearbook has a less dramatic but still positive effect—but playing on sports teams has little effect on whether someone later earns a bachelor's degree. And joining many other groups during high school, including scouting, 4-H and "hobby clubs," is correlated with reduced odds of earning those degrees.

But: Being the captain or MVP of a high school sports team or having a leadership position in a club or group is associated with increased odds of earning a bachelor's degree, suggesting that students should focus their extracurricular time and energy on one group to improve their odds of becoming a leader in that group rather than join lots of different groups.

Joining only one or two high school groups won't hurt students' chances of college acceptance. Contrary to the widely held belief, colleges almost always take a student who shows a deep interest in one or two areas over a student who dabbles in many.

HEADING TO COLLEGE

Three smart strategies as students transition from high school to college…

• **Don't take a gap year.** Taking a year off between high school and college might seem like a good way for a student to gain maturity and life experience, but research has found that it reduces the odds of earning a bachelor's degree from 72% to 56%. Those odds fall further still if, like many gap-year takers, the student fails to return to school after a single year. Once students get out of the habit of being students, they often find it hard to resume their studies.

• **Don't use community college as a steppingstone to a four-year school.** It seems like a savvy way to trim college costs—attend an affordable community college for two years, then transfer to a pricier four-year college for just two years to earn a bachelor's degree. But only around 20% of students who head to community college with this plan in mind actually earn their bachelor's degrees within six years. Students who take a detour through a community college on their way to a four-year degree are much less likely to reach their destination, regardless of academic performance in high school.

But: If the student's goal is to get an associate's degree or a certificate and not to transfer, a community college is a very good option, especially for students who have lower GPAs in high school.

• **Enroll in a college that has a high graduation rate.** Some colleges have graduation rates well above 90%…others below 20%. Schools' graduation rates can be found in college guidebooks or on the US Department of Education's College Navigator (NCES.ed.gov/collegenavigator) or College Scorecard (CollegeScorecard.ed.gov) websites.

IN COLLEGE

Four ways college students can significantly improve their odds of graduating…

• **Don't work more than 12 hours per week in paid employment.** If your plan for paying for college involves the student working more than this, you need a new plan. Every hour worked beyond 12 hours a week significantly reduces the odds of graduation, likely because it leaves the student with insufficient time for studies. On the other hand, working in a paid job 12 or fewer hours per week in college improves the odds of graduation, perhaps by teaching the student the value of work or forcing the student to become better at time management.

• **Live on campus.** Students who live on campus have a 77% chance of earning a bachelor's within six years…those who live off campus, around 48%. And 51% of students who live on campus graduate with a bachelor's degree within four years, compared with 24% of students who live off campus and 20% of students who live with their parents.

Campus life immerses students in the college environment, improving access to study groups and providing an atmosphere where almost everyone is focused on the goal of graduation.

- **Avoid transferring between colleges.** Changing colleges midway lowers the odds of earning a bachelor's degree within six years from 76% to 56%. Transferring can create unexpected complications—not every credit earned and prerequisite reached at the first college will be accepted by the new one, for example.

- **Earn 15 credits per semester.** Colleges and student-loan programs define "full-time student" as someone taking at least 12 credits per semester...but it typically takes 120 credits to earn a bachelor's degree. If you do the math, that means students need 15 credits per semester to graduate in four years.

WHAT PARENTS CAN DO

Saving for college is the single best thing parents can do to increase the odds that their kids will earn their bachelor's degrees—financial problems are among the leading reasons students drop out. *Four more ways parents can help...*

- **Join the PTA.** Belonging to and actively participating in the PTA when a child is in elementary, middle and high school increases the odds that the child will go on to earn a bachelor's degree by 17 percentage points, according to one data set. Students put greater value in their education when their parents are involved in the process.

- **Be open to a young child repeating kindergarten...but resist having him/her repeat later grades.** Students who repeat grades in elementary or middle school are significantly less likely than other students to go on to earn a bachelor's. But students who repeat kindergarten enjoy significantly improved odds of earning a bachelor's, perhaps because they end up being slightly more advanced than their classmates for the remainder of their academic careers. And unlike being held back in later years, repeating kindergarten tends not to point to long-term academic shortcomings.

- **Encourage pursuit of a master's degree** —even if a bachelor's is the goal. Students who plan to earn master's degrees earn their bachelor's degrees 74% of the time...while those who expect to earn only a bachelor's degree earn those degrees 58% of the time.

- **Don't divorce until graduation if possible.** Researchers have consistently found that students are significantly less likely to earn their bachelor's degree if their parents divorce or separate before they do so.

Buy Your Kid a Typewriter

They're still available in thrift stores and on Facebook Marketplace and other online sources, and the ink ribbons are easy to find. Kids love them because of the sensory experience, with the substantial feel of the keys, the clacking, the ding at the end of the row and the swoosh of the carriage return. Typewriters also instill good typing habits, since errors have consequences and force you to slow down and be precise. Plus, there's something to be said for having the finished product in hand when you're done typing instead of having to print.

LifeHacker.com

GOOD TO KNOW...

Going Someplace Crowded with a Child?

Snap his/her photo first. Having a photo of the child on your phone—especially one that shows what he/she is wearing—can help police and other security personnel find your child faster.

Also: For children old enough to follow instructions, establish a meeting point so that you know where to check if you become separated.

LifeHacker.com

Reading White Noise

Fuzzy letters may help children with learning disabilities. Children with attention problems, including ADHD, who read words with pixelated letters—called "visual white noise"—performed significantly better on reading ability and recall. The visual white noise had no negative effect on children who were already good readers.

Study of 80 11-year-old children by researchers at University of Gothenburg, Sweden, published in *Brain and Behavior.*

New Gen Z Trend— Ditching Smartphones

About half of the Gen Z generation (born between 1997 and 2012) report that constant connection to social media makes them sad, anxious and depressed. So a growing number are exchanging their smartphones for so-called "brick" phones—such as the old Motorola, Nokia and flip phones. Observers predict that this generation will migrate away from public platforms to private friendship groups.

HuckMag.com

Children with Autism Are Good for Cats

Children with autism often are given shelter cats as companion pets to help lower their stress and anxiety.

Recent study: Interacting with the child also had a positive effect on the cats. Levels of the stress hormone cortisol in the cats went down in the weeks after adoption and their weight increased—both signs that the cats

were less stressed and adapting well to their new homes.

Study by researchers at MU Research Center for Human-Animal Interaction, University of Missouri-Columbia, published in *Frontiers in Veterinary Science.*

Save Money on Veterinary Bills

As long as your pet doesn't need an expensive procedure immediately, shop around for the best price. Typically, you can find low-cost clinics at veterinary schools.

To find the veterinary schools in your state: Check the American Veterinary Medical Association (AVMA.org), and contact the schools directly to ask if they have a clinic.

ThePennyHoarder.com

Baby Talk Works

Want to Make Instant Friends With a Baby?

Imitate him or her. Scientists studying interactions between six-month-old babies and strangers have found that infants recognize when they're being imitated, perceive imitators as more friendly, and look and smile longer when adults imitate them than when they interact in other ways. Mimicking behavior seems to catch babies' interest and may play a role in social learning.

Study by researchers at Lund University, Sweden, reported in *PLOS One.*

Baby Talk Helps Infants Learn Speech

When adults speak to babies at a higher pitch and slower speed and with exaggerated pronunciation, it helps infants understand what is being said and learn how words should sound.

Study by researchers at University of Florida, Gainesville, published in *Journal of Speech, Language and Hearing Research.*

Do Not Let Dogs Play with Tennis Balls

The balls are not sturdy enough for sustained chewing—and if a dog swallows pieces of a tennis ball, it can cause an intestinal blockage. Chemicals used in making tennis balls also are dangerous to dogs. And excessively chewing tennis balls can damage the enamel of dogs' teeth. Safe chew toys should give a little to avoid hurting the dog's teeth but not be so soft that they can be ripped or torn apart. Avoid any flavors or coatings that might upset the dog's stomach. The size of the toy should be based on the dog's mouth and head—not too small or too large. Ideally, all toys should also be washable.

Consensus of veterinarians, reported at Lifehacker. com.

Catnip Protects Felines Against Mosquitoes

Nepetalactone, the psychoactive compound in catnip that makes cats euphoric, also keeps mosquitoes away. Mosquitoes are much less likely to land on cats that have rubbed themselves on catnip leaves…a finding that may pave the way for new insect repellents for humans.

Study by researchers at Iwate University, Morioka, Japan, published in *Science Advances*.

Is That Plant Safe for Your Pets?

Plants with milky sap…naturally shiny leaves…yellow or white berries…or that grow in an umbrella shape can be dangerous.

Examples: Amaryllis, calla lily, chinaberry, dracaena, elephant's ear, ficus, ivy, rubber plant and snake plant.

GardeningKnowHow.com

Better Dog Food

"House brands" from companies that make products for other companies and their own dog foods as a sideline—such as Tuffy's, NutriSource and PureVita—have strong safety records, healthful ingredients and reasonable prices. But pay attention to recall notices.

Example: Midwestern Pet Foods had two safety-related recalls—one for an *aflatoxin* contamination that killed more than 100 dogs. Affected brands included SportMix and Pro Pac. Avoid buying any food within six months of its "best by" date, which can be up to 24 months from the manufacturing date.

Nancy Kerns, editor, *Whole Dog Journal*, provider of dog-related guidance. Whole-Dog-Journal.com

Free Apps to Keep Your Cat Entertained

Friskies Catfishing 2—fish move around on the screen and when your cat swipes at one, the reward is a satisfying water sound. *Mouse for Cats*—first one mouse, then more and more, appear and squeak when tapped. *Mouse in Cheese*—3D mice peek out from the holes in a round of Swiss, squeaking satisfyingly when they're "caught" and getting faster with each round.

Catnip, a newsletter from Tufts University Cummings School of Veterinary Medicine.

Homemade Holiday Treats for Your Dog

Peanut butter bites—mix until stiff three tablespoons olive oil, one-quarter cup smooth peanut butter (salt-, sugar- and xylitol-free), one-quarter cup honey (not raw), two eggs, two tablespoons water, two cups whole wheat or rice flour and one-and-a-half tablespoons baking powder. Roll dough to one-half inch thickness and cut out shapes with a cookie cutter. Bake for 20 to 25 minutes at 350°F... then turn off the oven and leave the cookies inside the oven for one to two hours to harden. *Banana oatmeal cookies*—mix one-and-a-half cups whole wheat or rice flour, one-half teaspoon baking soda, one cup applesauce (sugar- and xylitol-free), one-quarter cup olive oil, three mashed bananas, one-and-one-quarter cup honey (not raw) and one-and-three-quarter cups uncooked quick oats. Drop spoonfuls of dough on a baking sheet about one-and-a-half inches apart...bake at 350°F for 10 to 15 minutes...then turn off the oven, leaving cookies inside for one to two hours to harden.

Recipes from *Our Doggie Desserts* by Cheryl Gianfrancesco, reported in *Dogster*.

Pet-Friendly Home Upgrades

Vinyl *hardwood flooring and/or stain-resistant carpeting* make cleanup of pet accidents easy. *Radiant floor heating* keeps pets comfortable in cold weather while keeping your feet warm and improving your home's energy efficiency. *A fenced-in yard* keeps your animal companions safe and other wildlife out and can boost your home's resale value. *A feline fortress* is an otherwise unused area of your home—such as space beneath stairs—where you can put scratching posts, carpeting and cardboard to make a den for a cat. *Smart*

dog doors are electronic and weatherproof, with automated controls linked to programmable collars or pet-safe microchips that unlock the flap while keeping your home secure.

Ally.com

Cold-Weather Cautions for Dogs

Most dogs enjoy chilly weather, but they need your help to stay safe and comfortable.

Salt-treated roads/sidewalks: Salt can sting a dog's feet and be toxic if ingested, so consider buying boots or use a paw coating such as Musher's Secret to keep paws from cracking. Always wash and dry your dog's paws when you get back home.

Coat: Most dogs do not need a coat if the weather is in the teens. But small, thin, short-haired and/or elderly dogs should wear a jacket—and watch for signs that the dog is getting too cold, such as shivering, moving more slowly, having cold ears and/or whining.

When your dog has had enough: If your dog is picking up his paws, sitting and/or refusing to walk, it means that he wants to go back inside. If you've been playing in the snow or if it's slushy outside, be sure to dry him off when you get back.

DogWatch. Vet.Cornell.edu

16

House and Garden Help

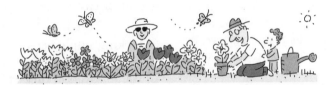

Surviving a Home Renovation

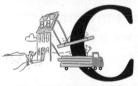

ontractors who can't be contacted...projects that don't progress...the privacy of home replaced by living in a construction site. When people picture home renovations, they typically imagine how nice their homes will be after the work is complete...and ignore how challenging life could be while that work is underway. Renovation inconveniences can be especially daunting now—building product shortages, shipping delays and contractors stretched thin in today's red-hot real estate market mean that many renovations are taking longer and costing more than expected.

Ways to make a home renovation as painless as possible...

CHOOSING A CONTRACTOR

Which contractor you choose and how well you communicate with him/her will have a tremendous effect on how unpleasant the project becomes.

•**Hire a contractor who specializes in your project and price range.** The contractor recommended by your friend might not be a good choice for you if your friend had his kitchen redone and you want your basement finished. Most renovation contractors earn the lion's share of their income from a specific type of job—but you might not realize that when looking at their websites and ads. Contractors generally claim expertise in a wide range of renovation projects to avoid missing out on potential clients.

So how can you confirm that a contractor has the proper specialization for your project? Tally up the photos on his website—often the largest number will be of the type of project the contractor does most. If website photos

Jim Molinelli, PhD, who has more than 35 years of experience as an architect and remodeler in Columbia, Maryland, and author of *Remodel Without Going Bonkers or Broke*. RemodelingProfessor.com

249

don't offer an answer, count up which types of renovations are mentioned in online reviews—you can't always trust that online ratings are honest, but when most reviews point to a particular type of renovation, that's likely the contractor's focus.

After discussing your project with promising contractors, ask how many jobs they do in a typical year...and what dollar volume they do each year. Contractors usually will disclose these figures because they like to brag about how successful and in demand they are. Divide the dollar volume by the number of jobs to get a rough sense of the typical job size. Choose a different contractor if that figure is not in line with what you had in mind.

•**Confirm that you will receive a "fixed price" contract.** This type of contract will establish the total price for the job—the contractor generally won't be able to bill you extra even if building-component prices rise or he encounters an unexpected construction complication. Fixed-price contracts usually do include a few exceptions—homeowners might be required to pay any costs related to the removal of termites, lead paint or asbestos discovered in the home...excavation cost overruns related to bedrock...extreme events such as wars or acts of God...and/or adjustments that the homeowners themselves make to the plans mid-project.

When you receive the contract, make sure it describes in detail the renovations that the contractor will complete and what is and isn't his responsibility, all in easy-to-understand language.

Don't hire a contractor whose contract lists little more than the price—that contract guarantees him the amount you are promising to pay but does not give you sufficient guarantees about what you'll get for that money.

A contract that lacks detail or lacks a fixed-price guarantee also could be a sign that the contractor lacks experience with this sort of work—he might be building wiggle room into the contract because he lacks confidence in his ability to price the job properly.

•**Be clear with your contractor—and yourself—about your primary goals for the renovated space.** Think through exactly what you want the renovated space to do for you and how much you're hoping to spend to achieve that. Reflect on the features and details you would like to include, then divide these into two lists—"needs" and "wants."

Example: "I *want* a six-burner cooktop, but I *need* a kitchen island with room for six stools." Keeping renovations on budget usually involves compromise so it's crucial to be clear with yourself and your contractor about where you are and are not willing to compromise.

When you consider budget, ask yourself not just *What do I intend to spend?*, but also *What is the absolute maximum I'm willing to spend?* If you cannot get everything you must have for your maximum price, consider walking away from the project. Check in with contractors in a year or two to see if costs have declined.

CHOOSING COMPONENTS

Picking appliances, bathroom fixtures and floor coverings might seem like the fun part of the renovation process—but your decisions could accidentally undermine the project.

•**Choose appliances, cabinets and tile as early in the process as possible.** These components are especially prone to delivery delays, so the sooner they're ordered, the lower the odds that your project will grind to a halt while workmen wait for them to arrive.

Also: Ask your contractor what other decisions he needs from you and when he needs them.

•**Order components locally.** The odds of project holdups increase dramatically when appliances and other key components are shipped from distant suppliers. Either buy from suppliers located close enough that you could rent a truck and pick up the items personally if necessary...or order appliances and fixtures through your contractor or subcontractors even if they charge more than online sellers. When you buy through your contractors, those contractors should take responsibility for finding solutions if there are delivery delays. When you order components yourself, any delivery delays likely will be considered your problem.

Keep a list of your second and third choices for each component in case your top pick becomes unavailable.

LIVING IN A CONSTRUCTION ZONE

Your home life is going to be disrupted during the renovation, but those disruptions can be minimized by taking these steps...

•**Construct a kitchen-and-bath plan for your construction-zone life.** Some homeowners tell themselves, *Having no kitchen is no big deal—it's an excuse to eat out...*or *Having no bathrooms is no big deal—there will be portable toilets, which is more than we have when we go camping.* That's delusional—living without kitchen and bathroom access is among the most unpleasant aspects of remodeling.

If your kitchen is being renovated, set up a temporary kitchen with your microwave, coffee pot and refrigerator. If there's no good way to reposition your full-size fridge, consider buying a small fridge for $100 to $200. Ideally set up this ad hoc kitchenette near a sink that will remain functional—a large mudroom sink is perfect. Or for $500 to $1,000, your plumbing contractor might be able to set up a temporary sink (or use the sink that is being discarded) in a room adjacent to the kitchen under renovation.

If you're having your bathrooms redone, your contract should specify that at least one bathroom will be fully operational—including hot water—when the workmen leave each night.

•**Get pets and possessions to safety.** Construction sites can be distressing and dangerous for pets because of all the power tools and strangers around. A panicked pet even could escape through a door left open by a workman and get lost or hurt in traffic. If your pet is unlikely to handle the hassles of renovation well, arrange for it to stay with a friend or kennel.

Possessions and furniture should be moved out of the part of the home being renovated. The odds of damage are significant even if everything is under drop cloths. If it isn't convenient to store these things in other parts of the home, have a portable storage unit delivered to your property.

•**Offer the contractor a workspace that works for you.** The section of your home being renovated isn't the only area that will become a construction zone—workmen will have to use power tools and stow materials in adjacent rooms and/or your yard as well. Ask your contractor if it would be convenient to use your carport or a garage bay as the work/storage space—that's often the space that best contains noise and leads to the least disruption for homeowners.

DIY Mistakes Homeowners Make

Danny Lipford, host of *Today's Homeowner with Danny Lipford,* a syndicated TV series now in its 24th season, and of *Today's Homeowner Radio,* which airs on 325 stations nationwide. He has more than 40 years of experience as a remodeling contractor based in Mobile, Alabama. TodaysHomeowner.com

Experienced do-it-yourselfers can handle a host of home projects, but overconfidence and other issues occasionally derail their efforts and lead to wasted time, wasted materials and damaged homes. *Veteran homeowners are particularly prone to a relatively small set of mistakes that they can learn to avoid, including...*

MISTAKE: Tackling projects that are almost impossible—or excessively risky—for amateurs. If even tiny imperfections will make the results look amateurish, hire a pro.

Examples: Finishing drywall and pouring concrete—amateurs are perfectly capable of performing these tasks, but only people who do this work full-time know how to make it look great.

What to do: Homeowners can hang drywall and do the prep work for cement, but most should hire a pro to finish the drywall and pour the concrete.

Exception: DIY is a viable option if the drywall or concrete is in an out-of-the-way location where aesthetics are not important.

Important: Always hire a pro for any electrical project where a mistake could cause a fire…any plumbing project that could result in major water damage…and any HVAC work that could ruin pricey HVAC components. "I think I can do it," simply isn't sufficient in these situations.

MISTAKE: **Rushing drying times.** Some tasks simply cannot be rushed. If you apply

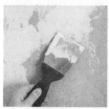

spackle, joint compound, paint or stain as part of a project, your next step is going to be to wait for hours or even days. If you paint spackle or apply polyurethane on stain that's not completely dry, the result is going to look terrible.

What to do: Read product packaging before you begin a project to determine recommended drying times, then factor these times into your project's schedule.

MISTAKE: **Not measuring twice before making tricky cuts.** Every DIYer has heard the advice "measure twice, cut once"—but

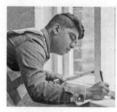

how many truly follow this advice every time? Two types of cuts are especially likely to go wrong—bevel and angle cuts, which are chronically cut in the wrong direction.

What to do: Measure twice with bevel and angle cuts even if you don't bother to do so with other cuts. This is especially important if the material you're cutting is expensive and/or you don't have much surplus on hand.

MISTAKE: **Not prepping the subfloor before installing vinyl flooring.** Installing vinyl flooring is well within many DIYers' abilities, as long as they don't make one common and critical mistake—failing to properly prep the subfloor. This step is easy to overlook when replacing flooring—the subfloor was fine for the prior flooring, so it stands to

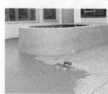

reason that it will be fine for the new flooring, too. But vinyl flooring shows subfloor ridges, dips and other imperfections much more than other flooring.

And once vinyl flooring is installed, there's little that can be done to fix subfloor issues without ripping up the flooring.

What to do: Before installing vinyl flooring, look for all imperfections by getting down on the subfloor with a flashlight and a long straight edge. Use subfloor leveling compound, which typically costs around $30 per gallon, and a floor sander, available for rent at many home centers, to correct any imperfections.

Warning: Don't just lay a piece of vinyl flooring over a subfloor imperfection to gauge whether that imperfection will show through. It can take up to a month for subfloor flaws to appear in the vinyl floor on top.

MISTAKE: **Sawing into a wall without knowing what's inside.** Cutting open a wall might be the simplest part of a repair or remodeling project, but it's also the part that can cause significant damage—it's easy to accidentally cut through wires or pipes inside the wall.

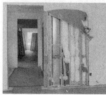

What to do: Before cutting, scan the wall with a stud finder that can identify not just studs and joists but also live electrical wires and both ferrous and nonferrous metal (a stud finder that warns only of ferrous metal won't detect copper pipes). These high-quality stud finders—sometimes called multiscanners or wall scanners—are available at home centers or on Amazon for about $50.

Problem: No stud finder can identify every potential hidden hazard, however—for example, flexible PEX pipes might not register—so before cutting into a wall, examine both sides of it for plumbing or electrical fixtures in positions that suggest wires or pipes might be inside the wall.

If the layout of the house allows, also examine the base of the wall you're about to cut into from the basement below…and/or the top of the wall from the attic above to see if there are any pipes or wires routed through that section of the wall.

If all seems clear, use a reciprocating saw with a short blade to cut a small pilot hole and peek inside. If this peek offers no cause for concern, you can use a more aggressive cutting tool to make the larger hole that the project requires.

MISTAKE: **Working without directions.** Experienced DIYers often disdainfully dispose of the directions when they are preparing to assemble furniture or install appliances—they consider following directions an insult to their DIY skills. But even if you already know how to assemble a bookshelf or install a ceiling fan,

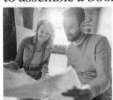

you probably don't know how to assemble or install *that* particular bookshelf or ceiling fan. The task might feature steps that must be completed in a specific and less-than-obvious order...or require screws, bolts or other hardware that have subtle differences and must be used in specific spots. A lockset might include bolts of different lengths, with different bolts used depending on the exact width of the door, for example.

What to do: Review and refer to the directions even if you're confident you don't need them. There is no reason not to. If the directions are hard to understand, see if anyone has posted a video on YouTube showing how to assemble or install the item—watching assembly steps often is clearer than reading them.

Cut Remodeling Costs by Scavenging

Architectural salvage and reuse stores, such as Habitat for Humanity's ReStores, offer gently used light fixtures, doorknobs, sofas and other household items. If you know a contractor, tell him/her what you're looking for—they typically throw away cabinets during kitchen renovations, even if they are in good condition.

Also: Drive around well-heeled neighborhoods and look through what people are throwing away. Keep an eye on online marketplaces such as Craigslist, eBay and Facebook Marketplace for great bargains. Act fast—desirable items tend to go quickly.

Roundup of interior designers reported at The New York Times.

Best Place to Find a Contractor Is Angi

Many Yelp reviews are fake...and Google searches can turn up scammers.

Better: Only bona fide customers are allowed to leave reviews of contractors on Angi (formerly known as Angi's List)—so you know they're legit. The site has a network of 230,000 professionals, and that number is growing.

Also: You can book the contractor you choose directly from the website or by using Angi's free app.

Komando.com

Hire the Right Plumber at the Right Price

Ed Del Grande, master plumber, home-improvement TV host and author of *Ed Del Grande's House Call.* EdDelGrande.com

Overwhelmed by the thought of finding a plumber—a good one who will do the work correctly and charge you fairly? *Here's how to make sure you don't get taken…*

• **When do you need a plumber?** If you're handy, you can probably fix a leaky faucet or replace a sink or a toilet by yourself. But you shouldn't tackle anything related to the home's main plumbing system. If the work requires you to turn off a single cut-off valve (below a sink, behind a toilet), DIY is fine…but if you need to cut all the water to the house, call in a pro.

• **Finding and vetting plumbers.** Online reviews can help, or ask friends or family members if they've dealt with one recently and would recommend him/her.

Or: Visit your local plumbing-supply store, and ask for recommendations.

• **Planning the job.** If a pipe has burst and your house is flooded, there's no time for planning. But in non-emergencies, first contact your city's or county's plumbing inspector—the person who ensures that local plumbing jobs are done correctly and up to code. Tell the inspector what you're planning to have done, and ask what permits are needed. Local codes vary—an insignificant job that requires no permit in one area could require one in another. The inspector will be your ally throughout the job, so pick that person's brain about what the work should entail so that when you talk to plumbers, you know the scope of the job and can push back if they suggest something excessive.

• **Bidding and estimates.** If you've already decided which plumber to hire, ask for an estimate. Most bill on a flat-fee basis rather than hourly.

If you haven't decided on a plumber, ask for bids.

Caution: Don't just go with the lowest bidder—learn the reasons behind exceptionally high or low bids. Two honest plumbers could disagree about what the job calls for, and hearing about diverse perspectives could be helpful.

• **Vetting plumbers.** Don't be shy about asking to see a plumber's license and insurance certificate. Plumbers work hard for such credentials and should be proud to share

them. A refusal to produce the documents is a red flag.

• **During the job.** Build rapport with your plumber by making him/her feel welcome—not like you want him out of your home as quickly and cheaply as possible. Most plumbers won't mind if you watch them work and ask questions.

Remember: Plumbers work in uncomfortable conditions. Offering a cold drink on a hot day, a coffee in the morning or hot tea on a winter night means a lot.

• **After the job.** If an inspector is involved, he/she will check periodically to make sure the work is being done correctly and will give a final sign-off. If the job was too small to require an inspector, ask the plumber to walk you through what was done and show you that everything is working. If anything goes wrong after the plumber has left, contact him immediately. Letting a problem go could make matters worse.

Heating Myths and Realities

*R*aising the thermostat does not heat your *home faster*—the furnace works at the same pace. *Keeping the temperature the same at all times does not cost less* than having it higher at some times of day and lower at others—turning down the thermostat for extended periods reduces fuel use. *Space heaters are not more effective than a furnace:* They can warm cold spots temporarily, but the electricity to run them costs a lot more than the natural gas usually used in furnaces—money is better spent fixing your heating system than adding space heaters. *Ceiling fans are not just for summer*—reverse the blades, and they help hot air circulate more efficiently in winter. Most fans should run counterclockwise in the summer and clockwise in the winter. *Fireplaces are not a good way to heat a home*—they seem cozy but actually cause heat loss in a home, and the wood they burn can be expensive.

FamilyHandyman.com

Heat Pumps: The New Way to Heat Your Home

Danny Lipford, host of *Today's Homeowner with Danny Lipford*, a syndicated television series now in its 24th season, and of *Today's Homeowner Radio*, which airs on 325 stations nationwide. He has more than 40 years of experience as a remodeling contractor based in Mobile, Alabama. TodaysHomeowner.com

Furnaces and boilers aren't the only options for heating a home today. In fact, they are not even the best options for most American households—they've been eclipsed by a device known as an air-source heat pump.

Heat pumps are not a new technology, but recent efficiency improvements made them the clear choice for the majority of homes. Heat pumps warm homes not by burning fuel but by taking heat from the air or the ground outside the home and transferring it inside… and in the summer, they can cool the home by transferring heat in the other direction. These devices can replace a home's furnace and air conditioning.

Heat-pump purchase and installation costs tend to be roughly comparable to those for high-efficiency gas furnaces and well below the combined price of a furnace and an air conditioner—though certain types of heat pumps can be very expensive. Some states and utilities offer rebates or tax incentives that further tip the balance in a heat pump's favor—enter "heat pump," "incentives" and your state into a search engine to locate these incentives.

Heat pumps are likely to produce lower annual heating bills, too—the average homeowner saves 10% to 20% compared with the cost of heating with a modern natural gas furnace…and potentially more if replacing oil heat or an old, inefficient gas furnace. These savings can be less impressive for households in the northernmost US—heat pumps are less efficient when outdoor temperatures drop below 15°F or so, because it's difficult for them to extract heat from such frigid air. Steep local electricity rates could curtail savings, too—heat pumps almost always are powered by electricity (although some gas models are available), though they use far less electricity than traditional electric heaters. *Three types of heat pumps…*

• **Air-source heat pumps transfer heat to and from the outdoor air, as their name implies.** They can be used with the ductwork originally installed for a furnace, which helps contain installation costs. Expect to pay $4,000 to $10,000 installed, depending on the size and efficiency of the system selected.

Drawbacks: Installation costs could be prohibitively steep if a home lacks ductwork, perhaps because it previously was heated by radiators. And as noted above, air-source heat pumps are less efficient in very cold parts of the country, though some of the latest models fare much better in extreme cold than earlier generations.

• **Mini-split heat pumps are much like the air-source heat pumps described above, except they don't require ductwork**—one component of the "split" system is installed on the wall or in the ceiling of each room to be heated/cooled…a second component sits outside. Because each room has its own wall/ceiling unit, mini-splits provide "zoned" climate control—homeowners can set different temperatures in different rooms, potentially reducing their utility bills without reducing comfort. Mini-splits also are a cost-effective way to heat and cool an addition put on a home or a garage or attic that has been converted into living space, because they can be added without upgrading the heating, ventilation and air-conditioning (HVAC) system that serves the rest of the building. Prices range from $2,000 to more than $10,000 depending on the number of units required, the efficiency of those units and other factors.

Drawbacks: The wall-mounted units are unattractive. Ceiling units are less obtrusive but don't fit easily into every ceiling. As with air-source heat pumps, efficiency can suffer in very cold temperatures.

• **Geothermal heat pumps exchange heat with the ground outside the home, not the air.** The temperature five to 10 feet underground generally stays between 50°F and

60°F year-round, which helps these systems remain extremely efficient even on the coldest days in the northernmost US. Geothermal heat pumps have few moving parts, so they tend to require few repairs and last an impressively long time—potentially 25 years, roughly twice as long as the typical furnace, air conditioner or air-source heat pumps. But the excavation required to install the underground components can push up-front costs from $10,000 to $25,000.

Drawbacks: You probably won't recoup the steep installation costs of a geothermal heat pump unless you remain in the home for decades. These systems are so efficient and long-lasting that they truly can pay back their high up-front costs over time, especially in very cold climates—but home buyers typically are unwilling to pay extra for homes that have geothermal heat pumps, so you'll lose out if you move.

Heat pump brands to consider: American Standard and Trane make the best heat pumps across all types, sizes and efficiency levels, though they tend to be pricey. Carrier is a good choice if you'd prefer to pay a little less for a heat pump that's almost as good as the top brands. Lennox and Bryant are respectable brands if controlling up-front costs is a higher priority than the unit's longevity—for example, if you expect to sell the property within the decade. Janitrol and Goodman heat pumps often are used because they tend to be the least expensive, although they are not built as well as others and may not last as long.

Do You Need a Generator?

Dan Mock, brand manager for Mr. Sparky, a national electrical services company.

The decision about whether to buy a home generator to be prepared for power outages—and which one to buy—can be confusing. *Here's what you need to consider...*

• **Cost versus risk.** Think of a generator as an insurance policy against outages. Weigh the costs against the risk of an event and potential consequences.

• **How common are outages?** To see where your state falls, check out MROElectric.com/blog/most-least-power-outages. For details about your local area, check your utility's website.

• **What are the consequences of a prolonged outage?** Can you get by without a CPAP machine? Will the pipes freeze and burst, costing you thousands in plumbing repairs?

• **Which generator should you get?** Home generators fall into three main categories...

• **Gasoline and/or propane-powered portable inverters** are called inverters because, while they generate direct-current (DC) electricity from burning fuel, they convert it to alternating current (AC)—what you have in your wall outlets. Inverters must be operated at least 15 feet away from the home, and you need an appropriate extension cord from the inverter to the appliance you need to power. A typical inverter generates about 3,000 watts, enough for a freezer or a small window air conditioner—but not both. You can run multiple inverters in tandem, but that's not very economical given the cost (about $550 for an off-brand model to $2,530 for the highly regarded Honda EU3000). A 2,000-watt generator running at half load will run about six hours on one gallon of gas or propane...a 3,000-watt generator, about four hours on one gallon.

Bottom line: If your needs are minimal and you want something plug-and-play, an inverter is probably right for you.

• **Gasoline and/or propane-powered portable generators** weigh more than 200 pounds and crank out DC electricity, so you can't just run a cord from the generator to appliances. Instead, an electrician will connect the generator to selected circuits in your switchbox—don't expect to run your entire house off a portable generator. They produce between 7,000 and 9,500 watts. You'll decide which circuits you can't live without, and an electrician will install a transfer switch to plug the generator into. You'll operate the generator at least 15 feet away from the house and run a dedicated cord to the transfer switch. Installing a manually operated transfer switch costs about $500...an automatic one, $1,500 or more. A quality generator should run for eight hours or more using a barbecue-sized tank of propane. You will pay around $800 for a bare-bones model and up to $2,300 for the premium Generac XG Series.

Bottom line: A traditional portable generator will provide about one-third your energy needs.

- **Standby generators are permanent installations placed on a concrete pad.** Typical wattage is 22,000 (or 22 kilowatts, enough to power the average house), with an automatic transfer switch so that the instant the power goes down, the generator kicks in. If you heat your home with natural gas, the installers will run a line to the generator and that will be your fuel source—otherwise you'll run off a large propane tank. Expect to pay $12,000 or more for an installed system (the Generac Guardian 24kW costs around $5,500...installation cost will vary).

Bottom line: If you can afford it, a standby generator offers total peace of mind.

Home Warranties—Never Worth the Money

Kevin Brasler, executive editor of the nonprofit online resource *Consumers' Checkbook.* Checkbook.org

---

The marketing goes right to your deepest fear—what if an appliance in your home fails? How will you afford to repair or replace it? Shouldn't you have full coverage against such losses? Don't buy into the home-warranty hype. *Here's why...*

- **Too many exclusions.** The things most likely to break—such as refrigerator ice-makers—usually aren't covered. Home-warranty companies have reduced the number of exclusions in recent years, but they've also raised premium costs.

- **Caps on payouts.** Say you buy a policy to cover your HVAC system. Payment often is capped at $1,500, which doesn't do much toward replacing a $7,000 heat pump, $4,000 central-air unit or $3,000 furnace. Still, isn't coverage for $1,500 a decent chunk of change? Sure, but not when you consider that the policy premiums usually are $600 to $1,000 per year. If you carry a policy for two years, you may have spent $2,000 for a $1,500 payout.

- **Service fees.** You will pay a $75 to $125 copay whenever the warranty company sends a technician to your home...and that's just to look at the problem, not to fix it. But the average appliance repair costs only about $150.

- **No choice of contractor.** You get no say as to who does the repair work. Among the thousands of Better Business Bureau complaints filed against home-warranty companies each year, a staggering number are related to shoddy work. And if a contractor makes your problem worse, the warranty company isn't responsible for the damage even if he/she was sent by the home-warranty company.

- **The numbers don't add up in your favor.** It never makes sense to insure against risks you could cover out of pocket. Insurers make sure that most policyholders pay in more than they take out, but at least with health and auto insurance, you're covered against catastrophes. With home warranties, by the time you factor in caps and service fees, the protection you're buying is minimal.

What to do instead: Establish an emergency fund. Take the $600 to $1,000 you would have sunk into a home warranty and bank it. Then when something goes wrong, pay a contractor of your choosing out of pocket. If you don't have an emergency fund, most contractors offer payment plans or you can take out a loan if necessary.

Caution: When you are getting ready to buy a home, you might be pressured by the real estate agent to purchase a plan or accept one in lieu of inspection. Ask for cash instead, and never waive the inspection.

How to Avoid Costly Water Damage

Danny Lipford, host of *Today's Homeowner with Danny Lipford*, a national television program that has aired for 24 seasons. Based in Mobile, Alabama, he has more than 40 years of experience as a remodeling contractor. TodaysHomeowner.com

The worst sound a home owner can hear is drip…drip…drip. Water damage is among the most common causes of homeowners' insurance claims. The biggest cause of water damage claims is leaks, drips and burst pipes that occur within homes. These are becoming more common in part because modern homes contain an increasing number of bathrooms and water-using appliances.

While this sort of water damage usually is covered by homeowners' insurance, insurers can deny claims that stem from failure to notice and correct a slow-developing problem.

Here are some of the most common mistakes home owners make…

MISTAKE: **Using rubber washing machine hoses.** These are prone to cracking and bursting.

What to do: If rubber hoses currently connect your washing machine to the water supply, upgrade to braided stainless steel. It's an easy do-it-yourself job, as long as you're able to move your washer to get behind it—just remember to turn off the water before removing old hoses. (Have a bucket ready because a small amount of water still might come out.)

MISTAKE: **Failing to check under sinks for drips.** Sometimes water damage isn't caused by a dramatic burst pipe but by a slow drip, drip, drip that goes unnoticed.

What to do: Every month or so open the doors of cabinets under sinks and glance inside for any drips and puddles. Take a sniff for musty odors. Look behind toilet bowls and washing machines for drips or puddles as well, and behind your refrigerator when you periodically pull it away from the wall to clean its coils.

When you look behind your washing machine, also remove anything that's fallen onto its water lines or drain line. Such things can stress lines, increasing the odds that they will burst. If your washing machine sits in a drain pan—this is particularly common when laundry rooms are upstairs—remove anything that has fallen into the pan. It's designed to be a fail-safe in case the washing machine leaks, but the pan itself could overflow if an item blocks its drain.

MISTAKE: **Failing to check on your air handler.** An air handler—that's the indoor component of a central air conditioner—typically has a pair of drain lines to cope with the water it removes from the air. The primary drain line is designed to drip whenever the air conditioner is in use. But most air handlers also have a secondary drain line that acts as an emergency backup—and if your air handler is in your attic, this line likely drips water in an easy-to-notice spot, such as near a door. The secondary drain line is in an obvious spot for a reason—if it drips, it means the primary line is blocked and you need to take action.

What to do: Determine where your primary and secondary air-handler drain lines are located, by following the drain lines leading away from the air handler or ask the HVAC pro who services your air conditioner. (The secondary line likely begins at a drain pan located under the air handler.) If your secondary line drips, use a wet/dry vac to suck any blockage out of the primary drain line. Or call an HVAC professional to clear the blockage.

To greatly reduce the odds of blockages, pour a cup of bleach down your primary drain line every three or four months to kill off algae that might be growing inside, potentially leading to a blockage. There should be an obvious spot to add this bleach—look for a cap or lid that can be flipped open to access the PVC pipe. When you do this, also confirm that the secondary drain line is firmly attached to the pan under the air handler—these sometimes come loose, leading to leaks.

MISTAKE: **Allowing water to sneak into gaps by tubs, showers or sinks.** A little water inevitably drips off of you when you step out of the shower or tub…or splashes onto the countertop when you wash your face at the bathroom sink.

What to do: Monitor the caulk around the perimeter of tubs, showers and sinks for cracks and gaps. If you see these, remove old caulk and replace it with a new bead of silicone caulk. (Leaving old caulk might prevent new caulk from sticking to surfaces on both sides.)

Also: Apply a bead of caulk behind the top edge of the trim rings that surround shower handles where they enter the wall. It's very common for water to get behind these and cause damage inside the wall.

MISTAKE: **Adding raised landscaping near the perimeter of the home.** Raised beds can cause water to pool against the side of the foundation, especially if the highest point of those raised beds is not directly against the side of the house. That pooled water eventually could seep into the home through tiny cracks.

What to do: Grade landscaping so that it encourages water to flow away from the foundation of the home, not pool against it. Gutter downspout extensions can help divert water away from the foundation as well, and they often cost less than $10.

MISTAKE: **Failing to maintain sump pumps.** Basements are the most vulnerable part of the home for water damage—anything from a failed water heater to a backed-up sewer line could cause water damage here. Basements vulnerable to flooding often have sump pumps designed to remove water—but those sump pumps are hidden away in the corner where home owners often ignore them.

What to do: Every three to six months, inspect the sump basin and intake screen and remove debris and obvious obstructions. Pour a bucket of water into the basin, and confirm that the pump works. If your sump pump has a backup battery, replace the battery every few years (or as directed by the manual).

EASY TO DO…

Easy Ways to Diagnose a Weak Toilet Flush

Simply dump a bucket of water into the toilet bowl and flush. If it flushes slowly, the problem is in the drain. If it flushes quickly, the drain is fine but the toilet itself has an issue.

FamilyHandyman.com

Clever Solutions for Tricky Home-Cleaning Tasks

Danny Lipford, host of *Today's Homeowner with Danny Lipford*, a syndicated series that recently aired its 500th episode. He has more than 40 years of experience as a remodeling contractor based in Mobile, Alabama. TodaysHomeowner.com

---

Do those hard-to-remove stains have you stymied? Are those hard-to-reach spots in your home backing you into a corner? And does your household garbage raise a stink? Well, rejoice. *There are simple solutions to many of the most challenging of your cleaning tasks…*

• **Stop trash can odors.** Garbage smells are unpleasant to human noses…and they can lure critters to your garbage can when you put the trash out.

Solution: To control odors in outdoor trash cans, spray the inside of the cans with ammonia diluted 50% with water, a disinfectant that's very effective at removing trash odors. As an added benefit, the smell of ammonia repels most animals, reducing the odds that raccoons or neighborhood dogs will get into your garbage. If animals are a recurring problem, spray the outside of the trash can with ammonia as well.

But the smell of ammonia can be overwhelming indoors. To prevent garbage odors with an indoor trash can, place a section of old newspaper flat on the bottom of the can below the trash bag, then another section into each new bag when it's placed in the can. The paper will absorb any liquids that drip to the bottom of trash cans and trash bags, a common cause of garbage odors. If newspaper alone doesn't solve the problem, also add one cup of scented kitty litter.

If the smelly trash can is inside a cabinet or closet, place a charcoal briquette or two inside this space. Charcoal is a wonderful odor absorber—more effective than even baking soda, the traditional bad-odor home remedy.

• **Remove pet hair from carpets and upholstered furniture.** Pet hair clings to carpet and fabric fibers so tenaciously that vacuums often cannot dislodge much of it.

Solution: Rake the rubber edge of a glass-cleaning squeegee (the edge intended to wipe water off windows) through your carpets. Pet hair clings to rubber even more than it does to carpet fibers, so most of the hair will be pulled up into clumps on the carpet surface where it can be easily removed by hand and/or a vacuum. For upholstered furniture, don disposable rubber gloves and run your hands over the fabric a few times to achieve the same result. The straight rubber edge of a squeegee won't work as well on furniture as on floors because furniture surfaces aren't as flat.

• **Remove grease residue from wood cabinets near your stovetop without damaging the finish.** Homeowners often resort to aggressive scrubbing and harsh chemicals to remove the stubborn grease residue that builds up on surfaces near stovetops. Unfortunately, those tactics can remove the finish from wood cabinets as well.

Solution: Spray cabinets with an "orange oil" cleaner featuring d-limonene, a natural chemical found in citrus fruits. D-limonene is an extremely effective degreaser that won't harm wood finishes. It's effective on tile surfaces, too.

Examples: Green Gobbler Orange Oil Concentrate ($26 for 32 ounces). Spray this on, let it sit for 10 to 15 minutes, then microwave a damp sponge for 30 to 40 seconds and use this to easily wipe away both the cleaner and the grease. Dry using paper towels.

• **Clear away cooked-on microwave stains with ease.** Stains inside microwaves can be especially challenging to remove because they become cooked on.

Solution: Combine one cup of water and one cup of white vinegar in a microwave-safe bowl, then toss in a wood toothpick or wooden coffee stirrer. Microwave this on high for four minutes, then remove the bowl from the microwave, using oven mitts or other hand protection to avoid burns. Don rubber gloves, dip a scouring sponge into this heated water/vinegar mixture, and use this to wipe away stains inside the microwave. The stains should wipe away easily thanks to the "steam cleaning" treatment the stains received when you microwaved the water/vinegar mix. Wondering why the wood toothpick or coffee stirrer was placed in the bowl? On rare occasions, water can superheat when microwaved, causing it to suddenly and dramatically boil up, potentially causing serious burns. A piece of wood allows bubbles to form along the sides of the wood, eliminating this risk.

• **Prevent water spots on glass shower doors.** Your shower keeps you clean—but how clean is your shower? In many homes, shower doors are a cleaning trouble spot requiring regular attention.

Solution: Clean your glass shower door using a plastic-bristled brush and a cleaning solution made from one cup of white vinegar mixed into one-half gallon of warm, soapy water. When you're done scrubbing, rinse off this solution, dry the shower door and apply a coat of windshield rain repellent before the shower is used again. Though designed for vehicle windshields, these products are equally effective at making water bead up and roll off glass shower doors before water spots form.

Example: Rain-X Original Glass Water Repellent ($6 for a 12-ounce bottle).

• **Clean the inside of lighting fixtures.** Some fixtures—especially outdoor fixtures—enclose their bulbs inside small glassed-in spaces. It can be a hassle to clean the inside surfaces of this glass if your hand doesn't fit inside. Removing the bulb can help somewhat, but even the socket could block access to part of the interior glass.

Solution: Buy a pair of two-inch-wide foam paint brushes—these can be obtained for about $1 apiece at a home or craft center. Spray one of these with glass cleaner, and reach this inside the fixture to "paint" the cleaner onto hard-to-access interior glass surfaces. When you're done, use the second brush, this one dry, to wipe away any excess cleaner. Do this with the bulb inside when the light is off and cold to avoid any risk of burning your hand or getting a shock…or remove the bulb temporarily (make sure the power to the socket is turned off).

• **Vacuum under a fridge.** Dust that gets under a refrigerator can stick to its condenser coils, reducing energy efficiency and potentially shortening the life of the fridge. A thin brush can remove some of this dust, but brushes often just push dust around the tight space under a fridge rather than remove it.

Solution: Use the cardboard tube from a used-up roll of gift wrap to create a thin extension wand for your vacuum. Poke small holes every three inches or so along the length of the cardboard tube on both top and bottom. Use duct tape to seal one end of this tube to the end of your vacuum hose, then squash the rest of the tube so it fits into the gap under your refrigerator. Every few months, slide this around under your fridge to suck up the dust underneath.

• **Dust ceiling fan blades.** Ceiling fans often are too high to dust by hand without hauling a ladder into the house or perching precariously on a chair.

Solution: Attach a paint roller to the end of an extender arm, as if you were planning to paint your ceiling. Wrap a dryer sheet around the roller cover, secure this sheet in place with a pair of rubber bands, then wipe the roller along fan blade surfaces on top and bottom. The roller is attached to the handle only on one side, so you can reach it around the blades to do the top. Dryer sheets do a wonderful job picking up dust.

Don't Ever Use These Products to Clean Your Wood Floors

Ammonia—it damages the wood's lignite (the substance that gives wood its rigidity). To cut through gunk, use Zep Hardwood and Laminate Floor Cleaner instead. *Oil*—a little oil isn't a bad thing, but too much makes floors slippery. Try Method's Squirt+Mop Wood Floor Cleaner. *A wet mop*—too much water runs down into the cracks and damages the wood underneath. A damp mop is always better. *Steam*—the porous wood will absorb the moisture, causing cupping. Mr. Siga Professional Microfiber Mop will get it clean without causing damage. *Soap*—it leaves a filmy residue, dulling the shine. Bona Hardwood Floor Cleaner makes for a quick-and-easy clean without the unfortunate after-effects of soap. Still looking for a shine? Mix one-quarter cup Pine-Sol with one gallon of water.

Reader's Digest. RD.com

Great Products to Organize Your Garage

Liz Jenkins, member of the National Association of Productivity & Organizing Professionals and founder of A Fresh Space, an organizing firm near Nashville. AFreshSpace.com

We ask a lot from our garages these days. Once just a place to park the car and lawnmower, garages have evolved into storage spots for everything from bikes and camping gear to bulk purchases of paper towels. They've become workshops and craft rooms. Some have even become refuges for people in need of a little personal space.

Fortunately, there are many products designed to help organize our garages.

Before buying any garage organization products: Drag everything out of your garage…dispose of items that you no longer need...sort what's left into categories—yard stuff, car stuff, camping and so forth...then determine how much storage space each category requires. If you feel overwhelmed at this idea, consider hiring a professional organizer. The website of the National Association of Productivity & Organizing Professionals (NAPO.net) is a great way to find someone in your area who can help.

Even if you decide to do it yourself, here are the best organization products...

•**Best way to hang items from garage walls.** *Elfa Easy Hang Top Track system*, available at the Container Store, consists of hori-

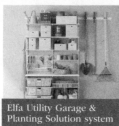

Elfa Utility Garage & Planting Solution system

zontal steel tracks that are screwed onto garage walls and have an extensive array of hooks, hangers, shelves and drawers in many finishes and materials. These components attach to the tracks to hold a multitude of garage items including ladders, extension cords, rakes, soccer balls and much more.

Advantage: You can reposition or replace the hooks and hangers if your garage storage needs change.

Prices: There are many components and combinations, but examples include $12.60 for a 32-inch length of track...$18.90 for an 80-inch length...$9.10 apiece for specialized hooks for ladders, lawn tools, cords and other items... and $21.30 for a hanging mesh storage basket appropriate for soccer balls and footballs. A full Elfa Utility Garage & Planting Solution system that includes enough track, hooks and other pieces to transform approximately seven square feet of garage wall space into versatile storage can be assembled for around $1,000.

Similar: *Rubbermaid's FastTrack Garage Rail Storage System* is comparable to the Elfa system but more widely available and generally less expensive.

•**Best way to hang items from garage ceilings.** The ceiling of a garage actually is an often-overlooked potential storage area. *Auxx-Lift's motorized overhead shelving* utilizes the space above parked vehicles. The chal-

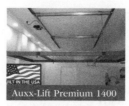

Auxx-Lift Premium 1400

lenge with storing things on shelves hung from the ceiling has always been that these shelves are tricky to access. But with this motorized unit you just push a button on a remote control, and a shelf that can hold up to 400 pounds will lower down to you or climb back up to near the ceiling. It's most useful in garages with ceilings at least 10 feet high. It must be mounted on a section of garage ceiling where it won't be in the way of the garage door when opened. The metal mesh and open side design make it easy to see what's on the shelf from below.

Price: $1,789 for the Auxx-Lift Premium 1400, which has a four-by-eight-foot shelf. Installation is about as challenging as installing an electric garage door opener. If you prefer to hire a handyman or contractor for the project, expect to pay for around two hours of his/her time.

•**Best way to store bikes.** *GarageSmart Universal Lifter* is a motorized lift that raises

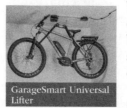

GarageSmart Universal Lifter

bicycles to near the garage ceiling at the touch of a button via a smartphone app—you don't need an electrician for installation.

Prices: $309 for the single-bike lift...or $369 for a multi-bike lift capable of holding three typical adult bikes. Installation can be done by most homeowners.

Beyond bikes: The company also offers a $329 Universal XL lift system for long items such as kayaks...and a $1,300 Truck Top Lifter that can lift a truck cap off a pickup.

•**Affordable durable shelving.** *Trinity freestanding metal wire shelves*, available at Costco, are the sturdiest freestanding shelves you can buy without spending a lot of money. They're available in a range of sizes, but the 24-inch-deep units are particularly useful for storing the large stuff found in many garages, such as big plastic storage bins, snow tires and warehouse club purchases of toilet paper and paper towels. They can be anchored to a wall for greater stability.

Price: $139.99 for a 24-x-48-x-72-inch four-tier unit...or $219.99 for a five-tier wheeled unit with similar dimensions.

●**If you think exposed shelving makes the area look cluttered,** *California Closets Garage Storage Cabinets* can hide stored items behind attractive, durable wood doors.

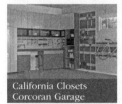
California Closets
Corcoran Garage

Price: Expect to spend $5,000 to $9,000 for a system large enough to cover one or two walls in the typical garage.

●**Most durable and affordable storage bins.** *Hefty's 72-Quart Hi-Rise Bins* are sturdy, sizable, stackable, inexpensive and moisture-resistant. They're made from translucent plastic, so you don't have to open them to see what's inside, and they're available at Target and other locations. You won't find a better big plastic bin for the price. Hefty bins are available in a range of smaller sizes as well.

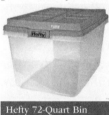
Hefty 72-Quart Bin

Price for one 72-quart bin: $13.79.

●**Best way to store tools.** *Craftsman's Rolling Tool Cabinets* are sturdier than competing tool storage units in their price range. They're constructed from steel, made in the US and feature drawers that are easy to open even when full of heavy tools because they glide on a ball-bearing system.

Price: $299 for the five-drawer 26-inch model. Other sizes are available.

●**Best way to stow golf gear.** *The Container Store's Heavy-Duty Golf Storage Rack* is made from durable steel and has room for two sets of golf clubs with shelves for golf shoes, balls and other equipment.

Price: $119.99.

Alternative: Millard's Golf Organizer is very similar and available on Amazon.

Price: $109.99.

Keep Your Car on the Road for 300,000+ Miles

Russ Evans, ASE Master Certified Automotive Technician based in Garretson, South Dakota. He is cohost of the syndicated automotive show *Under the Hood*, now in its 32nd season, which is broadcast on more than 240 radio stations and available on YouTube or as a podcast. UnderTheHoodShow.com

The average price of a new car recently raced past $46,000, a staggering sum that gives drivers more reason than ever to keep their vehicles on the road for as long as possible. Modern cars are capable of delivering a lot of miles—200,000...250,000...even 300,000 or more—but only if they're treated right. *Here are 10 ways you can increase the odds that your vehicle will live a long life...*

FLUIDS

The fluids that go into your vehicle can dramatically affect how long it lasts...

●**Choose the right oil.** Changing your vehicle's oil on schedule is among the most important things you can do to keep it on the road. If the owner's manual recommends oil changes every six months or 5,000 miles, don't wait any longer than that. The oil you choose is crucial as well—use the oil recommended in the owner's manual, even if it costs $75 to $100 for a full synthetic oil change or you can't use the same oil that's used in your household's other vehicles.

Warning: Do not assume that less expensive nonsynthetic oils are fine because you've been putting them in your cars for decades. Due to new environmental regulations, nonsynthetic oils don't protect engines as well as they used to.

●**Fill your tank with "Top Tier" fuel.** Use gas from pumps that feature a white, green and black label reading "Top Tier Detergent Gasoline." Top Tier certification means that the gas contains detergent additives that protect engines. Tests have confirmed that engines develop far less carbon deposits on fuel injectors, intake valves and other components when operated using this fuel.

To find stations that sell Top Tier gas: Use the search tool at TopTierGas.com. This type of gas is common at large chain gas stations…less so at independent stations.

Note: If you drive a diesel, the label will be white, blue and black and will say "Top Tier Diesel Fuel."

• **Don't ignore the transmission fluid—** even if it's almost impossible to check. If you search around for the transmission fluid dipstick under the hood of a modern car, you might be searching for a long time—many cars now have "sealed transmissions," which don't have dipsticks or any other way to easily check the fluid level and condition. But that doesn't mean the transmission fluid will last for the life of the vehicle. Check the maintenance schedule in the owner's manual— the fluid likely needs to be checked and/or changed at some point. I recommend that it be checked every 30,000 miles or sooner— and if there is any sign of leakage, it should be checked immediately.

Caution: These sealed systems can be tricky to access, so most car owners should leave this to the pros. Expect a mechanic to charge $100 to $200 to change the transmission fluid—that's a lot less than the $2,500 to $5,000 it might cost to replace the transmission altogether.

DRIVING AND OWNERSHIP HABITS

Some key things have more to do with daily use than with maintenance…

• **Keep it clean inside.** The messier a vehicle's interior, the shorter its life. Drivers who don't keep their cars clean inside tend not to maintain them under the hood either…but messes inside cars also can contribute to their demise. Food crumbs and packaging inevitably attract rodents that chew the vehicle's wiring, and the wiring of cars made this century often is coated with a soybean-based material that rodents find tastier than conventional plastic. Extensive wiring problems can easily end a car's life—not only is the wiring damage itself potentially expensive to fix…but if the rodents chew certain wires, it could trigger even pricier problems.

• **Don't tow or haul more than your vehicle's limit—or even close to your vehicle's limit.** To keep a vehicle on the road as long as possible, avoid towing and carrying significant weight as much as possible, and never exceed 80% of the weight that the manufacturer says the vehicle can carry or tow.

• **Let your car idle for a few minutes on cold mornings.** You might have read that modern fuel-injected engines don't need to be warmed up, and that doing so wastes fuel. It is true that warming up a car isn't as important as it used to be, but it still can take two or three minutes for oil to properly lubricate an engine on a cold day.

• **Drive conservatively.** The harder you push your car, the harder it's going to be to keep it on the road. Rapid acceleration and hard braking take a toll as well as increase the odds of accidents.

WHEN TO CALL IN THE PROS

Knowing when to take your car to a mechanic can make a major difference in how long it lasts.

• **Respond promptly to warning lights, drips or new noises.**

Warning lights: You don't need to immediately pull over or have the car towed if the dashboard warning light is solid yellow—but you should make an appointment with your mechanic as soon as possible, especially when a "check engine" light appears. If a yellow check-engine light is flashing, stop driving the vehicle immediately and have it towed to prevent further engine damage.

Caution: If a red lamp comes on, consult your mechanic right away. The longer you let dash lights linger, the greater the risk that a small problem will grow.

Drips: Take the car to a mechanic if any fluid other than water is dripping from it. A drip might be the result of a simple problem, such as a gasket that needs to be replaced… but the more fluid that escapes, the greater the odds that a major component will fail.

Exception: There is no need to take a car to a mechanic for dripping water—that's probably just condensation.

Noises: See a mechanic if your car starts making a sound it's never made before.

• **Have the timing belt changed on schedule.** In decades past, many cars had "non-interference engines" that would stop running if their timing belts failed but usually were fine once those belts were replaced. Most modern cars have "interference engines," which are more fuel-efficient than non-interference engines, but they often are destroyed if their timing belts fail because the pistons slam into valves. That makes replacing the timing belt on schedule among the most important maintenance steps car owners can take. Unfortunately, many car owners balk at the cost, which can be anywhere from a few hundred dollars to more than $1,000. Some maintenance schedules recommend timing-belt replacement as often as every 60,000 miles, though 90,000 or 100,000 miles is more common.

Exception: If your vehicle has a timing chain rather than a belt, this might not have to be replaced at all. Check your owner's manual.

• **Have a rust-proof undercoating professionally applied annually if you live in a rust-prone region.** Rust is among the greatest risks to cars' longevity in the northern US. Spray-on oil-based underbody coatings can greatly reduce rust damage.

Example: NH Oil Undercoating (NHOil Undercoating.com) is effective and widely available for a few hundred dollars.

air across whatever areas are wet for 12 to 24 hours.

If a garage is not available: Park in direct sunlight, and roll the windows down slightly.

Stubborn wet spots: Spot dry with a blow dryer, moving it around and taking frequent breaks so the dryer does not overheat. You also can use disposable moisture-absorbing desiccants or unscented silica-based cat litter. Leave desiccants in the car even after you think it is dry enough to continue pulling moisture out from deep in the upholstery.

LifeSavvy.com

Restore Dim Headlights

The lenses over headlights can become yellow or cloudy with age, reducing nighttime visibility.

What to do: Have your headlights professionally restored at a body shop for about $75 to $150, depending on the model of your vehicle. Or pick up a lens-restoration kit at an auto-parts store or online for about $20 to sand off the cloudy part of the headlight and apply a new protective coating. Both these options are temporary—the haziness is likely to return in a year or so.

More permanent option: Have the lenses replaced. Costs vary, typically $500 and up.

Consumer Reports. CR.org

Forgot to Close Your Car Windows and It Rained?

Start by sucking up as much water from the interior as possible using a wet/dry vacuum. Vacuum in a grid in one direction, then the opposite.

If you have a garage: Bring your car inside and use a high-velocity shop fan to blow

Easy Trash Can for Your Car

A large plastic cereal container makes a great garbage can for your car. It's the perfect size, and the opening is easy to pop open or seal shut.

OffbeatBros.com

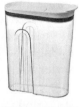

How to Recycle the Right Way

April Regan, sustainability specialist for USA Hauling & Recycling, Enfield, Connecticut. USARecycle.com

Did you know that every person in the US generates about five pounds of waste per day? Thankfully, many of us try to recycle as much as we can, but it can be confusing to know what you should recycle and what should just go in the trash.

Add to that all the misinformation floating around...and recycling may seem futile at times.

Reality: The more material we can recycle, the less waste we produce and the more we can preserve our natural resources.

WHAT TO RECYCLE

Recycling mandates vary by state, and rules vary by municipality. Check your town/city's website.

Example: Vermont is the first US state to require that people not put food scraps in their trash but instead use them for composting.

General rules: You can recycle magazines and newspapers...junk mail (including envelopes with plastic windows)...flattened cardboard boxes and packaging...office paper...phone books...paper bags...metal and aluminum cans...glass bottles and jars...and many plastics. Some towns and cities specify the types of plastics they accept, identified by numbers located inside a triangle on the bottom of an item.

Also: It is OK to recycle beverage caps—but only if they're screwed onto bottles. Small loose items can get caught in the sorting machines and are better put in a garbage can.

WHAT NOT TO RECYCLE

• **Plastic bags/packaging.** Never put these in your recycling bin, and don't bag your recyclables. Plastic bags can jam up recycling sorters.

Better: Switch to reusable bags for all your shopping.

266

EASY TO DO...

Secret to Cleaning Oven Racks

Frozen dish soap. Squirt liquid dishwashing detergent into ice cube trays, and freeze. Use the cubes to scrub oven racks—the grime will fall off easily. Dish soap usually contains enzymes to help break down food and grime. Freezing the soap allows it to act as an abrasive for additional oomph.

TikTok Content Creator @tanyahomeinspo, reported on LifeSavvy.com.

• **Boxes or bags with food stains...**and that includes greasy pizza boxes, which can contaminate the rest of your recycling.

• **Disposable cups.** Coffee cups and other cups like it are lined with polyethylene, which is not recyclable.

• **Shredded paper.** The paper's fibers are broken down by shredding, so it can't be remade into something else. Also, shredded paper sticks to other recyclables, making them unusable.

Better: Find out if your community or business sponsors regular shredding events that you can bring your paper to. If not, put shredded paper in your garbage bin.

Other things not to recycle: Foil and metallic paper...plastic-coated or wax-coated paper... Styrofoam...tissues or napkins...light bulbs... mirrors...Pyrex containers...pump spray nozzles...and aerosol containers.

Smarter Garbage-Disposal Use

Prevent sink smells by running the disposal for 30 seconds after food waste stops grinding and letting water run 15 more seconds after turning off the disposal. *It's OK to use the disposal if you have a septic system—* food scraps are mostly water, and homes with disposals do not need more pump-outs than ones without them. *Check the disposal's power* in your user's manual to know what it will grind—higher-horsepower ones can handle meat, bones, dairy and fibrous fruits and vegetables...lower-power ones (one-third horsepower or lower) are good only for food scraps.

FamilyHandyman.com

When Preparing Food in Advance, Make Parts of Dishes, Not Full Meals

You may not be in the mood to eat the same meal repeatedly and are more likely to order takeout or cook another meal—the point of advance food preparation is to avoid having to do that.

Instead: Make meal components such as curry, pesto and pasta sauces, and freeze in meal-sized portions. Then you can pick a curry portion, for example, cook some chicken and make rice, and have a complete meal much faster than making the whole thing from scratch.

Women's Health.

Chilis and Stews Need to Rest

If you eat a chili or stew the same day you make it, you're doing yourself a disservice. Instead, try refrigerating it, letting it get a good night's sleep, and reheating it the next day. The ingredients continue to undergo flavor-enhancing chemical changes long after you remove them from heat. Onions develop sugars, adding sweetness, while meats break down into amino acids that act as flavor enhancers, and starches such as potatoes and flour break down into flavorful compounds. And, as the concoction cools and then is reheated, it continues to evaporate moisture,

causing the seasonings to concentrate, making every spoonful a treat.

TasteCooking.com and LifeHacker.com

Easy Way to Speed Browning of Ground Meat While Keeping It Moist

Add baking soda to the meat before cooking. Use about one-third teaspoon of baking soda per pound of ground meat...toss the mixture...let it sit for 15 minutes...then cook it as usual, in a pan over medium-high heat. The meat will develop a thick brown crust, and the usual puddle of liquid will almost disappear. The ground meat will be more tender, too.

LifeHacker.com

How to Sharpen a Knife with a Coffee Mug

The bottom of most ceramic mugs (and plates and bowls) has an unglazed circle that makes a great knife sharpener. Hold the knife blade at a 15- to 20-degree angle and pull it along the edge of the unglazed ceramic a few times on both sides.

SeriousEats.com

Cooking Without a Recipe for Beginners and Pros

Sam Sifton, assistant managing editor of *The New York Times*, an "Eat" columnist for *The New York Times Magazine*, founding editor of the website and mobile app *NYT Cooking* and author of *The New York Times Cooking No-Recipe Recipes*.

You don't need to be an accomplished cook to succeed with the no-recipe recipes listed here. And each time you make one, it will taste even better than the last time.

• **Herbs and spices lead the way.** These ingredients can transform an egg, meat or vegetables into a triumph. Just taste as you go, and you will figure it out.

Hint: Eyeball a small amount of a dried herb or ground spice to see what one-quarter teaspoon looks like, and always start with a small amount.

Learn to balance flavor if you put in too much of an ingredient. It's all about maintaining balance between the tastes—sweet, sour, salty, spicy, bitter, astringent. That sauce is too sweet? Hit it with something salty, spicy, astringent or some combination thereof.

NO-RECIPE RECIPES

Black Bean Tacos

> Onion
> Olive oil
> Chile powder
> Canned black beans
> Lime
> Tortillas
> Cheddar cheese
> Crunchy lettuce
> Radishes

Sauté a chopped onion in a small pot with some olive oil, then sprinkle with chile powder, salt and pepper.

Add a can of drained black beans, and sim-

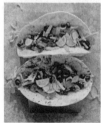

mer until hot. Drizzle the beans with the juice of a lime and set aside.

Serve on warm tortillas with a shower of shredded cheddar cheese, some chopped lettuce and slices of radish.

Roasted Fish with Soy, Ginger and Scallions

> Soy sauce
> Rice wine or dry sherry
> Ginger
> Scallions
> Fish fillets
> Neutral oil

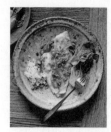

Heat the oven to 425°F, and put a sheet pan in to let it get hot.

Make a sauce in a small bowl—stir together a few tablespoons of soy sauce for every tablespoon of rice wine or dry sherry…a heap of minced or grated ginger…and plenty of thinly sliced scallions.

Optional: You could put some garlic in there, if you like, and a dash of hot chili oil or sesame oil.

Salt and pepper the fish.

Pull the hot sheet pan out of the oven, and pour some oil on it.

Add the fish to the hot pan carefully, put it in the oven, and roast for a minute or so, then paint the sauce onto the fillets and cook for a minute or so longer, until the fish has just cooked through.

Bananas Foster

> Unsalted butter
> Brown sugar
> Bananas
> Dark rum

Melt a lot of unsalted butter in a sauté pan with a big sprinkling of brown sugar. When

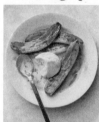

the mixture foams, add peeled and halved bananas, and sauté until lightly browned. Add a jigger of dark rum to the pan, and tilt it away from you. The stove's flame will ignite the alcohol (for electric stoves, you may need to ignite the alcohol with a match). Carefully spoon the sauce over the bananas until the flames go out.

Recipes in this article are reprinted from *The New York Times Cooking No-Recipe Recipes*. Copyright © 2021 by Sam Sifton and The New York Times Company.

No Air Fryer?

Make crispy fried foods in your oven! The secret is to use a roasting rack placed on a sheet pan—this allows hot air to circulate around the food.

How to do it: Preheat your oven to 450°F. Prepare your food—for example, for fried chicken breast, coat the chicken in flour, dip in egg and coat with panko breadcrumbs. Place the chicken on the rack, place the rack on a sheet pan, and put the sheet pan and rack on the middle shelf of the oven. Bake 15 to 20 minutes, until a meat thermometer reads 165°F.

Linda Gassenheimer, award-winning author of several cookbooks, including *The 12-Week Diabetes Cookbook* and *The Flavors of the Florida Keys*. Dinner InMinutes.com

---

DID YOU KNOW YOU CAN FREEZE...

Avocados...

Avocados can be frozen if you plan to unfreeze them for use in smoothies, guacamole or salad dressing. Freezing and thawing makes them unappetizing to eat on their own, but frozen avocados retain most of their nutrients and flavor if kept for no more than four to six months. Cut, mash or purée them before freezing. If freezing halves or pieces, brush the exposed flesh with lemon juice to reduce browning. To mash or purée, prepare the avocado by hand—you can add lemon or lime juice or seasonings but not vegetables such as tomato or onion. To use frozen avocado, thaw it at room temperature for about an hour.

Healthline.com

Whole Tomatoes...

Just put them in plastic bags, and store them in the freezer. The tomatoes will look fresh when taken out months later, although they will shrink and appear less appetizing as they defrost. But their skins will slip right off, and they are fine to use in sauce or anything else that involves cooking.

Mark Bittman, author of the *How to Cook Everything* series, writing at Heated.Medium.com.

Make Leftover French Fries Crispy Again

Place the fries into a nonstick pan, and heat over medium-high heat while tossing every 30 to 45 seconds.

Important: Each fry needs to stay in contact with the pan's hot surface to get crisp. Be sure to spread the fries out again after each toss. The heat removes moisture and reheats the oil in the fries to crisp them up.

Alternative: An air fryer also works well.

John "Chef John" Armand Mitzewich, American chef who publishes instructional cooking videos. FoodWishes.blogspot.com

---

Gravy Problems and How to Fix Them

Too salty—add a few tablespoons of unsalted butter or heavy cream...or simmer a potato in the gravy to absorb salt (remove the potato just before serving). *Flavorless*—salt, pepper, white wine, Worcestershire sauce, soy sauce, Parmesan cheese or dried thyme or sage all can add flavor (add sparingly). *Too thick*—whisk in heated chicken or turkey broth, or add a few dollops of heavy cream. *Lumpy*—pass it through the blender. *Too pressed for time*—buy a canned gravy and drop in some fresh sage stems as you warm it. Discard the sage before serving.

Real Simple.

Easy and Elegant Addition for Your Cooking: Brown Butter

This rich, nutty and deeply flavored sauce can be served over broiled fish or chicken, tossed with noodles and parmesan, or used in other creative ways. Put four tablespoons of unsalted butter in a small saucepan over medium heat for about 15 minutes. Stir, and scrape down the sides with a rubber spatula until the foam subsides and the butter turns brown.

To dress it up: In the last minute of cooking, add some finely ground nuts, chopped fresh herbs, mustard, vinegar or anchovies.

MarkBittman.com

Keep Mushrooms Mold-Free Longer

Remove the mushrooms from their plastic or cardboard container, and place them in a paper bag lined with paper towels. Roll or fold down the top of the bag so that it stays open, and put the bag in the refrigerator. This will keep the mushrooms dry and can help to prevent slimy mold for up to 10 days or longer.

Rachel Ng, food and travel writer based in Hawaii, writing at TheKitchn.com

Cream of Tartar Removes Stains in Your Kitchen

This familiar stabilizer and leavening agent for baking also bleaches. Mix a few tablespoons with hot water or hydrogen peroxide, and use it to clean aluminum pans, porcelain, copper kettles and even rusty drains.

Mary Jane's Farm. MaryJanesFarm.org

Less Is More with Laundry Detergent

Do not add extra laundry detergent in hope of getting clothes cleaner. The rinse cycles of modern washers are calibrated based

---

BETTER WAYS...

How to Store Cheese

Wrap in cheese paper (available online) or wax paper, and place in an unsealed plastic bag. Store in the refrigerator crisper (away from strongly flavored veggies) to avoid exposure to warm air when the door is open. Clean the refrigerator often to discourage mold spores. Don't freeze cheese—it alters the flavor and texture.

BHG.com

---

on the assumption that the correct amount of detergent has been used, and detergents are designed to mix with water in specific amounts. Also, hot water usually is not necessary—very hot water can be used when sanitizing is necessary, but in most cases, cold cycles are fine. Follow the directions on clothing labels.

Also: Beware of claims that certain products are "greener" for doing laundry. One reusable ball claims its "bioceramics" are as good as traditional detergents—but tests found it no better than plain water. Wool balls claim to be as effective as dryer sheets—but tests show they do not reduce drying time or wrinkles.

Roundup of experts on laundry products, reported in *USA Today.*

Better Than Woolite for Delicate Hand-Washables

Top product for washing delicate fabrics: Soak ($14), a no-rinse detergent that gently cleans wool, cashmere and silk. Other highly rated brands are Eucalan Fine Fabric Wash ($14), which is suitable only for wool because it contains lanolin…and Tide Plus Bleach Alternative High-Efficiency Liquid ($13/92 ounces), a good budget alternative that requires rinsing and is best for non-animal–derived fabrics because it contains the enzyme protease, which breaks down fibers in silk and wool. All are available at Walmart and other retailers.

Review of 22 detergents from Wirecutter.com, the reviews site of *The New York Times.*

Rethread a Drawstring in 60 Seconds

If the drawstring has pulled out of your sweatpants or hoodie, just grab a plastic straw and a stapler. Thread one end of the drawstring through the straw, then staple through the straw and the drawstring to keep the drawstring in place—it won't damage the drawstring. Thread the straw through the casing. The smooth surface of the straw is easy to feel through the fabric and won't snag on the material as you push it through. Finish by pulling the straw out the other end and removing the staple (and the straw).

ArtOfManliness.com

Inject Some Joy into Your Chores

Set a timer—finding that it takes only four minutes to empty the dishwasher can make the task seem less bothersome, and you'll be less likely to avoid it. *Create a ritual*—keep chores in perspective with a brief gesture of gratitude for the home you must clean or the family you must feed. *Let go of perfection*—accepting that a job is good enough can free you of some of the stress that accompanies chores. *Turn it into aromatherapy*—scented candles and cleaning products and powders that are scented can make household tasks more pleasant.

Ingrid Fetell Lee, founder of the Joyspotters Society, quoted on AestheticsOfJoy.com.

Smoking Marijuana in Your Home Is a Bad Idea

Whether you smoke for medicinal or recreational purposes in a state where it's legal, you could devalue your home by making a habit of lighting up there. Real estate brokers say residue and odors are hard to remove and are a turnoff even for fellow smokers, and they could take away up to one-quarter of your house's resale value. You also might run afoul of your community association or condo board.

Roundup of real estate and law experts reported at *The Wall Street Journal.*

Which Air Purifier Do You Need?

Caroline Blazovsky, nationally recognized as America's Healthy Home Expert and CEO and founder of My Healthy Home, LLC, which provides environmental solutions to homeowners, Whitehouse Station, New Jersey. HealthyHomeExpert.com

Indoor air quality isn't just a nice to have these days. But how do you determine which air purifier is best for your needs? *Here's how…*

•**Test your air.** *The Examinair* (Examinair. com, $400) is a DIY test that can reveal molds and allergens. You take an air sample, send it to a lab for analysis and get results in about a week. To find out if you are dealing with volatile organic compounds (VOCs) such as those in paint fumes and car exhaust, you will need to contact an indoor air-quality professional. You can find one at American Council for Accredited Certification (ACAC.org) or Indoor Air Quality Association (IAQA.org). Ask him/her about *IAQ Home Survey PREDICT* from Enthalpy Analytical (about $265 and up, Enthalpy.com/air/indoor-air/).

- **Remove sources of the contaminants.**

Examples: If your house has mold, it must be professionally remediated. If you're allergic to your pets, filtering the air won't help if you don't vacuum with a high-efficiency particulate air (HEPA) filter.

- **Find the solution for your contaminants.** The key characteristics when looking for an air purifier are particle size and method of capturing and/or killing the contaminant. The smaller the particle, the finer the filter needed to catch it.

Reminder: If your home is large and has more than one HVAC system, you will need one air purifier for each system.

- **Pet dander and pollen.** These large particles can be captured using a HEPA or, even better, ULPA (ultra-low-particulate air) filter. *AirDoctor 3000* circulates the air in a 1,274-square-foot space twice an hour using three-stage filtration to capture particles 100 times smaller than the HEPA standard ($629, AirDoctorPro.com). For basic HEPA, the *AprilAire Room Air Purifier* offers HEPA four-stage filtration ($399, Aprilaire.com).

- **Car exhaust, paint fumes, etc.** These VOCs can be removed using needlepoint bipolar ionization, which changes the electrical charges of tiny particles, causing them to clump and get caught in the filter.

Important: Check with the manufacturer that any unit you choose does not produce ozone. *GPS FC24-AC* is installed in your home's ductwork (typically, about $500 to $700, including installation) by an HVAC professional.

- **Wildfire smoke.** Smoke is a mixture of gases and large and fine particles, so it requires a multistage solution. *Intellipure Ultrafine 468* uses a six-stage VOC absorption filter and a patented filtration system. It can purify 1,200 square feet ($999, Intellipure.com).

- **Mold.** Mold spores are large particles that can be captured with a HEPA filter. The best purifier kills the spores using UV light. *Sanitaire* from Atlantic Ultraviolet ($1,257, Ultraviolet.com) is a standalone unit...or the *AeroLogic UV Air Duct Disinfection* system

(about $365 to $765, Ultraviolet.com) mounts inside an HVAC system, is more economical and can cover more space. For UV technologies to work, they need to be sized for your home. You will need an HVAC professional for sizing and installation.

When to Cover Your Outdoor AC Unit

Whole-house air-conditioning units are meant to be outside in all kinds of weather. Generally, it's OK to leave a unit uncovered in locales where it never snows. But you may want to cover the unit if it is close to trees, since sap, pine needles and leaves can get inside and trap moisture that will lead to rust and corrosion.

Also: If you're in an area that gets a lot of precipitation, covering it can help protect the inner chamber from multiple freeze/thaw cycles, which can deteriorate the unit.

Best: A cover designed to fit only over the top of the unit. Covers that wrap the entire unit can trap moisture and speed up rusting.

Warning: Never cover a heat-pump-style HVAC system that cools your house in summer and warms it in winter. Covering the portion that is outside the house can damage it.

LifeSavvy.com

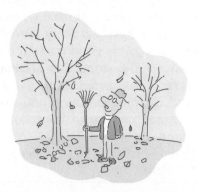

Brighten Weathered Aluminum Siding

Cleaning with a strong detergent solution can bring new life to faded aluminum siding. Mix one-third cup laundry detergent with two-thirds cup trisodium phosphate (available in stores such as Walmart and online), one quart 5% household bleach and three quarts water.

Note: Test the solution first to make sure your siding color won't be uneven when it dries. Avoid abrasive cleaners, which damage the finish.

The Old Farmer's Almanac. Almanac.com

Made for the Shade

Lawrence Winterburn, president of GardenStructure.com, a boutique designer/builder of outdoor wood structures in southern Ontario that sells plans to do-it-yourselfers worldwide. He has more than 30 years of experience as a master carpenter.

It's summer's backyard balancing act—how to enjoy a sunny day…without getting too much sun. Home centers offer a range of products and structures designed to provide backyard shade—but these often are shoddily constructed. *Here's how to choose the best shade-casting products without getting burned…*

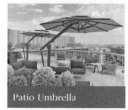
Patio Umbrella

•**Patio umbrellas** often are so cheaply constructed that they rip, bend or break during the first strong wind. Most also are small, forcing users to reposition themselves or the umbrella as the sun moves across the sky.

Better: A large, cantilevered umbrella is more attractive and functional—the post is to one side, not directly in the center where you want to position deck furniture. Pay a bit more for an umbrella made in North America or Europe. Look for a well-constructed unit designed for heavy commercial use. It will look nice and last many years.

Example: Poggesi's "Summer" 10-x-10-foot to 13-x-13-foot Italian designed-and-built cantilevered umbrellas. $3,920. PoggesiUSA.com

What to avoid: Umbrellas made in China by companies that sell primarily to the residential market.

•**Shade sails** are large triangular or rectangular pieces of canvas attached at their corners to posts or other fixed points to shade the area below. They're a stylish, summery shade solution—picture a ship's sail in your choice of colors moving gently in the backyard breeze. But like ships' sails, shade sails can catch a tremendous amount of wind, so they can be

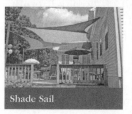
Shade Sail

difficult to take down when the wind picks up. To prevent wind from causing problems, attach the corners of these sails to strong pipes or posts set in hefty cement footings—at least one-third of the length of each pipe or post should be in the footing underground. If you want to attach a sail to your house, hire a contractor or engineer experienced with shade sails—otherwise, a strong wind could cause damage to your home.

For maximum durability, purchase a commercial-grade sail—one made of heavy Dacron for use on sailboats. Ask the company whether it offers an upgrade to this type of fabric.

Example: Shade Sail's Skyclipse 370 is better constructed than many other sails on the residential market. $1,150 for an 18-foot triangular sail. The cost of having the mounting posts professionally installed could add $2,000 to $5,000 to your bill. ShadeSails.com

•**Awnings** typically are mounted on the side of a home to shade adjacent outdoor areas under canvas and/or reduce the amount

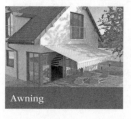
Awning

of sunlight that enters the home through windows. To prevent wind damage, most awnings can be easily retracted either manually or with a motor. Some even include sensors so they retract automatically in strong winds, a feature worth having.

Contact local companies that custom-make awnings. Work with one that has been in business for at least a decade and uses Somfy motors and systems, the most reliable in the sector. Awning makers that use quality components usually do quality work.

Also: Ask for an extended warranty. Expect to spend $2,000 to $6,000 for the awning and the installation, depending on awning size.

What to avoid: The poorly made awning kits sold at home centers.

• **Pergolas** are outdoor rooms without walls or complete roofs—vertical posts support overhead cross beams that block some

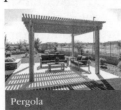
Pergola

but not all the sun. For additional sun protection, tinted polycarbonate panels can be added over the roof and drop-down shades to the sides. Vines such as bougainvillea, bower vine, clematis, grapes and trumpet creeper can be grown up and over pergolas for attractive natural overhead sun protection, though it takes several years for vines to grow sufficiently to provide shade. Ask a local garden store to recommend vines that will thrive in your area.

Alternative: Some pergolas have motorized louvered canopies on or under their roofs so that the amount of sun entering can be adjusted at the push of a button or pull of a draw cord.

Examples: Companies that sell well-made pergolas and pergola kits include Walpole Outdoors (WalpoleOutdoors.com) and Western Timber Frame (WesternTimberFrame.com). StruXure (Struxure.com) is the leading maker of pergolas with automated louvres.

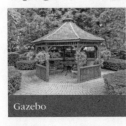
Gazebo

• **Gazebos and pavilions** are similar to pergolas except that they have full, finished roofs. As with pergolas, the kits sold in home centers generally are not as dura-

ble. Expect to pay a local contractor $7,000 to $20,000 for a well-made structure, depending on materials and size.

Example: Western Timber Frame offers gazebos and pavilions. WesternTimberFrame.com

Save Sawdust from Construction Projects or Tree Removal for These Hacks

Make a path—besides being aesthetically pleasing, a trail of sawdust through a wooded lot or garden can stave off erosion and prevent weeds. *Properly dispose of paint*—filling the bucket with sawdust and letting it harden allows you to toss the can in the garbage without running afoul of local-government regulations. *Fill gaps in wood*—take a portion of sawdust created from the wood you're trying to match, grind it to a paste and mix with wood glue to create a putty.

BobVila.com

Got Silverfish?

Signs such as chewed book pages and cardboard containers of flour, cereal and other sources of carbohydrate are clues of infestation by these silvery-colored insects whose bodies swing from side to side as they scurry away.

To get rid of them: Place sticky traps with pesticide in the glue in infested areas. Keep places where silverfish like to hide, such as under sinks and in closets, well-ventilated. Run dehumidifiers in rooms where you've seen the pests. Spread diatomaceous earth, a powder made of tiny silica particles, where you see silverfish and where they can enter your home, such as gaps around pipes. Try the natural insecticide pyrethrin or the synthetic permethrin—but be aware that both are extremely toxic to cats.

The Old Farmer's Almanac. Almanac.com

The Bugs You Want in Your Garden

Teri Dunn Chace, author of more than 35 gardening books, including *The Anxious Gardener's Book of Answers.* She lives in central New York. TeriChace Writer.com

While bugs, beetles and other creepy-crawlies are not welcome indoors, stay your hand when you spot them outside! The realization that not all bugs are bad is relatively new. In the past, gardening books and magazines touted remedies to rid your garden of insect pests, and garden-supply shelves were chock-a-block with sprays, dusts and granules intended to poison them. Nowadays we gardeners are learning to tolerate activity around and some damage to our plants in exchange for not upsetting the balance of nature. *Here is an overview of this fresh and important way of gardening...*

BEE HAPPY

Bees are the most important pollinators on earth. If they did not move pollen as they visit flowers—including in flowerbeds, window boxes, vegetable gardens, fruit trees and berry bushes—the food supply as we know it would collapse. No apples. No broccoli. No sunflowers. No pumpkins. You get the idea. Statistics on bee-population decline vary but are alarming. US National Agriculture Statistics, for example, report a 60% reduction since 1947. *To aid them...*

•**Grow plants whose flowers bees favor in order to feed and sustain them.** Bees generally prefer simple "single" open-form blossoms found on many native wildflowers and garden mainstays such as daisies, cosmos and coreopsis. Yellow, blue and purple flowers appear to be their favorites. Fluffy, full-pet-

aled (double) roses, hollyhocks, hydrangeas and marigolds are far less appealing.

Never hit, spray or otherwise tamper with a bee hive or a swarm. If it's in an inconvenient spot or it worries you, call a beekeeper to come move the bees.

•**Avoid using pesticides.** Though not the intended targets, bees are harmed or killed by many garden chemicals. Examine the fine print on the labels—the EPA requires cautions about potential harm to pollinators.

Also, do not buy seeds or plants that have been treated with neonicotinoids, which are "embedded pesticides." These have been shown to be a major culprit in bee deaths.

•**Make them a home.** Home gardens—unlike many agricultural or park settings, which often are subject to chemical sprays—

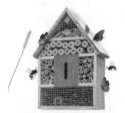

can be safe and healthy havens for bees. Native bees (which tend to be smaller than the familiar but non-native honey bees and chubby bumble bees) do not congregate in hives but can be accommodated by "native bee houses" mounted on walls, tree trunks or other spots. Some are quite cute, and it will help grow the bee population.

Fear not: These types of bees very rarely sting! You can buy bee houses from garden suppliers or online. Prices range from about $10 to $35.

OTHER "GOOD GUYS"

There are a lot of other insects busy in your garden...all good reasons to tolerate a little damage in order to respect nature's natural cycles and enjoy extra beauty.

•**Caterpillars.** Before you think about killing leaf-eating caterpillars, remember that they ultimately become moths and butterflies, which are valuable pollinators. A classic ex-

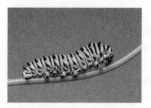
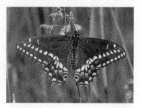

ample is the "parsley worm" caterpillar, which turns into a swallowtail butterfly.

• **Shimmering hover flies,** named for their ability to move in all directions like tiny helicopters, are voracious aphid eaters while in their larval stage, when they look like 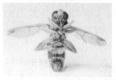 tiny slugs. Vegetable gardeners should welcome their assistance in ridding leafy greens, cucumbers, squash, potatoes and more of pesky, plant-sucking pests. Adult hover flies enjoy nectar and help pollinate many flowers.

• **Braconid wasps.** If you spot a destructive tomato hornworm covered with what looks like little grains of white rice, those are the eggs of braconid wasps. Don't interfere! These very tiny wasps will kill that hornworm and may even gain a foothold in your garden to 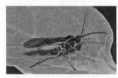 keep defending your tomato plants, although hornworms turn into sphinx moths, which are good pollinators.

• **Lacewings.** A beautiful little bug with light green wings, aptly called a lacewing, relishes mealybugs, aphids and other soft-bodied garden pests that may plague both flowerbeds and vegetable patches. In fact, it's possible to buy lacewings and release them into your garden, 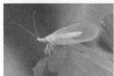 where they will settle in and become a valued part of your backyard ecosystem—a far nicer solution than deploying sprays.

MEET THE BEETLES

Of the many types of beetles in our yards, quite a few are valuable. Some play a role in soil health by aiding in decomposition via what they consume, digest and excrete. Certain beetles do this work in compost piles... others work on the bodies of dead rodents or birds in your yard.

Some beetles also eat other bugs. You may never notice night-hunting predaceous ground beetles, which go after caterpillars, grubs, grasshoppers and even snails and slugs, but they are common in most yards. Nurture them by leaving places for them to shelter in the daytime, such as out-of-the-way piles of leaf litter, logs or a pile of stones.

Most people do appreciate lady beetles, also known as ladybugs, which consume a lot of common garden pests, including scale insects and aphids. While it's possible to buy and release ladybugs into your garden, this is rarely successful.

Better: Attract a ladybug population to your yard by planting anything with a flat-topped multi-flowered head—they love these for the easy access to plentiful pollen. Dill, fennel, yarrow, sweet alyssum, angelica, carrot flowers and Queen Anne's lace are among their favorites.

You Can Help Conserve Native Bees

To combat the decline of bee species, the US National Native Bee Monitoring Research Coordination Network is asking everyday citizens to help monitor bee populations by sending in photos and descriptions of their sightings. Check USNativeBees.com for more information.

US National Native Bee Monitoring Research Coordination Network, USNativeBees.com

Deter Wasps with a Dryer Sheet in Your Mailbox

Mailboxes are a favorite place for wasps to nest...and mail carriers can get stung when they open the boxes and put in mail. The strong scent of unused dryer sheets repels wasps, discouraging nesting. Replace the sheet when the scent fades.

Advice from a postal worker on Reddit reported at LifeSavvy.com.

Better Way to Keep Your Lawn Lush

High-tech sprinkler-system controllers keep your lawn green while saving water. Rain Bird ST8-2.0 ($149) schedules and customizes watering and provides real-time reports. Orbit B-hyve Smart Hose Watering Timer ($72/Alexa and Google Assistant) meets Environmental Protection Agency standards for water efficiency, sends alerts for temperature changes and low battery, shuts off when it rains and increases or decreases watering based on temperature. RainMachine Touch HD-12 ($259) adjusts watering based on multiple Internet weather sources and can be customized for different areas of a lawn. Netro Spark ($150/Alexa and Google Home compatible) schedules watering based on variables such as soil composition, shade and local weather, and updates you on local water restrictions.

MansionGlobal.com

Enjoy Homegrown Veggies in the Fall

Teri Dunn Chace is author of more than 35 gardening books, including The Anxious Gardener's Book of Answers. She lives in central New York. TeriChaceWriter.com

Those of us who grow our own vegetables are accustomed to freshly harvested food, close at hand, delicious and healthy. As the gardening year winds down, we hate to think about going back to eating inferior grocery-store produce. No need! There are a number of tricks to delay that fate and keep the home-grown crops coming even in climates with snowy winters.

PROTECT VULNERABLE SUMMER CROPS

As temperatures drop in the autumn, the more tender vegetables (tomatoes, peppers, cucumbers with fruit still on the plant but not quite ripe yet) falter. You can lose them—and any unripe fruit still on the plant—to an early frost.

To get tender plants over the hump of a threatened early frost and productive on into the milder-weather week or weeks that often follow, there are several steps you can take to protect plants from the cold...

• **Water the garden in the late afternoon—** use a sprinkler so the plants get wet from top to bottom. This is an old orchardist's trick, leveraging the fact that plants freeze at lower temperatures than water. Wet plants often survive a frosty night, even if the water freezes and they become temporarily encased in an icy shell.

• **Cover plants with "floating row fabric" made of spunbonded polyester** (popular brands are Reemay and Agribon). This

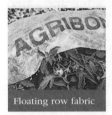

Floating row fabric

lightweight material lets in light, air and moisture so you can cover the plants (in groups or entire beds) as the weather gets colder for days or weeks on end, moving it aside only to harvest or provide supplemental water if the weather has been dry. This covering provides a few extra degrees of frost protection, which may be enough.

Drape the fabric gently over the plants, anchoring it in place on the ground with rocks, boards or wire wickets so autumn winds don't tear it loose or blow it away. You can buy it wherever garden supplies are sold, in rolls or precut sizes. (It's very affordable—for example, an 83-inch-wide, 50-foot-long roll is about $28.)

• **Shelter plants individually.** What you use depends on the size/height of the plant.

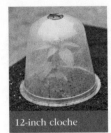

12-inch cloche

Tents of newspapers or up-ended cardboard boxes offer overnight protection to taller plants such as peppers and tomatoes. Plastic one-gallon milk jugs (bottoms cut off) can be placed over smaller plants such as strawberries. You want to protect the plants from the cold night but not let the next day's sunshine cook them. The best approach is to remove during the day and put them back on at night.

Or buy some of the plastic domes (cloches) sold by garden suppliers for this purpose. They look nicer! A set of three sturdy plastic 12-inch cloches—that is, 12 inches high and 13 inches in diameter—runs about $23 at Gardeners.com.

●**Try the Kozy Coat or Tomato Teepee.**

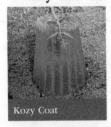

Kozy Coat

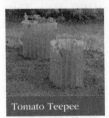

Tomato Teepee

Fill these vertical plastic tubes with water, and place over the plants (you leave them in place). The water inside will absorb heat during the day and radiate it back to the plants they're surrounding during the cold night. Buy from a garden retailer or catalog. They come in different sizes and often are sold in packs of three or six. A typical three-pack for 18-inch-tall plants usually is $30 or less.

VEGETABLES FOR FALL HARVESTING

If you've had more than enough tomatoes and peppers for one season, rather than extend earlier plantings, you can tear out your fading summer garden and pivot to fall crops…

●**Salad greens.** Try sowing lettuce, arugula, mesclun, spinach, Swiss chard and many Asian greens (tatsoi, etc.). They grow quickly from seeds directly sown into the garden and are fairly cold-tolerant and don't mind autumn's reduced sunlight. You can enjoy them before truly cold weather arrives. Use the frost-protection measures described above if winter comes early or you are trying to push your luck with successive sowings.

●**Cold-tolerant crops.** These can be started as seeds during the summer and then transplanted into the ground in fall to produce delicious crops before winter arrives. Good candidates include broccoli, cauliflower and scallions. Some farmers markets offer seedlings of these right when you want them, and some mail-order catalogs also offer seedlings for fall planting.

Pro tip: Source your fall-planting seeds wisely! Skip the standard choices in big seed catalogs or on seed racks in your area. Instead, browse the websites or catalogs of specialty seed companies in northern or high-altitude areas—areas with a short growing season. They select for good flavor and fast growth, and their offerings can just as easily be raised in less challenging, longer-season regions. Some of my favorite sources are Johnny's Selected Seeds (JohnnySeeds.com) and Pinetree Garden Seeds (SuperSeeds.com) in Maine… High Mowing Organic Seeds (HighMowingSeeds.com) in Vermont…and out west, Seeds Trust (SeedsTrust.com) in Colorado.

While many people do a spring crop of root vegetables such as carrots, beets and potatoes, I encourage a second round in late summer or fall. In both seasons, it is wise to start the plants indoors weeks before you plan to move them into the garden proper.

Alternatively, buy seedlings! Many garden centers and some farmers markets offer seedlings of beets, carrots and more in late summer and early fall. Parsnips and leeks have an even longer growing season and should be sown in late spring or early summer. Either set aside space for these, or fill empty parts of the midsummer garden.

Root vegetables can be harvested well into winter, especially when their rows are deeply mulched. Use mounded-up earth, leaf piles and/or bales of straw up to one foot thick. A little snow cover on top of that, when it arrives, does no harm. You'll notice that your fall-to-winter harvest often tastes milder and sweeter than the same crops grown in the heat of a summer garden. Spot-checking is the key to knowing when it's time to harvest. Then harvest as needed or harvest completely if the spot-check confirms they are just the size and flavor that you like.

The Right Way to Close Down Your Garden

Teri Dunn Chace, author of more than 35 gardening books, including *The Anxious Gardener's Book of Answers*. She lives in central New York. TeriChace Writer.com

How you care for your yard as the gardening year winds down can make all the difference for next year's garden. While there is plenty of advice about starting up a garden in spring, closing it down properly at season's end can be equally important. Moreover, not all of these tasks are intuitive. In fact, recent research has resulted in new recommendations. *Here are some best practices to follow…*

• **Timing is everything.** Pick your gardening days with care. Start too early in the fall, and your plants may not be ready to be "put to bed"—that is, they may not yet be on their way to winter dormancy. Tackle these chores too late, and you may discover frost damage on the plants or find yourself working in soggy or semi-frozen ground. Your best bet is to start preparing your garden for winter on a cool day in late fall, after at least one frost.

• **Get ready.** Just as a chef assembles supplies and ingredients before tackling a meal, you will work much faster and more efficiently if you lay out the tools and supplies you will need in a convenient place beforehand.

Tools to have handy: Shovel, spading fork, trowel, weeding tool, sturdy rake, wheelbarrow, pruners, loppers, garden hose and garden gloves.

Supplies to have handy: Large tarp, mulch, tomato cages, burlap or pieces of plywood for winter-shrub protection and grass seed.

Caution: Spare your back—don't bend at the waist! You'll be out of commission after just the first day. Instead, bend your knees… get down on your knees…or work sitting on a stool. If the ground is damp, kneel on a comfy kneeling pad or a scrap of carpet or cardboard.

• **Begin with cleanup.** Start with the biggest job in your yard, which almost always involves the annuals-filled flower beds and/or vegetable patch. Although these areas contain different plants, the job is essentially the same.

Lay out a tarp on the ground, or position a wheelbarrow close by. Toss all your discards here, and dispose of them when it's full or at job's end.

Yank out spent plants, even if they look like they still have some life in them. (Otherwise, you'll only have to return later.) Grasp each plant low to the ground so that you can pull out the roots. Use a trowel to extract stubborn root systems.

• **Separate debris.** *Make three piles…*
Ordinary plant debris goes straight to the compost pile or an out-of-the-way area, where it can safely decompose.

Disease- or insect-affected plants should be segregated and sent away with your household trash, so they don't survive the winter (in the form of spores or eggs) and return to plague next year's garden.

Nonorganic materials, such as plant tags, pots, ties and stakes, should be rinsed off and saved if they're still in good shape…otherwise toss them out.

• **Be careful about cutting.** For years, gardeners have been encouraged to cut down perennial plants to inches-high stubble in the fall. True, this results in a tidier look—but researchers have found that sparing the stalks and foliage confers valuable cold-hardiness (as it does with wild plants). Also, leaving flowerheads, such as those of coneflowers and black-eyed Susans, and ornamental grasses means that there will be some seeds for hungry birds to eat as they prepare to fly south or even to hunker down locally for the winter.

Resist the temptation to prune your shrubs, rosebushes, hedges or trees now. While some may have lost their leaves and pruning them may allow you to better assess their shapes or outlines, this is a bad time to prune because it exposes fresh-cut stems to cold damage…or it may encourage a plant to put out lush new growth that gets nipped by a frost.

•**Amend and mulch beds.** Rake over the cleaned-up beds as best you can. This not only gives your work a finished look, it may turn up a few scraggly annuals or vegetable plants that you missed.

Fall is a fine time to dig or till in some organic matter such as compost or shredded fallen leaves (to shred them, run a lawnmower over them). Leave these to "meld" or break down a bit in place over the winter months. The plants you install next year will benefit from the improved nutrition and texture they supply.

Finally, if you expect a cold winter or one without a good insulating snow cover, mulch all your beds. This task is best left until your ground freezes—doing it too soon can create a good habitat for unwanted rodents that may feed on plants. A mulch layer of several inches usually is sufficient. Leave mulch in place until the garden comes back to life next spring. It also will discourage early-spring opportunistic weeds from invading your beds.

Give any marginally hardy perennials extra mulch. A good trick is to carefully position a tomato cage over the plant and fill it all the way to the top with mulch or chopped-up fall leaves. Plan to remove it all when spring returns.

•**Don't forget your shrubs.** Now that you've removed faded flowers and vegetable plants, your shrubs—including rosebushes and hedge plants—need attention. You can and should send them into winter in good condition so they can return in glory next year. Assuming that there has already been at least one good hard freeze, it's also wise to take winter-protection measures.

Do not prune or shape these shrubs now, but do remove obviously dead, diseased or damaged branches with sharp clippers or loppers. After all, these plant parts are not going to revive.

Pests and diseases can linger in fallen foliage and other plant debris near the base of your shrubs. Rake out this material, and throw it away.

Finally, set the hose at the base of each shrub at a slow trickle for a while, long enough for a good deep soaking directly into the root system. This sends a plant into winter well-hydrated. Once the ground is fully frozen, water won't be able to get to the roots.

Some people wrap evergreens in protective burlap or make plywood teepees over them. Unless you live in a very cold area, this is not strictly necessary for their survival.

•**Do not fertilize.** Fall is never a time to give any plants, small or large, a dose of plant food. This only encourages fresh growth when they are naturally slowing and shutting down for the winter months.

•**Give the lawn a little attention.** Raking off fall leaves is the main order of business. But don't send this perfectly good organic matter away with the trash. Instead, make a mulch pile somewhere convenient or add it to your compost pile if there's room. To avoid matting, chop up fall leaves (it is easier when they're dry). Or you can chop them up in place with a traditional lawnmower or a mulching mower. They'll give the grass some measure of protection and nourishment.

Fall also is a fine time to do some lawn repair or renovation. The soil is still somewhat warm and probably drier than it will be in spring. Also, the air is cool, so watering and rainfall will be beneficial.

Remove scraggly, thin or damaged sod with a shovel or spading fork. Take it to your compost pile, but lay it in grass-side down so that it will break down instead of re-rooting.

Lightly dig in some topsoil or compost, and sprinkle new seed on the improved surface—not thickly, but as though you were salting food. Mulch lightly to protect the seeds from sun and birds, and water with a sprinkler every day for a few days, unless it rains. The idea is to keep the area damp but not drenched, so the patch can "take."

17

Tech Savvy

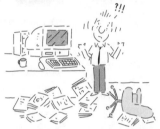

The Best New Consumer Gadgets from the Consumer Electronics Show

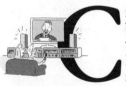

Circular smartphones, robotic cats, tech that tracks your toilet paper usage. Hundreds of unnecessary new gadgets in one place can mean only one thing—the Consumer Electronics Show. The annual convention where electronics makers unveil their latest products took place only online in 2021 due to the pandemic, but it returned to Las Vegas in 2022. *As in earlier years, hidden among the show's who-would-need-that gizmos and futuristic-but-far-from-the-market prototypes were innovative products…*

TV TECH

• **Ultra-portable digital projector.** *Samsung Freestyle* is a lightweight device that

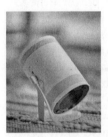

can project streamed high-definition video content onto a wall or ceiling. Earlier products like this tended to be bulky and suffer from picture-quality problems. The Freestyle weighs less than two pounds and can be plugged into an AC socket. You also can purchase a battery so that it can be moved from room to room or taken outdoors. It automatically focuses and levels its image. In fact, Freestyle will maintain its picture's rectangular shape even if it's aimed upward at a wall. It features 360-degree sound and responds to voice commands. Samsung.com

• **Astonishing TV picture quality at a colossal size.** *LG's G2 "Gallery Series" OLED*

Marc Saltzman, a technology columnist whose work appears in *USA Today*, among other publications. He is author of 16 books on consumer technology including *Apple Watch for Dummies*, now in its fourth edition. His radio show, *Tech It Out,* is syndicated on 279 US stations and available in podcast form. MarcSaltzman.com

TVs are available in an 83-inch size. OLED—short for organic light-emitting diode—is probably the best of the TV-screen technologies on the market. It provides wide viewing angles, excellent motion quality, bright colors and perfectly black blacks. With most TVs, black portions of the picture never seem truly black because backlight leaks through, but OLEDs don't have backlights—each pix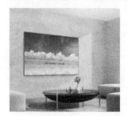el serves as its own light source. That also makes OLED TVs thinner, lighter and more energy-efficient. These LG OLEDs are an excellent way to create the immersive big-screen theater experience. These don't come cheap, though. The 83-inch TV costs $6,500. LG.com

•**TV remote that never needs new batteries.** *Samsung SolarCell Remote* debuted last year to help solve a chronic TV frustration—finding fresh batteries for the remote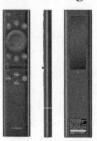 control when the old ones run down. This remote has a solar panel that can produce all the power it needs. That solar panel thrives if the remote is left in sunlight streaming in through a window…but even the light from indoor electric lights can be sufficient. This year's version of the SolarCell Remote is unlikely to run down even if it's left in the dark for days—it can also draw power from the radio waves generated by your Wi-Fi router. If all else fails, it can be charged via a USB-C port. This remote is now included with Samsung TVs. Samsung.com

KITCHEN AND BATH TECH

•**True touchless kitchen faucet.** *Moen Smart Faucet with Motion Control* isn't the first kitchen faucet that can be turned on with the wave of a hand, but this Moen takes touchless control even further—you can adjust the water temperature by gesturing left or right. Hands-free faucets are useful even in less-virus-focused times—no more trying to operate the faucet with an elbow when you need to wash dirty hands. This faucet

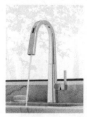 responds to voice commands when paired with an Alexa or Google Assistant smart speaker—even precise commands such as "two-and-a-half cups of 150° water." Prices start at $675. Moen.com

•**Tub system that runs a bath for you.** *Kohler PerfectFill* automatically fills your bathtub to your preferred depth and temperature upon your verbal command, with the help of Kohler's phone app. PerfectFill can maintain your desired temperature while you're bathing, too. The system is expected to be available sometime 2023 and is compatible with a range of Kohler tubs. Your budget will take a bit of a soaking, however—PerfectFill costs $2,700. SmartHome.Kohler.com

COMPUTER TECH

•**Massive tablet that fits in a modest-sized backpack or purse.** *ASUS Zenbook 17 Fold OLED* has a huge 17.3-inch screen that can be folded in half for transport—the less-than-four-pound tablet measures just 12.5 x 7.5 inches when folded. With its stunning OLED picture quality, it's the ideal tablet for streaming video. But it also comes with a wireless 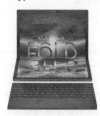keyboard so you can stand the tablet up and use it as a large and powerful laptop computer—it's equipped with the latest-generation Intel processor. If you don't want to cart that keyboard around, you can fold this Zenbook into an L-shape and use the lower section as a virtual keyboard. It's expected to reach the market by midyear. Pricing has not yet been announced. ASUS.com

•**Big laptop with a spare screen in its keyboard.** *Lenovo ThinkBook Plus Gen 3* has a 17.3-inch screen plus an additional eight-inch screen built into the right side of its keyboard. That second screen lays flat on the keyboard rather than facing forward when the laptop is in use, which makes it ideal for

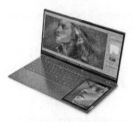

jotting notes with the help of the ThinkBook's stylus.

Example: You might jot notes or edits on a shared document while participating in a Zoom meeting on the laptop's main screen. The second screen also can function as a calculator and can mirror your smartphone. This laptop is expected to reach the market in 2023 with a starting price of $1,399. Lenovo.com

FUN AND GAMES TECH

• **Better bird feeder.** *Bird Buddy* is a bird feeder with a built-in digital camera and microphone to bring you closer than ever to the avian action. It saves photos of the birds that visit so you can see who flew in to enjoy your hospitality, and its artificial intelligence system

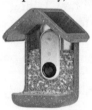

identifies breeds based on their appearance and songs. The Bird Buddy has a detachable battery module that lasts about a month between charges. It is scheduled to ship in the fall of 2022, but you can preorder one now at a discounted price of $189 or $259 with a solar roof attachment. MyBirdBuddy.com

• **Classic board games without all the bits and pieces.** *Arcade 1Up Infinity Game Table* is a freestanding touchscreen high-definition digital table that comes with virtual versions of more than 40 classic board games, including Monopoly, Scrabble and Yahtzee. Additional games can be downloaded for $3 to $10 apiece, including modern hits such as Ticket to Ride and Pandemic. Up to six people can play without ever searching for lost game pieces or having to clean them up when they're done. The table provides "haptic feedback"—a tactile response to increase the immersive experience when,

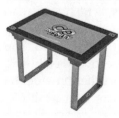

for example, you roll the dice—and its legs can be removed if you prefer to place this game table on another table. It's available with a price of $699

for the 24-inch model…or $899 for the 32-inch. InfinityGameTable.com

EYEWEAR TECH

• **"Reading glasses" that can read for you.** *OrCam MyEye Pro* is a lightweight device that attaches to one of the arms of a pair of eyeglasses. It helps a visually impaired wearer decipher words, objects and faces that he/she can't make out. OrCam has been working on this technology for years, but the latest MyEye Pro version represents such a significant step forward in speed and accuracy that it won an innovation award at this 2022's Consumer Electronics Show. MyEye Pro wearers simply say "Hey OrCam" to enable its voice assistant, then point it toward printed or digital text they can't read—the device will read it to them through a tiny speaker positioned

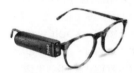

near the ear or through a paired Bluetooth audio device. MyEye Pro also can tell different denominations of money apart, for example. And if someone you know is standing in front of you, it could identify who he/she is. MyEye Pro is available for $4,250. OrCam.com

---

Can Your Smartwatch Save Your Life?

Michael Snyder, PhD, chairman of the department of genetics, and director of the Center for Genomics and Personalized Medicine, at Stanford University Medical School.

Thanks to "wearables" devices, you can collect medical data like heart rate and blood oxygen level that can help you determine a life-threatening illness before it becomes an emergency.

DETECTING COVID-19

We enlisted nearly 5,300 participants in a recent study, all of whom wore smartwatches, with most participants wearing a Fitbit, an Apple watch, or a Garmin device. In a previous study on Lyme disease, we had already discovered that average resting heart rate and skin temperature often increase days before an infection develops, and this study produced similar results. Up to 10 days before any kind of infection, there was a spike in the average resting heart rate. We also found that infected individuals walked an average of 1,440 fewer steps a day and slept 30 minutes longer than individuals who were virus-free.

Analyzing our data at the end of the study, we found that a smartwatch could correctly detect 81% of the people in the study who had developed COVID-19 about four days before their symptoms started and seven days before diagnosis.

Based on our research, we have developed an infection-detecting app that is now available on an array of smartwatches that can detect heart rate, including Fitbit, Applewatch, and Garmin. The app sends users a red alert about an elevated resting heart rate and a possible infection—though it's not yet able to tell the difference between an infection such as a cold or flu and a COVID-19 infection.

The Stanford Healthcare Innovation Lab is currently recruiting participants for a study on this app, with the goal of enrolling 10 million users. You can learn more about the study, and enroll, at Innovations.stanford.edu/wearables.

WEARABLES 101

Americans have already purchased millions of wearable devices—50 million smartwatches and 20 million other wearable fitness monitors—all of which can easily be adjusted to sense, record, and track health data. Other wearables either on the market or in development include rings, clothing such as smart socks, shoe inserts, contact lenses, and even e-tattoos.

●**Heart disease.** A wearable can alert you and your doctor to several signs of worsening cardiovascular disease that need attention. A faster average heart rate shows a decline in heart health, while low heart-rate variability is linked to worsening heart disease. Elevated

> In a study of 400,000 people, Stanford University researchers found that a smartwatch was 84% accurate in detecting atrial fibrillation.

blood pressure increases the risk for heart attack and stroke.

●**Atrial fibrillation.** In a study of more than 400,000 people published in *The New England Journal of Medicine* in 2019, Stanford University researchers reported that a smartwatch was 84% accurate in detecting this malfunction in the electrical system of the heart that can cause fatigue, shortness of breath, stroke, and sudden cardiac death.

●**Diabetes.** A continuous glucose monitor (CGM) is an effective and pleasant alternative to traditional finger sticks. I am a type 2 diabetic and wear a CGM, which is now available in a smartwatch. The CGM has allowed me to see which foods spike my blood sugar (they're not the same for everyone), and how taking a walk after a large meal is an effective method of post-meal glucose control. CGMs are also being used in veterinary medicine to help pet owners care for diabetic animals.

●**Immunosuppressed patients.** Measuring heart rate can detect life-threatening infections in cancer patients and people who are taking immunosuppressive drugs.

●**Other conditions.** As the technology continues to advance, people with chronic fatigue syndrome, where exercise can sometimes do more harm than good, will be able to tell exactly how much activity is good for them, and how much is too much. People with autism spectrum disorder will be able to see outburst patterns and do self-regulation exercises, in what we call a "just-in-time" intervention. People with major depressive disorder will be able to see if their physical activity levels are declining, a sign of worsening disease.

Think of wearables like this: Your car has more than 400 sensors, which you read through the dashboard. In fact, you can't imagine driving your car without a dashboard. You should have an equally effective dashboard, and wearables are the sensors that provide the data that you need to optimize your health.

There's an App for Tracking Coughs

Cough-tracking apps are useful monitors for many health problems.

If your chronic cough is caused by allergies, asthma, acid reflux, COPD or another health issue, an increase in coughing might mean that it's time to see your doctor or adjust your medication or that a particular location is an allergy trigger. Apps such as *Hyfe* (free for iOS and Android) and *Insubiq Cough Tracker* (free for iPhone) track coughing more accurately than patients can on their own.

Adithya Cattamanchi, MD, pulmonologist and professor of medicine, University of California San Francisco. UCSF.edu

Don't Repair Your Apple Device on Your Own

Apple announced that it soon will allow consumers to repair their own devices and buy official replacement parts and tools directly from the company.

But: Repairing computing devices requires technical skill. The slightest error can turn your phone's "simple" screen or battery repair into a recipe for an expensive paperweight. The repair program is mostly a PR exercise—Apple is embracing consumers' right-to-repair before legislators pass a law requiring it.

Mike Wuerthele is managing editor at the independent online publication AppleInsider.com.

Extend Your Apple Watch's Battery Charge

Disable "Always-On" display. Save power by instead choosing to wake the device by raising your wrist. Save even more battery life by choosing to tap the screen or press the Digital Crown rather than waking up the watch every time you move your arm. *Darken the display.* Using a dark watch face burns less energy, as does reducing brightness. *Disable some notifications.* Turning off the ones that aren't crucial will save battery life and possibly make you more productive. *Limit your calling.* Calls that last more than a few minutes are better made on the phone. *Use power-saving mode during workouts.* If you don't care about tracking your heart rate, this will save you some juice. *Be sure you're using Bluetooth.* If the watch and phone are communicating via Wi-Fi, you'll consume far more energy.

HowToGeek.com

Why You Should Clear "Cookies" from Your Phone

You likely remember to regularly clear cookies, which clog storage and bog down performance, from your computer but probably forget to do it for your phone.

To clear them: On an iPhone—go to "Settings," then "Safari," then "Clear History and Website Data." Tap the pop-up icon that reads "Clear History and Data." On an Android—open Google Chrome, and click the three vertical dots at the top right of the screen. From that menu, select "History," then "Clear Browsing Data." Next, select "Cookies and Site Data," and tap the upside-down triangle next to "All Time."

Note: Clearing cookies also clears your saved passwords—be sure to keep a list of passwords elsewhere—but doesn't affect any apps you have installed.

RD.com

Less Well-Known Voice Commands for Siri and Google Assistant

*T*urn on the flashlight—handy, for instance, if you're holding groceries while trying to unlock your door. *Add to my calendar*—this allows you to add events as you think of them, rather than trying to remember to add a date later. *Set a timer*—your digital assistant can set a timer for cooking or doing anything else that needs to be tracked for a specific amount of time. *Silence my phone*—can save you the embarrassment of having your phone ring during a business meeting or a church service. *That wasn't for you*—what to say if you accidentally trigger the digital assistant when you didn't mean to. Otherwise, the digital assistant may start recording your conversation by default.

Komando.com

"Live View" Helps You Find Your Way

*N*ew augmented-reality feature on Google Maps can help users find their way through malls and airports.

"Live View" works with your smartphone's camera to show where you want to go, locating stairs, escalators, stores, restrooms, ATMs and more. The feature is available currently for malls in Chicago, Long Island, Los Angeles, Newark, San Francisco, San Jose and Seattle, and more locations will be added soon.

USAToday.com

As Good as Microsoft Word—and Free

*F*ocusWriter creates TXT, basic RTF and basic ODT files without distracting tabs,

Android Apps Updates

Easy Way to Cancel Unused Android App Subscriptions

Simply deleting an app that you don't want won't keep you from being billed for it.

Instead: From your phone, go to the Google Play store and tap on the icon for your account. Choose "Payments & Subscriptions"... then select "Subscriptions." You'll see a list of the apps to which you're currently subscribed. Select any you don't want, and click on "Unsubscribe."

The process is similar on a desktop: Go to Play.Google.com. On the left, click "My subscriptions." To delete a subscription, select it and then choose "Manage" and "Cancel subscription."

Komando.com

Android Users—No Need to Close Apps!

There is a common but mistaken belief that apps on Android phones should be closed once you've finished using them—rather than letting them run in the background—to help improve battery life, reduce data usage or just generally speed up the phone. But the Android operating system is designed to have lots of apps running in the background...and apps will close automatically if the system needs more operating power.

Reality: Closing apps manually can hurt your phone's performance. It takes more power to start up an app that has been closed than it does to switch open one that was in the background.

HowToGeek.com

bars and document options. *Google Docs* is similar to Word but available only online. *WPS Docs*, the online version of WPS Office Writer, is compatible with Word and supports DOC, DOCX, TXT, HTM, DOT and DOTX file formats. *LibreOffice* has most of the features of Word—you can open and edit documents made in Office programs and save files in Office formats. *FreeOffice TextMaker* can open and create DOC and DOCX files and allows files to be saved as PDFs. *Jarte* is no-frills, based on Microsoft WordPad and supports Word document formats, Rich Text and Plain Text and lets you export documents as PDFs or in HTML. *WordGraph* is a small-size word processor that handles most file types and can export documents to PDF files.

Komando.com

Wish You Hadn't Upgraded to Windows 11?

No worries—you can still go back to Windows 10.

If you upgraded in the last 10 days: Go to "Settings," then click "System," then "Recovery." You'll see a button labeled "Go Back," which will roll back the recent update and you'll be able to use Windows 10 again.

If the "Go Back" button is grayed out or you upgraded more than 10 days ago: You'll have to reinstall Windows 10 manually. Go to Microsoft.com/en-us/software-download/windows10, and follow the prompts.

HowToGeek.com

Online Tech-Support Scam

Crooks are buying ads that appear as results when consumers Google-search a company's technical-support number. The ads show a fake number, and if you call it, a scammer tries to get access to your money. This happens with online retailers such as Amazon, as well as e-mail providers, airlines and hotels.

Self-defense: Don't use Google—go directly to the company's site to look for customer service or technical support. Don't use Alexa or Siri—they can inadvertently give you a scam number. Look closely at the URL—if it has misspellings or other oddities,

it may be a scam. Don't pay for what should be free—routine customer-service inquiries don't cost money. Don't give remote access to your computer—scammers could do real damage to your finances and identity if you let them in.

Roundup of fraud experts reported on AARP.org.

Tools for Deleting Your Tweets

It's possible—though cumbersome—to delete Tweets on Twitter's platform, but these third-party apps make it simple. *Semiphemeral*—set this free tool to automatically delete old tweets according to your criteria, with flexibility to make exceptions. *Circleboom*—bulk-delete or filter using search terms. Free for 200 tweets, but $24 a month beyond that. *TweetDelete*—mass-purge based on words or phrases or the age of the tweet. Zap 2,300 for free, or shell out a onetime $15 fee and delete up to your entire history. *TweetDeleter*—uses robust search tools to deep-six up to five tweets per month or pay $5 monthly to erase 3,200 tweets per month. *TweetEraser*—its premium service lets you keep copies of tweets you delete. Free with ads for a single account, or $7 monthly for unlimited search filters on multiple accounts.

ConsumerReports.org

How to Remove Your Info from Those People-Search Sites

If you're uncomfortable having your personal data exposed on sites such as PeopleFinders, Spokeo, Whitepages and ZoomInfo, check each site to find out its opt-out requirements (letter, phone call, etc.). If they ask for personal information in order to process your opt-out, proceed with caution (for example, redact your driver's license number if they ask for a copy). You also can pay a service to do the job for you. *DeleteMe* scrubs your information from more than 30 sites and starts at $129 annually. *PrivacyPros* removes data for one person from more than 170 sites for $999 a year. *OneRep* removes you from more than 150 sites for $100 per year per person or $180 per family of up to six people.

Consumer Reports.

How to Find Someone's E-Mail Address

Start with a simple search. *Example:* Enter "Jane Doe" + "email" into a search engine—using quotes tells the search engine to look for that specific phrase, rather than returning results for every single "Jane" and "Doe." Also try + "gmail.com" or + "Hotmail.com" or another e-mail provider to the search. If the person you're looking for is on Facebook, Twitter or LinkedIn, send him/her a direct message through that service. If you know where someone works, make a guess as to his/her e-mail address. Companies typically have formulas for employee e-mail, such as John.Smith@TheCompany.com, or JSmith@TheCompany.com. WhitePages.com and other directory sites may not give you an e-mail address, but they can sometimes provide addresses and phone numbers you can use to make contact.

Komado.com

How to Spot Manipulated Photos

If something doesn't seem right, it probably isn't. Unnatural lighting and an absence of wrinkles and pores often signal airbrushing. If background lines that should be straight are bent, someone may have expanded part of the picture to make it look bigger (like bulging biceps). Copying and pasting repeatedly can make a crowd look larger or a landscape more impressive. Look for an idiosyncratic detail, and see if it appears elsewhere in the composition. Mismatched or missing shadows are another giveaway.

Also: Two websites, "Image Edited?" and "FotoForensics" analyze pictures for manipulation. A reverse Google Images search could uncover trickeries revealed by other digital sleuths.

HowToGeek.com

Where to Move Your Taskbar

Move your taskbar to the side of your computer screen for better viewing. When it's on the bottom of your screen, the taskbar takes up more of your viewable space—plus, the important portions of most websites are in the center. Placing the taskbar off to the side puts it where your eyeballs aren't. (Left or right side is personal preference.)

HowToGeek.com

18

Travel and Leisure

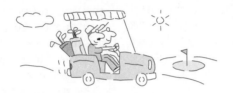

Delightful Destinations Near Small Airports

Some of the best—and delightfully unexpected—travel destinations are conveniently reached by smaller airports. Here's how to venture off the beaten track and enjoy a getaway in a region with sights and activities for adventure lovers and relaxation seekers alike.

•**New York's Long Island MacArthur Airport.** If beach time, wine-tasting and farm-to-table dining sound like an ideal escape, fly into this airport in Islip, New York, and explore eastern Long Island (DiscoverLong Island.com). It is only two hours from New York City, but it feels much further away. Home to the celebrity-laden Hamptons, Montauk and Fire Island, this summer and fall playground has rental beach houses and cottages as well as charming inns and B&Bs. Situate yourself on the North Fork to enjoy 70-plus

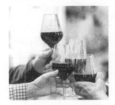

vineyards around Jamesport, Mattituck and Southold as well as the restaurant scene in Greenport. The manicured, shop-lined villages of the Hamptons on the South Fork are an easy drive away. Or head further east to Montauk for fishing, watersports, horseback riding and hiking. If you want something more low-key, hop a ferry from Bay Shore, near the airport, and escape to car-free Fire Island, where beach house rentals are plentiful and bicycles are the best way to explore the towns of Ocean Beach, Fair Harbor and Kismet. MacArthur Airport (MacArthurAirport.com) is served by American, Frontier and Southwest.

Donna Heiderstadt is a travel expert based in New York City who has visited nearly 100 countries and traveled to all seven continents. During her 25 years writing about travel, her work has appeared in Travel AndLeisure.com, Fodors.com, ShermansTravel.com and RobbReport.com.

• **Michigan's Pellston Regional Airport.** Fly into this northern Michigan airport to enjoy summer and fall adventures on and around the magnificent Great Lakes. The region is best-known for car-free 3.8-square-mile Mackinac Island (MackinacIsland.org), home to the circa-1887 Grand Hotel and historic Fort Mackinac (shown at left). The nearby

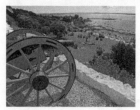

coastal town Petoskey (PetoskeyArea.com) offers pontoon boating, scenic walks and the chance to stumble on pebble-shaped fossilized Petoskey stones. Venture further north to the Upper Peninsula's dense forests and rushing waterfalls (UpTravel.com) to explore breathtaking Pictured Rocks National Lakeshore (NPS.gov/piro) and remote Isle Royale National Park (NPS.gov/isro) as you kayak, fish and hike along Lake Superior's shores. The latter, located on an island and accessible via ferry, is one of the top 10 least visited national parks. Pellston Airport (PellstonAirport.org) is served by Delta.

• **Florida's Destin-Fort Walton Beach Airport.** Florida has 1,358 miles of coastline, but if you're looking for sugar-white sand and emerald-hued Gulf of Mexico water, it's hard to top the Beaches of South Walton (Visit South

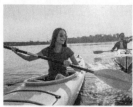

Walton.com), a 26-mile stretch on the Florida panhandle encompassing a series of resort enclaves that include Rosemary Beach, Seaside and WaterColor. All feature stellar rental homes, restaurants with outdoor dining (fresh Gulf shrimp and oysters are specialties), galleries filled with artwork, several state parks, bike rentals and watersports. Blackwater River State Park, located one hour northwest, offers river kayaking and birding. About 100 miles west, just over the Alabama state line in Gulf Shores (GulfShores.com), the spectacular beaches continue, along with activities such as golf, zip lining, kayaking and canoeing along the Coastal Alabama Back Bay Blueway and bird-watching on Dauphin Island (TownofDauphinIsland.org).

Destin-Fort Walton Beach Airport (FlyVPS.com) is served by Delta, Allegiant, American, United and Southwest.

• **Idaho's Friedman Memorial Airport.** Sun Valley (SunValley.com), located at an elevation of 6,000 feet just outside the town of Ketchum, may be known as a skier's paradise, but from June to October, the 400 miles of trails on and around Bald Mountain of-

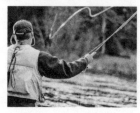

fer hiking and biking amid wildflower fields set beneath clear blue skies. Other pursuits include fly-fishing, horseback riding, tennis and golf—followed by a relaxing spa treatment or soak in nearby Frenchman's Bend or Sunbeam hot springs. Outdoor summer concerts and pottery-making classes are artsy alternatives, while Ketchum's downtown is a lively place to stroll amid shops and galleries before enjoying dinner. Take a scenic drive through the lunarlike volcanic landscape of Craters of the Moon National Monument and Preserve (NPS.gov/crmo), located just 76 miles away (caves and some trails are closed through 2021). Friedman Memorial Airport (IFlySun.com) is served by Delta, United and Alaska Airlines.

• **Texas El Paso International Airport.** Landing in far west Texas offers access to three national parks and endless open spaces. The spectacular mountains, canyons and sand dunes of Guadeloupe Mountains National Park (NPS.gov/gumo) are 105 miles east. Just 30 miles further north, amid the cacti and

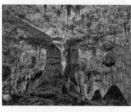

wildlife of New Mexico's desert landscape, you can experience the subterranean drama of Carlsbad Caverns National Park (NPS.gov/cave)—shown at left. If that's not quirky enough, Roswell, New Mexico (SeeRoswell.com), a mecca for all things extraterrestrial (including a UFO museum and planetarium), is 103 miles north of Carlsbad, and the gypsum dunes of White Sands National Park (NPS.gov/whsa) are 195 miles northwest back toward El Paso. You also can drive three hours southeast of El Paso to Marfa, Texas (VisitMarfa.com), an isolated artists' outpost with the motto "tough to get to; tougher to explain." El Paso (ElPasoInternationalAirport.com) is served by American, Delta, United, Southwest, Frontier, Alaska Airlines and Allegiant.

•North Carolina's Wilmington International Airport. There's something for everyone, from beach bums to botanists to film buffs, around Wilmington (WilmingtonAndBeaches.com). This city, set on the Cape Fear River, features a historic downtown plus easy

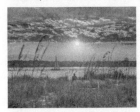

access to three island beach towns—Carolina Beach, Kure Beach and Wrightsville Beach. Green-thumb types can admire plant and bird species in 67-acre Airlie Gardens (AirlieGardens.org) or explore the Nature Conservancy's Green Swamp Preserve, home to the carnivorous Venus Flytrap. Love wine? This is one of the largest wine-producing areas in the US (NCWine.org). And if parts of Wilmington look familiar, it's because the TV series *One Tree Hill* and *Dawson's Creek* were filmed here. Wilmington (FlyILM.com) is served by American, Delta and United.

•Oregon's Roberts Field—Redmond Municipal Airport. For fresh air, spectacular views and lots of active sports—kayaking, fly-fishing, hiking, whitewater rafting—head to Bend, Oregon (VisitBend.com). For after-adventure thirst-quenching, visit the 22 breweries on the Bend Ale Trail. Outdoor enthusiasts have myriad choices within a two-and-a-half-hour drive—Crater Lake National Park (NPS.gov/crla) to see the deepest lake in the US and enjoy miles of hiking trails

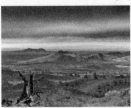

(shown at left)...54,000-acre Newberry National Volcanic Monument, home to lava flows and geologic formations... McKenzie Pass-Santiam Pass Scenic Byway, an 82-mile loop with volcanic peaks...and the High Desert of Southeast Oregon to experience its Painted Hills and wild horses. Red-

mond (FlyRDM.com) is served by American, Boutique, Delta, United and Alaska Airlines.

•Iowa's Eastern Iowa Airport. This airport in Cedar Rapids (TourismCedarRapids.com) is a gateway to Midwestern fun, especially in summer and fall when festivals abound (TravelIowa.com). Movie and baseball fans can drive 75 miles northeast to the *Field of Dreams* movie site (FieldOfDreamsMovieSite.com) in Dyersville. History buffs,

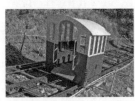

handicrafts collectors and beer lovers can head 19 miles southwest to the Amana Colonies (AmanaColonies.com), seven 19th-century villages founded by German immigrants where you can watch artisans at work in their shops and enjoy savory wursts paired with local brews and wines. Head 85 minutes east to sample life on the Mississippi along the Great River Road National Scenic Byway with its panoramic overlooks and charming towns. Stop in LeClaire on a Saturday for an excursion on the Riverboat Twilight (RiverboatTwilight.com) and Dubuque to ride the Fenelon Place Elevator (FenelonPlaceElevator.com), the world's shortest, steepest funicular railway (shown above), offering views of three states. Cedar Rapids (FlyCID.com) is served by Allegiant, American, Delta, Frontier and United.

Have a Perfect Picnic

Ashley English, the Candler, North Carolina–based author of 11 books, including her "Homemade Living" series as well as *A Year of Picnics: Recipes for Dining Well in the Great Outdoors*, where you can find recipes for all the dishes mentioned here. SmallMeasure.com

The idea of a picnic always sounds like fun, but it takes a bit of planning for the reality to live up to the dream. We asked Ashley English, author of *A Year of Picnics,* for her best suggestions to plan a perfect picnic any time of year...

•**Scout out the location in advance.** Note if there's access to a bathroom and what the terrain is like, especially if you have guests joining you.

•**Check the weather right before heading out.** It's always good to know what you might be dealing with, and plan accordingly. Bringing along an umbrella or an extra sweater can go far toward ensuring picnic success.

•**Wear the right shoes.** A sprained ankle or a stubbed toe can ruin your entire picnic.

•**Let go of your expectations, and appreciate the experience for what it is.** Don't let a few ants or raindrops make you lose sight of that. Some of the most memorable experiences occur when things go sideways. Roll with the punches, and the picnic will be more pleasant, both in the here and now and when it's reflected upon later.

A few more ideas to make your picnic truly memorable…

•**Get in gear.** The only "essential" gear needed on a picnic is something to transport the food. Whether you opt for a classic rattan picnic basket, an upcycled vintage suitcase, an insulated cooler, a backpack or even an apple crate is entirely up to you.

The same goes for the serveware—cups, plates, bowls and flatware can be purchased new or, my preference, sought out at thrift and estate sales or even online sites such as Etsy and eBay. I love using metal and wood utensils for picnicking, but I'm not averse to the occasional bit of ceramic ware or even glass if the destination isn't particularly far from where you will park your car (the added weight and delicate nature of such materials can make them difficult to carry).

Reminder: Bring along sunscreen and bug spray.

Set the stage for your picnic…

•**For a romantic picnic.** What makes a picnic romantic isn't necessarily the glasses or the flatware. It's the overall atmosphere—bring along cozy blankets and a cushy pillow (or several). The foods should appeal to both picnickers.

•**For a family/kid-friendly picnic.** Bring utensils and dishes that can withstand wear and tear—enamelware is perfect. Include foods that you know kids will enjoy. That doesn't mean chicken nuggets and apple slices…but this is not the time to make children try pâté or blue cheese.

•**Go with the season.** Any time of year is ideal for picnicking, so long as you dress for the weather and serve foods that exemplify the season—consider chilled soup, such as Gazpacho, for warm weather and hearty stew in fall, for instance.

•**Safety always.** Make sure that picnic foods are kept at safe temperatures, especially perishable items, regardless of the time of year.

When preparing foods that will be served cold: Let them reach room temperature before storing them in the refrigerator. Then, when you're ready to head out for your picnic, pack ice or, even better, reusable ice packs into the bottom of the cooler, and place the food containers on top of the ice layer.

Pack any food to be served warm in thermos-type containers, and carry them separately in an insulated bag.

At the picnic: Keep the cooler lid closed whenever you are not getting anything out or putting something into it, and store it in a shady spot.

At home: When the picnic's over, you will know that leftovers are safe to consume if there is any ice left in your cooler. If the ice has all melted, the food may have spoiled and should not be eaten.

•**Select the menu.** A grazing board is easy to prepare and delicious any time of year. Pack up a medley of fruits, charcuterie, cheeses, nuts, veggies, chips, crackers, spreads and pickles, and perhaps a little something sweet such as cookies, and you've got all you need to create a memorable meal outdoors.

For a full summer menu, I love "Fruta Picada," a Mexican street food of fresh melons topped with a salty/spicy seasoning blend, and a cold veggie and/or meat salad, such as Israeli Couscous Feta & Herb Salad or Chimichurri Chicken Salad. For a cool and refreshing beverage, try Jallab, a popular drink in the Middle East made with pomegranate juice concentrate and a honey simple syrup, and served with golden raisins and pine nuts.

For fall, consider warming, robust foods that fill you up. I love Dijon Mustard Pork Chop Sandwiches, Roasted Root Veggie Chips and Pumpkin Whoopie Pies with a Grape Juice Spritz or a mug of Smoky Chai.

Stay in a Castle...in the US

Blog.Cheapism.com

Airbnb, TripAdvisor and Vrbo list castles where you can "live like royalty" at least for a night!

Check out: *Thornewood Castle*—a "haunted" 500-year-old gothic castle in Tacoma, Washington, brought to the US from England in 1907 (check TripAdvisor.com for prices and availability). *Gothic Castle on a Hill*—located on a private lake in Rindge, New Hampshire, has easy access to miles of hiking trails (Vrbo.com). *Williamswood Castle*—in Knoxville, Tennessee, has its own pub, splendid river views and borders a nature preserve. There also is a moving bookshelf that hides a secret staircase (Airbnb.com). *Highlands*

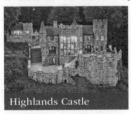
Highlands Castle

Castle—in Bolton, New York, overlooks Lake George and offers boating, hiking, biking and other activities, with plenty of shops, museums and restaurants nearby (Airbnb.com). *La Chambre Bleue*—in Sonora, California, has an on-site vineyard and theater and is one hour west of Yosemite National Park and other tourist destinations (Airbnb.com). *Texas Hill Country Castle*—in Burnet County, west of Austin, is surrounded by more than 100 acres of forest. Luxury indoor amenities include jacuzzi tubs and a game room (Airbnb.com or Vrbo.com). *Graystone Castle*—in Arlington, Washington, is halfway between Seattle and the Canadian border and features a movie theater, game rooms, spa and other amenities (Airbnb.com or Vrbo.com).

Space: The Hot New Travel Destination

Rachel J.C. Fu, PhD, chair and professor, department of Tourism, Hospitality and Event Management (THEM) at University of Florida, Gainesville, where she also is director of the Eric Friedheim Tourism Institute. HHP.UFL.edu/about/departments/them

The hottest travel destination right now isn't the tropics—it is heading off the planet and into space. In October 2021, William Shatner, famous for his iconic role as Captain James T. Kirk in *Star Trek*, became the oldest person to go to space. The 90-year-old actor described it as, "The most profound experience I can imagine."

Space tourism got its start about 20 years ago when investment manager Denis Tito spent a reported $20 million to visit the International Space Station for eight days via a Russian rocket. The industry has been growing since then.

Major space tourism companies planning or already selling rides into space include Blue Origin, headed by Amazon founder Jeff Bezos...SpaceX, from Tesla founder Elon Musk...and Virgin Galactic, started by Virgin Atlantic airlines founder Richard Branson. At the moment, Virgin Galactic is the only one publicly offering flights, and a ticket costs an astronomic $450,000 per person. But if space tourism catches on—and there is every indication that it will—more companies will come onto the scene, which means more competition and more affordable tickets.

Space tourism isn't too different from the space travel you have already seen. Blue Origin and SpaceX use traditional rockets to launch a small capsule into the sky, which then descends and decelerates with parachutes and lands in the ocean. Blue Origin has sent its rockets as far as 62 miles above the Earth's surface, passing the Kármán line—considered the boundary between Earth's atmosphere and space. (The Federal Aviation Administration, US military and NASA consider 50 miles above Earth the beginning of space, but the Fédération Aéronautique Internationale sets that border at 62 miles.) And SpaceX has sent four tourists on a three-day vacation orbiting 367 miles above the Earth.

Virgin Galactic does things a little differently. Its spacecraft starts off on a runway and is carried aloft by another aircraft. When the carrier aircraft reaches about 50,000 feet, the spacecraft is released, fires its rockets and ascends to the edge of space. Once it reaches this height, passengers can unbuckle themselves and enjoy a few minutes of weightlessness. Then the craft returns to Virgin's Spaceport America in New Mexico, making a gliding landing on a runway just as the NASA space shuttles did. Virgin's flights generally take passengers about 50 miles above Earth, and the round-trip takes about 90 minutes.

IS IT SAFE?

Space travel may be safer than you imagine. The rockets and spacecrafts are based on American and Russian models with years of design and safety precautions behind them, and NASA has been using private companies—including SpaceX—for cargo flights to the International Space Station for about a decade.

Of course, travel to space has an inherent and unavoidable element of danger. In 2014, a prototype spacecraft from Virgin Galactic broke apart after launch due to a copilot error, killing one pilot and injuring another. But tragic accidents such as these always produce waves of innovation and even greater focus on safety. Both Richard Branson and Jeff Bezos flew on the maiden voyages of their respective spacecraft, demonstrating a huge amount of trust in their machinery and personnel.

COUNTDOWN TO LIFT-OFF

Before your space flight, you will need some training. Some companies train passengers for as little as one day...some for as long as six months. You'll need a very different level of preparation if you're going to ride a rocket up to the edge of space and come right back down—a trip that lasts maybe 90 minutes—compared with a multiday orbital trip, for example.

Preparing for G-force: You may have seen astronauts in movies and TV shows blasting off with pained expressions because of the intense gravitational force (G-force) from the launch. But lift-off is not as bad as you might imagine—in fact, you are more familiar with G-force than you might think. You experience it every time you quickly accelerate your car or when your commercial airline flight takes off. A rocket's lift-off is certainly more intense and lasts longer, but if you're reasonably fit, you can handle it.

During training, you may ride in a centrifuge—a circular device that spins quickly, pinning you against the wall—so you will be accustomed to increased G-force. You even may have enjoyed a ride like this at an amusement park.

Another way to prepare for zero-G: Scuba diving. Achieving neutral buoyancy underwater is somewhat similar to zero-gravity—in fact, NASA has long used underwater training for its astronauts.

Getting ready for zero-gravity: When you are in a zero-G environment, the normal rules of motion do not apply—or at least they apply in a very different way than what you're used to. We have spent our entire lives tied to the Earth by gravity, so suddenly being free of this normally inescapable force requires a new way of moving. For example, when you are on Earth, if you want to get to point A from point B, you know how much force to use. But when you are in space, you'll need to push off from the floor or wall to "fly" across the cabin or get close to a window.

First-timer mistake: Pushing off with too much force and hitting your head on the ceiling or wall.

The rest of the training likely will consist of safety briefings, emergency drills, mission simulations, instructions on communications and general flight procedures.

LESS EXPENSIVE OPTIONS

More affordable than going into space—or even a good training session if you are planning to get up there—is a reduced-gravity flight. This takes you far up into the atmosphere, where the pilot performs a series of *phugoid maneuvers* (essentially steep dives and climbs). The plane—often a specially fitted Boeing 727, Airbus A310 or something similar—climbs up, like that first hill when you're riding a rollercoaster, then descends at a very steep angle. This steep descent lets you experience weightlessness for about a minute before the pilot levels out the plane and then takes the craft up again to repeat the process. These flights provide the closest thing to going into space but for a fraction of the cost—usually from about $7,500 per person.

Companies that offer these flights: Air Zero G (AirZeroG.com), Space Adventures (SpaceAdventures.com) and Zero Gravity Corporation (GoZeroG.com).

Another option: Instead of retrofitting an aircraft or inventing a new kind of ship or rocket, the company World View is planning to use a balloon to lift passengers into the sky, which provides a much gentler ride. It has performed more than 100 ascents into the stratosphere—about 100,000 feet off the ground, or nearly 20 miles—and expects to take its first tourists up by 2024. Ticket prices are expected to be about $50,000 per person for a six-to-eight-hour flight. World View is offering this trip as part of a destination vacation package—you will spend five days before the flight exploring and enjoying Amazonia in Peru...the Northern Lights in Norway...the Pyramids of Egypt...the Grand Canyon...the Great Barrier Reef off the coast of Australia...the Great Wall of China...or the Serengeti in Kenya.

"Takeover Tours" Offer Safe Group Travel

Donna Heiderstadt is a travel expert who has visited nearly 100 countries and traveled to all seven continents. During her 25 years writing about travel, her work has appeared at TravelAndLeisure.com, Fodors.com, ShermansTravel.com and RobbReport.com.

If you want to get away but don't feel comfortable spending most of your time traveling with strangers, consider private-charter travel—so-called takeover tours—where you know everyone in your group and choose to travel with them. (Note that tours are subject to change.) *Exciting possibilities...*

If Italy tops your list: Perillo Tours offers private guided trips of nine to 14 days for 12 to 20 travelers. PerilloTours.com/italy/private-tours

Lots of friends and family? Charter Uniworld's 124-passenger S.S. Bon Voyage on the Dordogne and Garonne rivers in the Bordeaux region of France...or 126-passenger S.S. La Venezia on Italy's Venice Lagoon and Po River. From $2,600 per person in 2022, based on 124-person capacity plus airfare. Uniworld.com

Other options: Explore from a private base, such as a vacation rental, by contacting small group tour operators about private day-trip bookings within the region and searching online for specialized tour companies (for hiking, river rafting, culinary exploration or cooking classes).

Road-Tripping with Your Best Buddy

Nancy Kerns, founding editor-in-chief of *Whole Dog Journal*, a monthly publication offering advice on responsible dog ownership. Whole-Dog-Journal.com

Most dog owners are eager to take their pets on vacation with them. It is fun to travel with Fido, and more places now allow you to bring along well-behaved dogs.

But it also can be limiting and requires planning, so it's important to know what you're getting into. *Here are some tips from* Whole Dog Journal *editor-in-chief Nancy Kerns...*

BOOKING A DOG-FRIENDLY VACATION

When searching for motels, hotels, Airbnbs and other accommodations that will welcome your pet, ask the following questions...

Are there fees for dog(s)? Are there weight, size or breed limitations? How many dogs are allowed per room? Can you leave the dog in your room unattended? Does your dog have to be crated when you're not in the room? Are there designated pet-relief areas nearby...and off-leash dog parks in the area?

Best: Check out booking apps such as *BringFido* and *BarkHappy* for other pet owners' experiences at accommodations as well as discounted rates.

PREP YOUR DOG

Before you commit to a long drive, make sure your dog is able to relax in a moving vehicle.

Important: Teach the dog to ride in the backseat of your car—front-seat airbags can be deadly to pets.

•**Take the pet on two-hour test drives.** Before getting in the car, always walk the dog so he has had a chance to empty his bowels and bladder and is not restless in anticipation of an opportunity to do so.

•**If the dog shows signs of car sickness or anxiety,** try one of these approved stress-reducing products…

•Adaptil Calm collar ($24.99, Adaptil.com) for around the neck or Adaptil Travel spray ($24.99), which is applied to the seat or crate where the dog sits in the car. These were developed to mimic a pheromone emitted by lactating female dogs to calm your pet and reduce barking, chewing, whining and whimpering.

•Anxiety Wrap ($34.95, AnxietyWrap.com) or ThunderShirt ($39.95 and up, ThunderShirt.com) both apply gentle, constant pressure around the trunk of the dog's body, which has a calming effect on many dogs.

•ThunderCap ($19.95, ThunderShirt.com) is a sheer hood that allows the dog to see only shapes and reduces arousal from outside stimuli. This helps dogs that are triggered into a frantic state by what they see outside the car windows.

•**Try playing dog-friendly music in the car.** "In the Car" features classical music specifically geared to the anxious dog ($20 to $39.98, iCalmPet.com). Available as a download, CD or microSD memory card.

•**Ask your vet for medication to calm your dog if the products above don't help.**

Also: If you're planning to take your dog on a hiking, canoeing or kayaking vacation, do some test runs first to make sure your pet feels comfortable with these activities. That means trying out a doggie life vest for water sports and bringing along a first-aid kit for cuts and scrapes on the trail.

Behaviors to encourage: Teach your dog to walk loosely on a leash—a leash will definitely be required at times…come when called (in case the dog gets off leash)…and calmly greet human and canine strangers.

Also: Your dog should be crate-trained—there are many instances when the pet may need to be confined while traveling.

Examples: In the car…at hotels when you go out for the day or for meals…and at campsites.

CAR EQUIPMENT AND DOG GEAR

Although most states do not have laws requiring dogs to be restrained in vehicles, it makes good sense for everyone if you do. *To make the trip pleasant for you and your dog…*

•**Place the dog in a crate that is strapped to child-safety seat anchors** or cargo anchors (such as those in the back of an SUV or wagon). A loose crate is no better than a loose dog!

Best: Crash-tested car kennels—these are different from typical household crates, which have been shown to fly apart in crash situations. These crates are more expensive than house crates (with the larger sizes costing the most), but dogs in them have survived accidents that totaled the cars they were strapped into.

•**If you don't have an SUV or you need a less expensive option,** restrain your pet with a specially designed dog harness that attaches to a seat belt.

Best: A recent review of car harnesses by *Whole Dog Journal* found the Sleepypod Clickit Terrain Plus ($126.49, Sleepypod.com) to be the safest harness on the market.

Other good choices: Ruffwear Load Up Dog Car Harness ($79.95, RuffWear.com)… Kurgo Impact Car Dog Harness ($78.95, Kurgo.com)…and EzyDog Drive Dog Car Harness ($125, EzyDog.com).

Note: All but the Ruffwear Load Up Harness have a leash attachment so you can walk your dog from the vehicle to your destination, but these harnesses are not for long or frequent walks.

• **Pack essentials for your pet**—water, food and food bowls...poop bags...the aforementioned pet first-aid kit...medications your pet takes regularly...brush and tick-remover tool...dog bed or blanket...crate...and an extra collar or harness and a leash.

Also remember: Proof of rabies and other vaccinations.

• **Make sure the dog has a well-fitted collar with an ID tag that displays his name and your current cell-phone number.** Also, every dog should be microchipped, with the chip registered to your current phone number, in case the collar comes off.

Avoid: Retractable leashes. Your dog can get into trouble with oncoming vehicles or aggressive dogs faster than your ability to restrain him. And those long cords can cut into any body part they come into contact with.

• **Bring toys and chews for the dog to play with both at your accommodations and when the pet is awake in the car.**

CAR SAFETY AND TRIP TIMES

You know you should never leave your dog in the car while you go into a store or restaurant or sightseeing. Even with the windows open, the car can quickly heat up to a temperature that is deadly to a dog. Likewise, cold weather can be dangerous. And there's always the danger of your pet being stolen. *Also...*

• **Do not let your dog stick his head out the window while the vehicle is moving.** Dirt, debris and objects can fly into his eyes, nose or mouth. If your dog loves the wind in his fur, purchase a safety product for your car window.

Example: BreezeGuard (starting at $375/pair, BreezeGuard.com), powder-coated raw steel mesh screens (not unlike a security screen door) that fit in the car window so your pet can feel the breeze without sticking his head out (or being able to jump or fall out).

• **Limit daily drives to seven to eight hours for your own enjoyment and the dog's.** Plan to stop every few hours to walk and interact with your dog.

To facilitate fast stops: Teach your dog to eliminate on cue using a command such as, "Get busy" or "Go potty." Offer a food treat when the dog complies.

DOG PARKS, BEACHES AND RESTAURANTS

Booking a dog-friendly accommodation is just half the equation of traveling with your pet. Next, research whether you can bring your dog to attractions, restaurants, galleries, trails, beaches and parks.

Important: Dogs are not allowed on trails at some national parks and must be accompanied by their owners in campgrounds.

Good news: With the emphasis on outdoor eating these days, dogs are welcome at more restaurants and venues than ever before, but check out these opportunities before you arrive.

Some accommodations will allow you to leave your pet in the room, usually restrained in a crate, while you go out. Be sure your pet is okay with being left alone and in the crate, or he may try to get out or howl for hours.

Outstanding Audiobooks

Robin Whitten, founder and editor of *AudioFile Magazine*, which reviews audiobooks. She has served on the board of directors of the Audio Publishers Association. AudioFileMagazine.com

---

If it has been a while since you listened to an audiobook, you might be in for a surprise. Over the past decade or so, audiobooks have undergone a renaissance, not just in terms of dramatically increased popularity but also in how they're being produced. Turning on an audiobook today can mean opening your ears to original music, casts of actors, archival recordings and sound effects. With so much value being added, many of today's audiobooks are far superior to their original versions. *Here are six that fit that description...*

The Only Plane in the Sky: An Oral History of 9/11 by Garrett Graff. This impressively sourced recollection of the day our world was forever changed features the gut-wrenching stories of hundreds of survivors, first responders and witnesses. Transcripts are read by actors, who convey the intensity without allowing the emotion to become insurmountable. The result is a gripping, astonishing piece of living history.

More Myself: A Journey by Alicia Keys. As we learned from Carole King's *A Natural Woman*, one of the joys of listening to a singer read her own memoir is hearing her break into song. Alicia Keys follows suit, but in telling her story of gradual self-realization, she brings in a who's who of friends to comment on her personal odyssey, including Oprah, Bono, Michelle Obama and Jay-Z.

Lincoln in the Bardo by George Saunders. Saunders's trippy, groundbreaking work combines the supernatural, the historical and the intensely emotional, as it follows Abraham Lincoln's dead son into a purgatory-like state. It is as bizarre as it sounds, but it's a remarkable achievement of imagination and humanity. The audiobook turns up the dial, with performances by a jaw-dropping army of stellar talent that includes Susan Sarandon, Nick Offerman, Ben Stiller, Julianne Moore and 162 others.

Firekeeper's Daughter by Angeline Boulley. One of the great joys of literature is delving into a culture that isn't yours—but all those unfamiliar words, names and sounds can get in the way. This young-adult thriller is set in an Ojibwe (also known as Chippewa) community, and narrator Isabella Star LeBlanc, of the Sisseton-Wahpeton Dakota tribe, is the perfect guide, effortlessly delivering Ojibwe names and phrases and making us feel at home.

The Bomber Mafia by Malcolm Gladwell. Gladwell is an amazing researcher and podcaster, and he brings those talents to bear in the audio version of his engrossing behind-the-scenes history of the advent of precision bombing during the Second World War. His polished narration is accompanied by sound effects, original interviews, music and archival clips.

Four Hundred Souls edited by Ibram X. Kendi and Keisha N. Blain. Kendi and Blain gathered up the works of 90 writers to cover each five-year period of more than 400 years of African American history, from the landing of the first slave ship in Virginia in 1619 to

the present. A kaleidoscope of stories, poems, sketches and vignettes shows dazzling proof of the immense variety of the Black experience in America, and the incredible voices of more than 85 readers—including Phylicia Rashad, Soledad O'Brien and Leslie Odom, Jr.— bring the spirits of the past back to vivid life.

Beware of the Rental-Car Toll Trap

Christopher Elliott, a consumer advocate who writes "The Travel Troubleshooter," a syndicated newspaper column. He also is a columnist for *The Washington Post*. Elliott.org

Toll roads can take a bigger toll than you expect in a rental car. Rental agencies often impose fees of $4 to $6 per day for the transponders that let customers use cashless toll lanes. Opt out of that per-day fee, and you might be charged $10 to $15 for each cashless toll you incur—in addition to actual toll charges. Avoiding cashless tolls isn't always easy—some toll roads and bridges no longer accept cash. *Three potential solutions…*

•**Stay off toll roads.** Select the "avoid toll roads" option in your phone's map app when driving a rental car. If that isn't feasible, avoid cashless tolls. One way to do that is to check PlatePass.com—click "view map" for the area you're visiting. Toll roads/bridges that don't accept cash are marked with asterisks.

Warning: If you intend to pay tolls in cash, ask the rental agency how to shield or disable the car's transponder. Otherwise the transponder—and you—could be billed even though you paid cash. Request and save receipts for tolls paid in cash in case you're billed.

•**Choose a rental company that charges reasonable toll fees.** Car-share company Zipcar has no toll fees—it passes along only actual toll charges. (Zipcar membership costs $9 per month or $90 per year—$8/$80 in Boston and Washington, DC—plus a onetime $25 application fee, but its usage fees may be comparable to car-rental companies depending on the time and distance of your trip.)

The others: Alamo, Avis and Enterprise charge $3.95 to $5.95 per day, sometimes with a per-rental cap of $19 to $30. Details vary by company and state—search "tolls" on the company's website before booking.

Worth checking: Will this fee be applied for each day of the rental…or only for days when tolls are incurred?

Dollar, Hertz and Thrifty offer the electronic toll-payment system PlatePass, generally for $10 to $30 per day depending on location, which includes the cost of any toll you go through.

•**Bring your own transponder…maybe.** First, confirm that your transponder works where you're headed—E-ZPass works throughout much of the northeastern US and some parts of the Midwest, but most other transponders work only in a small number of states. (You could buy the correct transponder for your destination, but it might be as expensive as a rental-car company's toll fees.)

Contact the government agency that issued your transponder to confirm that it can be used in rental cars—not all programs allow this. Or you might have to add the rental's plate number to your transponder account, a potential hassle.

Reminder: Position your transponder directly under the rental's windshield when passing through cashless tolls—you'll face rental company fees if it fails to register.

driver misjudged the motorcycle's distance and speed. And motorcycles require longer braking distances than cars.

Best practice: Assume that a motorcycle is approaching faster than it looks, and use your turn signals so that motorcyclists know what you're up to. Bikers especially love it when you flash your lights or give them a wave to let them know you see them.

•**Riders sometimes "lane filter."** Filtering, or "lane-splitting," is when motorcycles keep moving between lanes of stopped cars. Motorcyclists do it for a few reasons—to get where they're going (If you could slip between the cars, wouldn't you be tempted?)… they fear being rear-ended by an inattentive driver…and stopping over hot pavement without air-conditioning can be unpleasant. And part of California's reasoning for legalizing lane filtering is that it reduces emissions.

Best practice: Whenever you're in stop-and-go traffic and contemplating a lane change, check your mirrors for motorcycles before pulling out.

•**They like to stay together.** Recreational riders often travel in a pack.

Best practice: Treat the group like it's one vehicle. If you want to pass, pass the whole group. If you want to let it pass, let all the riders go by.

Share the Road with Motorcycles

Nicholas P. Just, Highway Safety Office program manager for the Connecticut Department of Transportation and program manager for the Connecticut Rider Education Program, the state's mandatory motorcycle course for new riders. Portal.CT.gov/dot

Love them or hate them, motorcycles have as much right to the roads as cars and trucks. *Knowing a bit about them will help keep your interactions with them safe…*

Even when we notice motorcycles, judging their speed of approach is difficult. Crashes often occur when a driver makes a left turn across the path of a motorcycle because the

These Boots Are Made for Hiking

Philip Werner, a former New Hampshire wilderness guide who is founder and editor of the hiking website SectionHiker.com.

What could be better than hiking through a beautiful wooded area… or up a mountain trail…on a bright sunny day? Lots of people are discovering the joy of hiking these days. But before you hit the trail—any trail—make sure you have the right footwear to hike safely and comfortably. *Things to consider when you are shopping…*

•**Style of hiking shoe.** Matching the type of shoe to the distance and terrain is critical for both enjoyment and safety.

Trail runners are essentially running shoes with a more rugged sole for unpaved surfaces. They're especially lightweight, so they are good for longer distances on smooth terrain. If you don't plan on trail running, a lighter-duty hiking shoe provides a little more structure but with minimal weight—good for well-groomed trails.

Above-the-ankle stiffer-soled boots have more support and structure for uneven grass, gravel or rocky terrain. An in-between low boot option called "mids" offers protection from debris without the bulkiness of a full boot. Getting rocks between your sock and shoe is a common annoyance with low-sided hiking shoes, unless you wear them with gaiters that protect the lower leg.

Other hiking footwear features worth considering: A sturdy toe box or internal shank can provide foot protection, especially when hiking over rocky terrain. And the weight of the shoe or boot can affect how fatigued you become on long hikes—every ounce adds up when you are walking 10,000 steps or more on a five-mile hike.

•**Material.** Different materials are appropriate for hiking in different seasons and conditions. Footwear made mostly or entirely from synthetic materials are lighter and more breathable, allowing heat to escape and your feet to breathe. Footwear that feature mesh panels is especially breathable and potentially very light, but unless they're made with GORE-TEX or a similar material, they won't be waterproof. If you hike early in the season, when snow may still be on the ground or winter runoff is filling streams, you will need waterproof boots to keep your feet dry. Leather provides great durability but can be more expensive and heavier than synthetics and must be properly treated to be waterproof.

•**Comfort.** Some people like the sensation of having their toes splay out with each step, as they do when walking barefoot. Others prefer a tighter toe box to contain their feet. No matter your preference, make sure there's some room in front of your toes—otherwise your feet will feel cramped when you hike downhill and you can bruise your toes and toenails.

Best: When trying on hiking shoes, walk up and down an incline. Outdoor-gear stores often have a ramp set up for customers to test the fit.

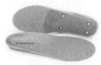

•**Arch support.** Support is always critical with hiking shoes, but it is especially important if you're prone to the painful condition plantar fasciitis or other foot conditions.

Helpful: If the hiking boots or shoes you like don't provide enough arch support, add a pair of Superfeet insoles (about $50).

•**Distance and difficulty.** The longer or more challenging the hike, the more solid and protective the shoe should be and the more important its weight becomes.

BEST HIKING FOOTWEAR

The best hiking footwear options—all available for men and women...

Best trail runners: **Salomon Sense Ride 4s** are excellent off-road running shoes. They 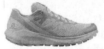 provide all-terrain grip... are lightweight—about eight ounces...breathable...and provide a reasonable amount of underfoot cushioning. $120.*

Best value shoes and mids: **Merrell Moab 2 Ventilator Shoes and Mids** hold their own when compared with pricier footwear. They're durable and provide stability and protection without sacrificing cushioning and comfort. Mesh panels make the Moab 2 breathable and quick to dry, but they are not appropriate for snow or wet patches. 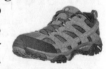 Available as a hiking shoe or a mid and in wide and standard sizes. $110 for shoes...$120 for mids. A waterproof Moab 2 also is available for men and women in shoe and mid styles. $135 for shoes...$145 for mids.

Best mids for waterproof comfort: **KEEN Targhee III Waterproof Mid** combines the

*Prices are manufacturers' price for men's shoes. Discounted prices are available.

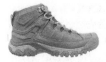

traction and support of a hiking boot with the flexibility and comfort of a hiking shoe. The exterior is mostly leather, which provides stability and a shoelike feel. Additionally, the leather is waterproofed and there is an internal waterproof membrane, but they are not particularly breathable—your feet may get hot on summer hikes. The toe box is roomy, and they are built off KEEN's traditional wider footwear form. $165.

Best boots for protection and support: **Salomon Quest 4D 3 GTXs** are fantastic hiking boots that provide excellent stability, traction, water-resistance and durability. You can feel confident wearing these boots even on long jaunts through the wilderness. They're strong and protective but also light and comfortable, with GORE-TEX membranes that keep out water without sacrificing breathability. $230.

Best combination of style and performance: **Zamberlan Vioz GTXs** provide the traditional look of Italian-made leather hiking boots. They're durable, waterproof and comfortable, but as with other leather boots, they're expensive…heavy— more than three pounds per pair…and not especially breathable. $310 to $360 depending on style.

What Not to Wear for Air Travel

Jewelry and anything with a lot of metal— jewelry, the nails in high heels and clothing with large metal decorations will slow you down at security checkpoints. *Anything tight*—bodies swell during flight, making restrictive clothing (including a too-tight bra) uncomfortable. *Revealing clothing*—planes are cold, skimpy clothes may be offensive in some countries, and evacuation slides, if needed, are uncomfortable on bare skin. *Fragrance*— it can trigger allergies in nearby passengers.

Long and Short Airport Layovers

Best Ways to Get Through a Long Airport Layover

If you have at least eight hours, leave the airport and do some sightseeing. Plan enough time to get back to the airport and through security before your flight leaves.

For shorter layovers: Camp out in a lounge—they usually have showers, free food and plenty of comfortable seating. Some lounges require membership, but some may be available through your credit card, or you can check the apps *LoungeBuddy* and *PriorityPass* for lounges that you can pay to use for the day.

Or: Look for a seat in a café or bar close to power outlets.

Even better: Find a sleep capsule. Usually found only in larger airports, they are tiny places to relax and catch a nap. Some are like micro-sized hotel rooms.

Harry Guinness, photography expert and writer, writing at LifeSavvy.com.

Avoid Missing Your Connecting Flight

Short layovers for airport connections usually will work when the tickets are booked through airlines. Because the airline personnel know just where your first flight will land and how far you will have to get to your second one. Even a 45-minute layover at a busy airport can work out—and some airlines schedule layovers as short as 30 minutes at selected airports.

But: Bookings cannot account for problems such as weather delays or aircraft maintenance issues.

To be on the safe side: Aim for a two-hour buffer between flights even if the airline says a shorter one is available. Plan a three-hour buffer if you need special services, such as a wheelchair. And if you are flying internationally, give yourself a four-hour window for your return to the US and a connection to your next flight—because customs delays can be lengthy.

Roundup of experts on air travel, reported in *The Washington Post*.

High heels, flip flops or slides—they can slow you down and come off in an emergency. Lace-up shoes are the safest choice. *Synthetic fibers that do not breathe*—they can be uncomfortable during your flight and dangerous in case of fire. Natural fabrics (cotton, wool) are better than synthetics such as polyester and nylon.

Roundup of flight attendants, reported at RD.com.

Save on Roundtrip Airfare

Save money by buying separate one-way tickets for a roundtrip. One-way tickets on domestic flights generally are half the price of a roundtrip. Booking separate tickets on different airlines may allow you to find bargains…and might get you better flight schedules and more comfort for at least half the trip.

Example: Book one ticket on a cheaper, no-frills airline and get a somewhat more comfortable seat on a different carrier for the other half of your trip.

HuffPost.com

Get More Legroom When You Fly

The online flight-booking service Google Flights lets you compare the prices of flights from different carriers. Check out the "Legroom for Google Flights" browser extension available on the Chrome Internet browser. Adding this extension to your search will display the legroom, carry-on restrictions and amenities for flights.

TravelAndLeisure.com

Keep Your Phone Working When There's No Service

If you're on a road trip, your phone can keep helping you navigate even when you're in a dead zone.

Best: Download or sync data beforehand. *Google Maps* or the free *Here WeGo* app for iOS and Android allow you to download maps of specific areas before your trip. (Test the apps to make sure they work offline by switching to Airplane mode while Wi-Fi is off.)

Nicole Nguyen, personal-technology columnist for *The Wall Street Journal.*

Stay Connected While Traveling Overseas

Get an international phone plan with your cell-phone carrier—offered by all major carriers. *Buy a local SIM card*—available at phone stores and some supermarkets, plans run from $5 to $25 a month for several gigabytes of data. *Switch to Google service*—Google Fi has offered cell-phone service for a few years, which is compatible with its phones or some unlocked phones. Check if your phone is compatible on the Google Fi site (Fi.Google.com). Its $70/month Unlimited Plus plan will give you access to data in more than 200 locations.

The Wall Street Journal.

Best Hurricane Tracking Apps

Storm Radar (The Weather Channel)—lots of map customizations and animations. Free with ads. The free app *Hurricane: American Red Cross* lets you track loved ones who may be in harm's way by monitoring the location of anyone in your contacts list. Also displays shelters within impact areas. *My Hurricane Tracker*—a bare-bones tracker with forecasts, updates and alerts. Free with ads. *NOAA Weather Radar*—provides map overlays for rain, radar and satellite images. Free for one week—subscriptions start at $2.99. Hurricane season for the Atlantic is from June 1 through November 30.

Lifewire.com

19

Create Your
Success Story

Secret System for Success: Reverse Engineering

Before Stephen King was one of America's most successful novelists, he used to copy comic books panel by panel, according to his son. Before Apple was one of the world's most innovative companies, it launched the Macintosh by adapting user-friendly computer interface concepts previously developed by Xerox. Before Chipotle was one of the country's most successful restaurant chains, it was modeled after the Tex/Mex restaurants already popular in California.

Conventional wisdom holds that great success springs from breakthrough ideas, natural talent and/or endless practice. But when you examine how success actually happens, you often see something quite different—many massive successes are the result of taking some-thing that already has been proven to work and using it as a springboard or roadmap.

Copying elements of prior successes is not the same as stealing other people's ideas—it's finding inspiration in those ideas...learning lessons from them...and/or filtering new ideas through a framework or format that is a proven winner.

Nor does copying inhibit creativity. A 2017 study published in *Cognitive Science* found that the work produced by artists becomes more creative when those artists first spend time copying the works of other artists. Counterintuitively, the process of copying helps people unlock their own new and original ideas. What does inhibit creativity is getting stuck in one's own head and ignoring outside influences.

Ron Friedman, PhD, social psychologist and author of *Decoding Greatness: How the Best in the World Reverse Engineer Success*. He is founder of ignite80, which translates research in neuroscience, physiology and behavioral economics into practical strategies, Rochester, New York. RonFriedmanPhD.com

But transforming existing ideas into personal successes requires more than imitation—it's also necessary to dissect the source of inspiration, pulling it apart to understand what truly makes it work. Engineers call this process of carefully examining the construction of someone else's product "reverse engineering." *And you can use this process to reverse engineer your own success...*

STEP 1: Collect ideas, items and examples that you consider great. This could be a collection of physical objects, such as a shelf of your favorite books if you're a writer...or a bulletin board covered in wonderful logos if you're a graphic designer...or a digital collection, such as a Pinterest page, featuring photos of beautiful gardens if your passion is gardening.

These collections will serve as inspirational reference tools. Having examples of greatness on hand, either physically or digitally, is much more effective than trying to recall them—the human brain isn't as good at recalling details as people like to believe it is. As productivity consultant David Allen noted, "Your mind is for having ideas, not holding them." What's more, it's surprisingly common to discover something new when you refer back to a work of brilliance, even if you already have examined it many times.

STEP 2: Identify differences between the great and the less-than-great. When you see something that falls short of greatness in your area of interest, ask yourself, *What's the difference between this and the examples of greatness in my collection?* Sometimes these differences are obvious. *When they aren't, here are two strategies to figure it out...*

● **Change the format.**

Examples: If comparing the items on your computer screen doesn't make the differences clear, maybe you could print them out and look at them on paper...or find images of them from different angles...or view the items in person...or take them apart...or read other people's reviews or descriptions of them.

● **Quantify it.** Distilling things down to numbers often makes it easier to spot differences.

Examples: Why do people find Apple's website more appealing than Samsung's? Maybe it's because Apple's tends to have many fewer words and details, something that may become obvious when you compare word counts.

Why did the book The DaVinci Code *outsell so many other thrillers?* Maybe it's because it had more chapters but fewer words per chapter than most, creating a sense of pace.

What made one speech successful while another failed? Quantify the transcripts—maybe the first speaker told more stories and jokes and didn't bog down listeners with as many facts.

STEP 3: Create a template. Write a "reverse outline" based on an existing work of greatness. Outlines most often are created as frameworks for projects not yet begun. A reverse outline describes an already completed work. That reverse outline can serve as a framework for the new project you have in mind.

To create a reverse outline: Simply write out the elements or steps that together form the work.

Example: If your goal is to create YouTube travel videos, find a travel video that you consider great and break it down shot by shot. For each shot, note details such as length, camera angle, subject matter and background music. Then follow this same format, shot by shot, but with a different travel destination.

Step 4: **Evolve the existing idea.** Researchers at Harvard University analyzed which medical research proposals win grants. They discovered that the more novel a proposal was, the less likely it was to receive funding... but they also discovered that successful proposals usually did contain a small amount of novelty. In other words, groundbreaking originality is generally not the path to success—it tends to trigger fear or confusion—but neither is outright mimicry. As fictional advertising executive Don Draper said on the TV show *Mad Men,* "It's derivative with a twist. That's what they're looking for."

Exception: Outright copying can be OK if something is only for your private use.

Example: If you find the living room of your dreams on someone else's Instagram page, there's no harm in re-creating that exact living room in your home.

Among the ways to evolve an existing great idea…

•**Relocate the idea to a new place.** Starbucks is a Milan espresso bar relocated to the US. Chipotle, as noted earlier, found success by offering Tex/Mex food in parts of the US where Tex/Mex was uncommon.

•**Apply the great idea to a different topic or type of product.**

Examples: Absolut vodka set itself apart from other vodkas by calling attention to the distinctive shape of its bottle in advertisements. A few years later, the same formula was successfully used to launch a new gin, Bombay Sapphire—its bottle was an eye-catching blue. Chef David Chang's massively popular pork buns are an Asian dish, but Chang uses flavors and textures that evoke memories of an American comfort food—the BLT—which greatly improves the odds that the meal will resonate with US customers. A restaurant featuring a completely different cuisine could follow that same strategy.

•**Re-create the item using different eyes and hands.** Maybe the existing concept will be transformed into something substantially new and different simply because you made the new version yourself. Or maybe you could bring in someone from a different background, discipline or department to give it his/her take. The Marvel superhero movies are formulaic, but they have remained fresh and successful in part because the producers bring in new directors who previously worked outside of the superhero genre.

Beat Distractions by Making Work Fun

Distractions are a temporary way to avoid the stress of doing tedious and unpleasant tasks. But becoming distracted only puts the tasks off—increasing the stress later, especially if you must meet a deadline. Instead, find things that are interesting and therefore enjoyable in the tasks themselves by paying super-close attention to what you are doing.

Example: Mowing the lawn is a form of drudgery, so use the time to figure out the best path for the mower to take. Or calculate how long it took to do the job last time and try to beat that time. Focus intently on some element of a tedious job that you can try to do better, faster or more thoroughly—or something about it that makes you curious, such as why grass grows the way it does—and you can have fun considering small, even trivial, elements while getting the bigger job done.

Nir Ayal, author of *Hooked: How to Build Habit-Forming Products* and *Indistractable: How to Control Your Attention and Control Your Life.* He was previously a lecturer in marketing for Stanford Graduate School of Business. NirAndFar.com

BETTER WAYS…

How to Quit a Job Gracefully… and Leave Your Bridges Intact

The way you leave a job is how you will be remembered. *Schedule a meeting with your boss* to explain that you are leaving—preferably in person, or by phone if that is not possible. This shows respect, keeps your options open and could lead to a positive reference. *Write a resignation e-mail*—it should detail some of the best things you have done for the company and express your appreciation for the skills you learned on the job. Ask HR if there are specific elements that need to be included in your resignation letter. *Assure the company and your manager that you will tie up loose ends before your last day.* If you can't complete a project, check that whoever takes it over has what they need from you to be able to finish it.

Grow.Acorns.com

You Sent in a Job Application—Now What?

Unless the application instructions explicitly say not to follow up, contacting the employer a day or two later by phone, voicemail or e-mail can help you stand out from the crowd. Be professional and never pushy.... restate your interest in the position, and remind the recruiter of your qualifications... thank him/her for reviewing your application and say how much you're looking forward to talking again.

Best days for following up: Tuesday through Thursday. Mondays are usually busy transition days, and calls and e-mails sent on Fridays often can get missed and buried over the weekend.

FlexJobs.com

Prep for Your Job Search

For better job searching, try this two-day prep...

DAY 1: **Triple-check your résumé for accuracy.** Arrange your virtual interview space. Position some interesting objects around for conversation starters. Set up your voicemail message. Review your LinkedIn profile, and consider the online job-search sites Handshake and Simplicity.

DAY 2: **Reach out to friends, former colleagues and other contacts** for e-mail connections with potential employers and contacts for references and cold-mail inquiries. Practice a quick personal presentation that highlights your background, interests and specific focuses for each company you are interested in.

Reminder: Rehearse personal anecdotes that show who you are for appropriate points during an interview.

Advice from recruiters and hiring managers, quoted in *The Wall Street Journal.*

Career Certificates for In-Demand Jobs

Career certificates could replace traditional college degrees by teaching skills to help job seekers find employment quickly. The certificates could be obtained by taking courses that last just six months, not the four years or more needed for a traditional college education. Google is planning to offer programs for getting certified, taught by experts working in fields such as project management, data analysis and user-experience (UX) design. Prices for the new courses are not set yet, but they are likely to be in the $50-a-month range, based on similar existing offerings. That would make it possible to obtain a career certificate possibly for as little as $300. Google also plans to offer 100,000 need-based scholarships for students pursuing the certificates.

Inc.com

The Hottest Career Paths Don't Require College

Katie Fitzgerald and Stacy Whitehouse, director of communications and membership and senior associate for communications and state engagement, respectively, of Advance CTE, Silver Spring, Maryland. CareerTech.org

When the US Bureau of Labor Statistics (BLS) ranked professions by projected growth this decade, wind-turbine service technician landed at the very top of the list. It isn't shocking that pros in the red-hot renewable-energy sector will be in demand, but it is notable that the career projected to have the greatest growth in the 2020s does not require a college degree. Most wind-turbine techs enter the field with a certificate from a technical-school program.

Historically known as trade, technical and/or vocational programs, today's "career and technical education" (CTE) programs focus on making students career-ready by combining a standard academic curriculum with hands-on experiences and job-specific skills.

GET TO WORK, NOT INTO DEBT

The usual path to professional success in the US has long included a bachelor's degree and, often, postgraduate education—but that path no longer is as secure as it once was. More than one-third of college grads end up underemployed, taking jobs that don't require a four-year college degree, according to research by the Federal Reserve Bank of New York. Plus, many college graduates begin their working life buried under tens of thousands of dollars of student loan debt.

CTE programs can get students into the workforce faster and at a fraction of the cost. A typical four-year private college charges about $1,160 per credit hour...the typical four-year public college, $315...while the typical area technical center charges just $2 per credit hour for skills-based classes. The number of credit hours required to earn a certificate in a CTE-related career path is significantly lower, too. And CTE programs generally take no more than one to two years. Today most CTE programs are aligned to a rigorous national curriculum and are approved at the state level.

IT ISN'T JUST AUTO REPAIR

Modern CTE programs offer instruction in 16 "career clusters" including manufacturing and construction trades...health sciences... finance...business...science, technology, engineering and mathematics...information technology...transportation, distribution and logistics...the arts...and even the law. A CTE program doesn't make someone a lawyer, but it can train students for in-demand legal roles such as paralegal or court reporter. The emphasis is providing real-world skills that are useful to employers. See page 308 for some of today's most attractive CTE career options based on projected job growth and earnings.

Bonus: Many programs involve work-based apprenticeships that provide real-world experience as well as a foot in the door with employers.

Some CTE students go on to earn four-year degrees, but many enter the workforce armed with a certificate earned in a year or less...

or a two-year associate's degree. These students are not necessarily finished learning. CTE programs are designed to provide "stackable skills," meaning that students can enter the workforce quickly but have opportunities for additional training that opens additional doors.

Example: A student could earn a firefighting certification...take a job as a firefighter...and later complete a program in fire science to become a fire inspector.

CTE courses are offered at multiple institutions including community colleges and area technical centers, though many students start by taking CTE classes in middle and high school. In some areas, there are high schools that focus on CTE programs—career academies, vocational high schools and trade high schools. To find CTE programs in your area, enter "CTE" or "area technical center" and the name of your state into a search engine. If you want to know which programs near you are highly regarded, ask local employers who hire people in the field you are considering for their recommendations.

GREAT TRADE AND
TECH SCHOOL CAREERS

Classic CTE careers such as plumber, electrician and HVAC/refrigeration mechanic and installer remain as viable as ever, with median annual salaries of $50,000 to $60,000 because the home-building and home-repair sector is flourishing. But there are plenty of other CTE careers worth considering.

Washington state's Career Bridge website (CareerBridge.wa.gov) is a good example of tools provided by states to investigate career options. It features details about in-demand professions and earnings potential, a quiz to help students identify careers that match their interests and more. It also has details about specific CTE programs for students who live in Washington state.

Or consider the following careers, which offer impressive earnings and/or are in great demand...and don't require a four-year college degree but rather a relevant certificate from a CTE program or, in some cases, a two-year associate's degree from a CTE program...

•**Radiation therapist.** These medical professionals administer treatments to cancer patients. Demand is strong—the BLS expects a 7% increase in jobs this decade. A two-year degree typically is sufficient to qualify, though licensing requirements vary by state. *Median pay:* $86,850.

•**Radiologic or MRI technologist.** Radiologic technologists take X-rays and other scans…while MRI technologists operate MRI scanners. Job growth of 7% is expected this decade, and an associate's degree generally is sufficient. *Median pay:* $63,710.

•**Respiratory therapist.** These health-care pros work with doctors to help patients who have difficulty breathing due to asthma, emphysema or cystic fibrosis. They connect patients to ventilators and perform respiratory procedures such as chest physiotherapy. Demand for respiratory therapists is expected to increase by 19% this decade. An associate's degree generally is required. *Median pay:* $62,810.

•**Aerospace engineering and operations technologist or technician.** These professionals operate the equipment used to develop and produce new air- and spacecraft. Jobs are expected to increase by 7% this decade and typically require an associate's degree in engineering technology or certificates in relevant topics such as machining, computer programming and/or robotics. *Median pay:* $68,570.

•**Wind-turbine service technician.** The BLS projects that 61% more people will be employed maintaining wind turbines in 2030 than in 2020—the highest growth rate of any profession. Comfort working at great heights is necessary. *Median pay:* $56,230.

•**Court reporter or simultaneous captioner.** Court reporters type up transcripts during trials, and simultaneous captioners do the same for live events such as TV programs and press conferences. The ability to type accurately at high speed is necessary. Requires postsecondary education but less than a two-year degree. Licensing requirements vary by state. The sector is expected to grow by 9% this decade. *Median pay:* $61,660.

•**Computer-support specialist.** These pros provide assistance with computer problems to individual computer owners or as in-house tech support staff for organizations. Demand is strong—8% growth is expected this decade. Additional education could lead to a variety of career paths across IT including management, computer software engineering and computer programming. An associate's degree or tech-school certificate in a computer-related field often is sufficient. *Median pay:* $55,510.

•**Paralegal or legal assistant.** It typically takes seven years of post-secondary education to become a lawyer—four years to earn a bachelor's degree, followed by three years of law school. But to support lawyers as a paralegal or legal assistant generally requires only a two-year associate's degree in paralegal studies. These professions are in great demand, with 10% job growth expected this decade. *Median pay:* $52,920.

•**Licensed practical or licensed vocational nurse.** Students generally can qualify for these entry-level nursing positions by completing a one-year state-approved CTE program. The profession is expected to grow by 9% this decade, and with additional education, these entry-level nursing jobs can be a stepping stone to more lucrative health-care roles such as registered nurse or nurse practitioner. *Median pay:* $48,820.

•**Solar photovoltaic installer.** Increased interest in renewable power is boosting demand for solar panel installers almost as dramatically as it is for wind-turbine techs—there are expected to be 51% more jobs in this field in 2030 than in 2020. This requires just a high school diploma and one year of on-the-job training. *Median pay:* $46,470.

•**Air traffic controller.** No profession requiring only an associate's degree pays higher median annual wages, according to the BLS. Students hoping to enter the field typically attend an "Air Traffic Collegiate Training Initiative" program—there are several dozen across the US (FAA.gov/jobs/students/schools). On the downside, air traffic controller is a high-stress profession that's projected to experience only modest 1% employment growth this decade, potentially making it difficult to land jobs. *Median pay (as of 2020): $130,420.*

A COVID-Related Résumé Gap Won't Hurt Your Job Hunt

Résumé gaps ordinarily make employers wary about applicants' motivation and skills. But the pandemic was an extreme situation. And with today's hot job market, 2020–21 gaps aren't taking candidates out of contention. Provide a simple explanation such as "employer shut down due to COVID." Gaps of two years or longer remain problematic, however—take relevant classes so that you have something to fill these.

Tami Forman, chief executive of Path Forward, a New York City–based nonprofit that helps people return to the workforce. PathForward.org

Don't Let Bad Body Language Undermine Your Job Interview

Mark Bowden, founder and president of Truthplane, a communication training company based in Toronto. He is author or coauthor of several books about body language including *Truth & Lies: What People Are Really Thinking.* Truthplane.com

You could say all the right things during a job interview, but if your body language sends the wrong message, you won't land the job. Interviewers might not consciously hold your body language against you, but they will form opinions about you based on cues from how you move and hold your body without even realizing that they are doing so. The way you carry yourself or make gestures could leave interviewers with a nagging sense that you won't fit in, can't be trusted or won't hold up under pressure. Even people who normally have no trouble making strong first impressions sometimes flub job interview body language because the pressure affects how they hold themselves.

Smart body language strategies for job interviews…

•**Move decisively as the interview begins.** There often are moments of uncertainty immediately before a job interview officially starts.

Examples: Should you walk into the interviewer's office or wait at the door to be invited in? Should you extend your hand for a handshake or wait until a hand is offered? Should you take a seat or wait to be asked to sit? Which seat should you take?

It's normal to hesitate for a second as you consider these options—you don't want to do the wrong thing. But your body language will reflect that hesitance, creating an impression of someone who's indecisive or anxious—you might make stuttering movements…your eyes might dart around…or your stride might falter. First impressions are lasting impressions, so this momentary uncertainty could damage your chance of landing the job before the interview even begins.

Instead, decide in advance what you will do or make a fast choice in the moment, then move forward with confidence. Occasionally, you might make a wrong choice, but there usually is no wrong choice—often the reason it isn't clear what to do in situations such as these is that any reasonable option is acceptable.

Warning: Move with purpose and confidence from the moment you arrive at the company's premises—even in the parking lot. Some employers ask receptionists, assistants and/or security guards their opinions of interviewees because they want to find out what job candidates are like when they don't realize they're being evaluated.

Example: I know a corporate president who goes up to interviewees at her company's reception desk and asks whether they would like a coffee without disclosing who she is.

•**Make hand gestures with open palms at navel height.** Hand gestures below navel level seem disengaged and passionless. Hand gestures much above navel level can make us seem overwrought. Gestures at approximately navel level strike the proper balance when sitting or standing—they seem calm and focused.

Symmetrical gestures—gestures that feature the same movement from both hands and arms—are best. Gesturing with one arm and not the other (or gesturing differently with each arm) sends a mixed message that the interviewer's brain might struggle to interpret. That mental struggle could leave him/her feeling uncertain about how to read you—even though he won't realize that your arm gestures are the reason for this feeling. Also, when you gesture, open hands are better than fists, which seem aggressive.

Bonus: The interviewer might not be the only one who interprets your navel-height, open-hand arm gestures as a sign of calm focus—your own mind might receive the same message. Studies have found that our body language and facial expressions are not just a result of how we feel but also can influence how we feel.

•**Sit up—not forward or back—in your chair,** and position the chair properly. Leaning forward can seem overly aggressive, and leaning back seems disengaged. If seated at a table, position your chair so that your torso is approximately the width of a hand with fanned-out fingers from the table's edge. That's close enough that you won't seem disengaged to the interviewer…but not so close that your navel-level hand gestures, described above, will be hidden beneath the table. People tend to feel nervous when they can't see what strangers are doing with their hands.

When not gesturing, place your hands on the table…or in your lap if you're not seated at a table. Do not cross your arms across your torso, which seems defensive and closed off.

•**Weed out nervous tics and things that look like nervous tics.** Repeatedly touching your face…swinging a leg or foot…tapping a finger…and/or licking or biting your lips can send signals of anxiety. If you're prone to leg or foot swinging, position both feet flat on the floor rather than cross your legs when seated. If you're a finger tapper, fold your hands

loosely together. If you're a lip licker, apply a little lip balm before the interview—you're less likely to feel the need to lick moist lips. Anything you can do or think to calm yourself should cut down on these nervous tics, too.

•**Make extended eye contact.** Conventional wisdom holds that if we make too much eye contact, we'll seem threatening and off-putting. In truth, there's no such thing as too much eye contact. Prolonged eye contact sends the message "you're of interest to me," which is a positive message during a job interview. The trouble comes when people accidentally pair extended eye contact with aggressive body language such as leaning forward in one's chair or making closed-fist hand gestures—the combination of aggression and deep interest is indeed off-putting.

Tip: If you're being interviewed by more than one person at the same time, share your eye contact equally among the interviewers. Our natural inclination in job interviews is to give most of our eye contact to the person we believe is highest in the corporate hierarchy or who seems most positive toward us. But that person might not be the key decision maker when it comes to filling the job.

•**If you write something down during the interview, explain why you're writing.** Think about how uncomfortable it feels when an interviewer jots something down during the interview—is he/she writing something good about me? Something bad? The uncertainty can trigger anxiety. If you jot something down during an interview, you could be making the interviewer feel similar discomfort—and making interviewers uncomfortable is never beneficial.

Example: The interviewer stresses something about how the corporate culture differs from the culture of other companies in the sector. You could respond, "That's a good point—I'd like to jot it down," as you pick up your pen and pad.

Warning: Do not hold a pen and pad throughout an interview. That can make you seem like someone without ideas of his own who just writes things down that other people say. Holding objects also makes it difficult to gesture symmetrically with open hands, as described earlier. If you wish to keep a pen and pad handy, set them on a table in front of you or on the chair next to you...or leave them next to your seat in a pocket of your portfolio or bag where you can reach them quickly if needed.

•**Send a strong parting message.** As the interview progresses, be on the lookout for signs from the interviewer that the interview is over. Most interviewers make this clear by standing up and/or thanking the candidate for coming in, but others send subtler signals that they are ready for it to be over...and become frustrated when these are not heeded. Subtle signals could include checking the time repeatedly...asking the interviewee if he/she has any more questions...or long silences. If you suspect the interview might be over, ask the interviewer, "Is there anything else I can provide to you?"

Reminder: Your palms may get a little sweaty during a job interview. So when you rise from your seat at the conclusion of the interview, subtly brush your palm against your pants leg or skirt to dry it off before the final handshake.

Virtual Trainers Are as Good as Real People

People who worked with virtual trainers to learn leadership skills in a completely virtual environment or one combining digital and real-world elements improved their skills just as much as those who worked with trainers in a real-world setting.

Study of 30 people by researchers at University of Canterbury, Christchurch, New Zealand, published in *Frontiers in Virtual Reality.*

Want to Work with Animals?

These jobs don't require a degree: Dog walker and pet sitter—check sites such as Rover.com to find clients...doggy day care attendant...animal trainer...or service dog trainer. Volunteer at a shelter for dogs or cats...work for a cat café—a place where cats can hang out and socialize or wait for adoption while humans get their caffeine fix. Bake pet treats and food for a local pet bakery or food company—or start your own company.

ThePennyHoarder.com

Prevent "Zoom Fatigue"

Turn off the computer camera to reduce the energy drain caused by having virtual meetings all day long. Employees' stress levels rise when they are constantly on camera because they are concerned about how they come across visually and about distractions, such as kids coming into the room. These concerns not only increase fatigue but also make employees less engaged in the meeting topics.

Study by researchers at University of Arizona, Tucson, published in *Journal of Applied Psychology.*

Freelancers: How to Decide What to Charge

Start by checking the local going rate for similar services. Take into account materials and preparation time as well as the time you spend actually doing what you do. *Factor in taxes and insurance costs.* A flat-rate per session/project or a weekly rate for a certain amount of work is preferable to hourly rates, which penalize you for working quickly and efficiently. As you improve and build a client

Secret to Artistic Success

Successful creative people seem to follow a pattern—years of study in their field of interest (exploration) followed by intense, narrow focus (exploitation) on what they learned.

Example: Artist Jackson Pollock spent years investigating other art techniques, such as drawing, print-making and surrealist paintings, before he hit it big with his drip paintings. Exploration could be perceived as potentially leading nowhere…but it seems to increase the likelihood of stumbling upon a great idea. Narrow focus, on the other hand, can be thought of as something that would stifle creativity—but when it follows exploration, it is a consistent way to find your hot streak. Interestingly, neither exploration nor exploitation on their own lead to artistic success.

Study using artificial intelligence to compare the careers of artists by researchers at Kellogg School of Management, Northwestern University, Evanston, Illinois, published in *Nature Communications*.

base, it's reasonable to increase your fees—10% to 20% annually is common. Although you may lose some jobs, don't undervalue your work. *Present your skills clearly* to potential clients to justify what you charge.

Example: Explain that you are able to finish a project more quickly than others because you have been doing such work for 10 years.

ThePennyHoarder.com

Don't Send an E-Mail That You'll Regret

Lashing out in an e-mail is almost always a bad idea, especially since recipients usually read a negative slant into most e-mails they receive anyway—so even if your note is neutral in tone, it may be perceived as negative.

Better: *Write your e-mail, but don't send it* until you've taken a 10-minute stroll. When

you return, you'll have greater clarity about how to word your feelings constructively. *Sleep on it.* Letting it all hang out in a draft of your e-mail can be a good emotional outlet. The next day, with new perspective, you can edit it down to something reasonable and productive. *Get help.* Ask a trusted friend or colleague to review your e-mail and let you know if it comes off the way it should.

LifeHacker.com

Pushing Back When Others Overstep Your Boundaries

Terri Cole, licensed psychotherapist based in Averill Park, New York, and author of *Boundary Boss: The Essential Guide to Talk True, Be Seen, and (Finally) Live Free.* You can take her free boundary quiz at BoundaryQuiz.com. TerriCole.com

Nosy neighbors…critical spouses…friends and colleagues who cross the line. Life is full of "boundary breakers"—people who ask intrusive questions, take advantage of your goodwill and make hurtful comments. Whether their behavior is malicious and intentional…or just clueless and insensitive…it causes a lot of stress. And until you can communicate your boundaries in a calm, honest manner, these people will continue to make assumptions about what's acceptable to you and, more often than not, they will get it wrong.

Over the past 25 years, psychotherapist and author Terri Cole has coached thousands of clients on how to deal with boundary breakers. *Here are her strategies for fighting back…*

FOUR STEPS TO ESTABLISH BOUNDARIES

I use a four-step process created by psychologist Marshall B. Rosenberg, PhD, founder of the Center for Nonviolent Communication. Practice these steps with small boundary breaches before you move on to the bigger problems.

Example: You gave a neighbor a spare key to your home for emergencies, and now he uses it to occasionally borrow your garden tools and equipment without asking. *What to do…*

STEP #1: State the issue. Use factual language. "The other day you used your spare key to borrow my lawnmower."

STEP #2: State your feelings. Don't assume the other person's motivations or anticipate his/her reply. Simply discuss how it affects you. "I thought the mower had been lost or stolen. I couldn't mow my lawn, and I was frustrated when you told me a day later that you had taken it."

STEP #3: Make a simple request in a nonconfrontational way, and attach a mutual benefit to it. "In the future, if you want to borrow something of mine, please check in with me first so I can continue to let you have my key."

STEP #4: Suggest a shared agreement. This engages and enrolls the other person into taking equal responsibility for the success of your new boundary rule. "Can we agree that if you're interested in borrowing any of my things, you will text me before you let yourself in?"

FOR THE SPUR-OF-THE-MOMENT

Sometimes when your boundaries are violated, you don't have the time to calmly reflect on what's going on and use the four-step process. Instead, you need the right language and real-time strategies to quickly establish limits and prevent tensions from escalating.

• **Nosy questions.** You don't owe explanations or answers for every inquiry about your love life, family or finances. *Ways to respond…*

• Promise to answer the question on your terms when you're ready. *Example:* A relative asks how serious you are about the new person you're dating. *Your reply:* "I'd rather not discuss that right now. When I have news I want to share, I will let you know."

• Use humor (accompanied by a wink). You gently deflect the question while getting across the message that you are not interested in sharing. *Example:* A friend asks how big a raise you got at work. *Your reply:* "Trust me, not even close to what I am worth!"

• Respond with your own question. This shifts the dynamic instantly, turning the spotlight onto the other person and causing him to lose interest in what he just asked. *Example:* An acquaintance asks your age. *Your reply:* "Why would you want to know that?"

Alternative: Reply with a question on a different subject. *Example:* A neighbor asks if your son has found a job since he was laid off. *Your reply:* "Let me put that on hold. I keep meaning to ask you if you are enjoying your new grandchild."

• **When you're asked to do something that you don't want to do.** It can be difficult to say no when the other person is in a jam or sincerely just wants to spend time with you. You may not have a specific reason to turn her down but don't want to hurt her feelings—so you may end up reverting to what I call an "auto-yes," even when it means letting someone else's needs trump your own. *Other ways to respond…*

• Buy yourself some time. If you need to figure out what you want, be honest and show gratitude for the effort the person is making. *Example:* A friend invites you to dinner. *Your reply:* "That's very nice of you to offer. Thank you for thinking of me. I'll have to check my calendar and get back to you."

• You can use the same diplomatic approach to turn down an offer. *Example:* A friend asks you to volunteer for an event. *Your reply:* "Sorry, I have other commitments this weekend. I hope the event is a grand success, and I'm sending you good vibes."

• Use "no/but." *Example:* A friend suggests going out to eat. *Your reply:* "I'm going to say no to dinner, but I'm planning to go to the gym later if you'd like to come." *Or:* A colleague wants help with a project that's beyond the scope of your interest or responsibility. *Your reply:* "I can't, but once I finish up my current project, I'll circle back to see if there's some way that I can support you."

• **When someone is overly critical of you.** Comments that are rude or thoughtless can undermine your self-esteem and confidence. *Ways to respond…*

• Avoid putting yourself in the line of fire if you know the other person has a tendency to be judgmental. *Example:* Your father asks if you got your hair cut. Don't set yourself up for an insulting comment by asking, "Do you like it?" *Instead, just reply:* "Yes, I did."

• Use a "qualifier" before you share news or a personal dilemma with someone who tends to be a "fixer"—"I'd like you to simply listen without offering advice or criticism. Just a compassionate ear."

• Offer more context about what you need from him/her before you share—"I love that you are always game to help me. What I need right now is for you to listen and have faith that I'll come to the answer on my own."

• Shut down the "I'm just being honest" comments. Some people feel it's their duty to tell you how unflattering your outfit is or how badly you've messed up your marriage. *Your reply:* "I don't recall asking you for your thoughts." *Or:* "What you call honesty, I call you giving unsolicited and unconstructive criticism. Please don't."

BOUNDARY-DESTROYERS

You may have people in your life who simply refuse to respect your boundaries no matter how patient and skilled you become at setting limits and communicating your needs. They even may be so good at emotional manipulation that you find yourself apologizing to them!

Trying to reason with "boundary-destroyers" is a dead end. *Instead…*

• **Cut them off…or at least limit your time with them.** If someone is not emotionally trustworthy, you still can love and care about him—just less frequently and from further away.

Say: "We seem to argue more than we get along. I need a break because it's not healthy for me to continue this friendship."

Or: "I wish you all the best, but this relationship is really hard on me. I don't think we should be in contact until the family holiday party next year."

Important: It may not be possible to distance yourself from some boundary-destroyers—perhaps parents or colleagues. In these situations, adjust your expectations and accept that the relationship will be one-sided and offer the person very limited satisfaction. Conduct yourself in a calculated way to keep relative peace. Don't share important or emotional issues…and stop trying to defend yourself in conversations or change the other person's mind. Even boundary destroyers find it hard to argue or manipulate someone who always agrees with them.

Jobs with the Best Chance of Promotion

Product management, including strategy and road mapping, has an internal promotion rate 149% above the national average.

Other jobs with promotion rates above the national average: Marketing, including digital and e-mail marketing (94%)…program and project management, involving cross-functional team leadership (51%)…accounting (47%)…human resources (44%)…business development (26%)…finance (18%)…sales and consulting (13% for each)…purchasing (12%).

Study by LinkedIn's Economic Graph team, reported at Grow.Acorns.com.

Help Out Online from Your Couch

Nonprofits' websites and apps offer online opportunities to do good. *Be My Eyes* pairs sighted individuals with those who are visually impaired to assist with tasks through live video calls. *CareerVillage* volunteers provide career guidance and/or post–high school life advice for young people. *Smithsonian Digital Volunteers* help transcribe historical documents—birth certificates, letters, books, etc.—so they can be accessed online. *Tarjimly* needs multilingual volunteers to help refugees and immigrants translate job applications, e-mails and other documents. ZSL Instant Wild volunteers help monitor animal populations by checking photos from motion-triggered wildlife cameras.

LifeSavvy.com

20

Safety Survey

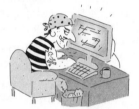

Are You Ready for the Next Disaster?

To be ready for a disaster, you need to develop a useful set of skills and, perhaps more importantly, work with others in your neighborhood to tap into their skills. *Here's what you can do to help yourself, your loved ones and your community to survive a disaster…*

TRACK NEIGHBORHOOD RESOURCES AND NEEDS

It's almost impossible to master every emergency skill to be prepared for every possible scenario. But if you coordinate with your neighbors, the group can be better prepared than any individual household on its own. *Before there's an emergency, compile a neighborhood list or map of…*

• **Who has medical training?** Know where doctors, nurses and emergency medical tech-

nicians (EMTs) live in your area, even those who have retired.

• **Which local stores, gas stations and pharmacies have backup generators and/ or plans to remain open during outages?** Encourage these businesses to develop such plans for the safety of the community. If you own a business that could be valuable during a disaster, explore how you could keep your business operational, especially if it provides vital goods or services.

Even better: Consider investing in a dual-fuel portable generator that will run on either propane or gasoline so that you can keep your own refrigerator and other essential appliances running during a power outage.

Jesse Levin, founder of Tactivate, which applies the principles of entrepreneurship and military special operations expertise to proactive emergency readiness and disaster response operations, based in Connecticut. Tactivate.com

Example: Champion 3400-Watt Dual Fuel portable generator for propane or gas ($1,339).

•**Who will have power when there is no power?** Note which neighbors have generators and/or solar panels and storage batteries. Ask if they would be willing to allow neighbors to charge cell phones, flashlights and other necessities.

•**Who will have water?** Everyone should keep a supply of water available in case of emergency. If your neighborhood gets its water from private wells, not a municipal utility, determine which neighbors can keep their pumps running during a power outage, and ask whether they would be willing to share water.

•**Who can communicate?** If one person in the neighborhood has a ham radio or satellite communications device, he/she can serve as a link for other neighbors when phone lines and cellular systems fail.

•**Who has an ATV or snowmobile?** When the roads are blocked, these could be the best way to reach a town or hospital.

Also: While you're tracking resources in your neighborhood, note who has special health or mobility needs. Check in on these neighbors during disasters, and/or arrange for other neighbors to do so.

STOCKPILE SKILLS...NOT JUST SUPPLIES

The bandages in that emergency kit are unlikely to save anyone's life during a disaster.

What will make a difference: Knowing basic emergency medical care...recognizing threats before, during and after the disaster... and being able to navigate your local area when roads are blocked. Just having these skills will help you remain calm and productive during a disaster. People who feel unprepared may burden other people, which only adds to the problem and lengthens the time it will take to get back to normal. *Skills you will need...*

•**First-aid training.** Obtaining your EMT certification and volunteering with your town's EMT service are wonderful ways to prepare for disaster while also serving your community. Basic EMT certification requires about 120 hours of training—probably more time than you can commit.

Instead: Consider an emergency medical training course offered locally or online.

Examples: Base Medical (Base-Medical. com) offers online and in-person wilderness first-aid and first-responder courses starting at $195. Or call the local chapter of the American Red Cross to find out if there are courses you can take. At minimum, you should know how to stop bleeding, stabilize broken bones and tend to head and neck injuries.

•**Advanced driving and basic automotive repair.** In a disaster, you might have to drive on icy roads, over obstacles or even off-road. You may have to change a tire or jump-start your car because road-side assistance can't reach you.

To prepare: Consider taking a driving and vehicle-repair course.

Examples: Northeast Off-Road Adventures (NYOffroadDriving.com) offers classes that teach off-road driving and maintenance. Prices start at $225. Overland Experts (Over landExperts.com) offers off-road driving classes, starting at $275.

•**Local navigation.** Would you know how to get around your area if the main roads were blocked?

To prepare: Learn the lay of the land. Your laptop and a Wi-Fi connection can provide a wealth of geo-location information. Study your environment. Satellite views and topographic maps may show hiking trails in case you must abandon your car.

For a flood: If roads are blocked, it might be better to shelter in place and get as high as possible—but don't go into an attic unless there's a way to get out.

If you're on an island: Keep an eye on the weather, and figure out in advance when to leave and where you'll go.

•**Situational awareness.** Military personnel are trained to identify potential threats and remain alert to everything happening around them, especially during emergencies. Those skills can be tremendously valuable during any disaster.

To prepare: Read the book *Left of Bang: How the Marine Corps' Combat Hunter Program Can Save Your Life.* Or check the website of former Marine Yousef Badou (Emergence Disrupt.com), which offers situational awareness training.

● **Chainsaw and generator operation and repair.** Chainsaws and generators can be tremendously useful after an event…when you are facing the real disaster challenges. Know how to use, maintain and repair these tools, since your local repair shop probably won't be accessible. Take a small-engine repair class at a local technical school. Read the safe-use and maintenance sections of the tools' manuals. Watch YouTube videos about using and repairing these tools.

STAY IN TOUCH

A cell phone is, of course, valuable during an emergency—it works even when phone lines are downed. But what if the local cellular system is knocked out? If you have no way of communicating, you might miss crucial updates and/or evacuation orders…you will be unable to summon assistance if you're trapped or injured…and you and your loved ones might not be able to contact each other.

To prepare: Consider buying and learning to use one or both of these backup communication tools…

● **Garmin inReach,** a portable device, lets you send and receive text messages via satellite—it doesn't rely on the local cellular network. The unit itself starts at $349.99, and

---

More from Jesse Levin…

What to Keep in Your Emergency Bags

You should keep two kinds of emergency bags packed and ready to go—an everyday carry bag (EDC) and a go bag for more prolonged emergencies. *What to pack…*

For Your EDC
● Portable secondary power source.
Example: Goal Zero Flip 36 power bank
- Individual first-aid kit
- Garmin inREACH Mini satellite communicator
- Leatherman Charge + multitool
- Headlamp and a small flashlight
- Small notebook and pen
- Pocket knife
- Computer thumb drive to back up and share/save important files
- Small dry-bag
- Ultra-compact rain jacket and travel blanket
- List of emergency contacts
- Drivers' licenses, passports

For your go bag
● Small, waterproof pouch with critical documents (passports, insurance cards, ID cards, medical records, medications list, copies of passports, list of important phone numbers and cash)
- Critical medications
- Small water-purification system

● Protein bar(s), beef jerky or other form of energy that will not spoil
● Small tent, sleeping bag and pad/hammock
● Map(s) of local area, compass and GPS
● Small collapsible .22-caliber rifle for hunting, depending on legality and location
● Flashlight/headlamp
● Small camping stove with fuel pod
● Kettle or small cooking kit
● Fixed blade knife
● Thermal layer and change of socks and underwear
● Backup batteries for devices
● Head covering and gloves
● Medical kit and supplies
● Satellite phone, ham radio or two-way satellite pager
● Collapsible bladder for water storage
● Fire kit, fire starter, matches, lighter ferro rod and emergency tinder
● Signaling device(s)—a chemlight, mini strobe light, signaling panel/mirror
● 25 feet of paracord
● Small camp towel and packable soap or baby wipes

annual service plans start at $143.40. Discover. Garmin.com/en-US/inreach/personal

• **Ham radio**—two-way long-distance communication via radio waves—doesn't depend on cell towers or phone lines. Handheld, battery-powered devices are available for less than $100.

Reminder: Learn to operate it, and obtain a license so that you can use it legally.

Example: Ham Radio Prep's online classes start at $35. HamRadioPrep.com

PREPARE FINANCIALLY

Readying your finances for a disaster can reduce your physical risk. People who are worried that a fire or flood might ruin them financially may be distracted, reducing their ability to focus on their safety and that of loved ones.

Steps to take: Speak with your insurers about your homeowners, life and health insurance coverage. Ask them how well you would be covered if there was a disaster. Are there gaps that could leave you financially vulnerable? Could these gaps be filled by purchasing riders or additional policies, such as flood insurance or an umbrella policy?

Also: Be sure to have enough money in an emergency fund to cover your insurance deductibles and expenses during and after a disaster.

Lightning Danger

Don't shower or bathe during a thunderstorm. Lightning from a storm up to 10 miles away can travel through the ground, following the path of your electrical wiring or plumbing. From the first signs of an approaching storm until at least 30 minutes after thunder has stopped, avoid anything involving plumbing (i.e., faucets, dishwasher, washing machine, toilet)…appliances that plug into outlets…and using a landline telephone.

Advice from NOAA's National Weather Service and Centers for Disease Control and Prevention.

Shelter-in-Place Necessities

Creek Stewart, survival instructor and host of the Weather Channel's *Could You Survive?* with Creek Stewart. He is author of *The Disaster-Ready Home: A Step-by-Step Emergency Preparedness Manual for Sheltering in Place.* CreekStewart.com

Don't overlook these disaster-preparation steps…

• **Buy a kerosene or propane space heater.** Home centers sell kerosene space heaters capable of warming up to 1,000 square feet, typically for around $150. A propane space heater also might serve this purpose, though these typically are designed to warm smaller areas. Kerosene and propane can be stored for years in a garage or shed—but whatever heater you select, confirm that it's safe for indoor use.

Example: Mr. Heater Little Buddy Heater runs on propane and is a cost-effective, fuel-efficient option for heating small rooms, recently $74 on Amazon.

• **Buy a portable stove that runs on twigs.** An incredible little device called EcoZoom Dura Rocket Stove (EcoZoom.com) generates enough heat from burning twigs to boil water or cook a meal. There's no need to stockpile fuel—just collect twigs from your yard or neighborhood as needed. Prices start at $119.99.

• **Create an emergency toilet.** A lack of functioning flush toilets can very quickly become a major problem. One affordable, effective solution is to buy five-gallon buckets and an "emergency five-gallon bucket toilet seat" (enter that phrase into Amazon to find numerous options for under $20). Store a few garbage bags of sawdust, too—lumber yards and home centers often provide free sawdust upon request. When your home's toilets are inoperable, put an inch of sawdust in a bucket, snap the seat on top, then add an additional inch of sawdust after each use. When a bucket is full, put a cover on it and transfer the toilet seat to another bucket. Stow filled buckets in the garage or yard until you can dispose of them safely.

•**Buy a solar generator.** Many households have a portable gas-powered generator for emergencies. Those can be valuable...but gas can be difficult to obtain during an extended disaster, so it's also worth buying a portable emergency solar system. A small system can charge essentials such as phones and flashlight batteries, while a larger system can power appliances.

Example: Goal Zero Solar Kits (GoalZero. com) start at $429.95, though prices climb into the thousands for more substantial systems.

•**Stockpile medicines.** Ask your doctor to adjust your prescriptions so that you have on hand several months' supply of drugs you take regularly. Explain that you don't want to risk being without medicine in a disaster. This might not be possible with controlled substances, such as opioid pain medications, but with most drugs it's a reasonable request. Use a "rotation" strategy (whenever you use up medicine, replace it with emergency supply, then replace the emergency stock) to prevent stockpiled medicines from expiring.

Could the Building You Live or Work in Collapse?

Mehrdad Sasani, PhD, professor of civil and environmental engineering at Northeastern University in Boston. His research focus is the collapse of structures and structural integrity. Northeastern.edu

---

The tragic collapse of Champlain Towers South, a 12-story condo in Surfside, Florida, in June 2021 triggered sympathy...and concern. Are other US high-rise buildings at risk as well?

Short answer: US high-rise buildings are at extremely low risk of collapse—but there always is some small probability of failure.

It has not been exactly determined why the Surfside collapse occurred—in probability a combination of factors, including improper constructions of neighboring projects...not a single flaw in the structure itself.

What is known is that certain signs may appear when a concrete high-rise is in danger, and some high-rises are at greater risk than others.

Here's what to watch for and what to do if you live or work in a concrete high-rise or if you're considering moving into a condo or an apartment building...

WARNING SIGNS

You don't have to be a structural engineer to identify the following potentially serious high-rise safety concerns. It's especially important to watch for these issues if your building was built before 1989 and near the ocean, two outstanding risk factors in the Champlain Towers South disaster. But everyone who lives or works in a high-rise should be on the lookout.

•**Cracks in the concrete.** If you look for cracks in structural concrete, you're going to find them—they're almost inevitable. While some concrete cracks are perfectly normal and not at all dangerous, others point to possible problems.

Rule of thumb: In general, sloping cracks on walls or beams—from around 30 to 60 degrees—are potentially more troubling in structural concrete than cracks that are largely horizontal or vertical. These types of cracks can point to shear or compressive failure, which are more dangerous in concrete structures. Also, cracks that are wide and/or widening, are more troubling than those that are stable and extremely thin.

What to do: Every so often, look for cracks, particularly sloping cracks, in concrete columns, beams, floors and walls. In some high-rises, you will have to visit the garage or underground parking area to find exposed concrete. If you spot cracks, purchase a concrete crack gauge online—they cost less than $20—and use it to measure the width of the cracks. A crack wider than about 0.016 inches is a concern, particularly if it is active or widening. Alert the building manager or condo board, and/or call in a structural engineer for an assessment if you have the power to do so. Monitor the width and length of cracks to determine if they're growing.

•**Small sections of peeling or flaking concrete.** This is called "spalling," and it could be a serious problem or no problem at all, depending on why it's happening. Sometimes sections of concrete flake off because the rebar inside the concrete is corroding—corrosion causes rebar to expand, pushing away the surrounding concrete. But sometimes spalling occurs without corrosion and is superficial.

What to do: If spalling exposes rebar previously hidden inside the concrete, examine that rebar. If it's visually corroding, alert the building manager or contact an engineer—more corroding rebar could be hidden inside the concrete, putting the entire building at risk. If there's no visible rebar or the exposed rebar shows no sign of corrosion, there's nothing significant to worry about. Just have the cover concrete repaired.

•**Crushing or crumbling concrete.** This often is a sign that concrete is failing under compression. It occurs most commonly in vertical columns but also can occur at the top or bottom of beams. Crumbling was spotted by residents of a six-story Singapore building before it collapsed in 1986.

What to do: As above, notify the building manager or a structural engineer.

•**Sloping floors.** This can be a warning sign that the floor is failing. Fortunately, it's probably failing slowly, giving everyone sufficient time to respond.

What to do: If the slope is slight—only noticeable because round items roll across the floor, for example—and not rapidly increasing, notify the building manager or an engineer. But if the sagging is obvious and growing worse at a noticeable rate, consider moving out until a structural engineer confirms that the building is safe.

•**Loud sounds.** If a high-rise's structure is the source of these sounds, that could mean there's a very serious problem and could point to imminent failure. But it can be difficult to identify the source of sounds in a large building—was that noise rebar fracturing…a nearby car backfiring…or something dropped by an upstairs neighbor?

What to do: Ask your neighbors if they know the source of the sounds before jumping

to conclusions. If you suspect that the building structure is the source, consider vacating until an engineer declares it safe and/or a nonstructural source of the sounds is identified.

•**Significant weight recently added to the building.** While some collapses occur because the building's capacity to support weight has decreased, others occur because additional weight has been added.

Example: A 16-story Boston apartment building under construction collapsed in 1971 in part because of the construction weight on its roof.

What to do: If a new penthouse, heavy air-conditioning unit or other substantial weight has been added to your high-rise, that's a good time to monitor concrete for the problems described above—and make sure that the added weight was approved by an engineer.

Stay Safe at Home When You've Lost Your Sense of Smell

Jay F. Piccirillo, MD, professor of otolaryngology—head & neck surgery, vice chair of research, and director of the Clinical Outcomes Research Office at Washington University School of Medicine in St. Louis. Dr. Piccirillo is editor of *JAMA Otolaryngology–Head & Neck Surgery*.

In January 2021, a teenager in Waco, Texas, made headlines for saving her family from a fire ravaging their home. Her loved ones all were recovering from COVID-19 and had lost their sense of smell. She was the only one who had not contracted the virus. The rest of her family couldn't smell the smoke, and they had no idea that a blaze ignited as they slept.

Anosmia—the technical term for loss of the sense of smell—is a pervasive problem for those who have had COVID-19. A study published in January 2021 in *Journal of Internal Medicine* followed more than 2,500 patients seen at 18 hospitals across Europe who had the olfactory dysfunction. Surprisingly, this long-term symptom mostly affected people with a mild form of the virus—85.9% of that group self-reported it, while only 4.5% of those with a moderate form and 6.9% of those most severely afflicted listed it. While 95% of all participants had their smell returned at a six-month follow-up, it's crucial to take defensive steps to protect your well-being while waiting for your senses to return to normal. *These precautions are also important if your sense of smell has weakened due to other reasons (other illness, side effect from medications)...*

●**Install a gas detector.** Though not as common as smoke detectors, these devices alert you to a gas leak by sounding an alarm and flashing lights—a lifeline when your nose can't pick up the usual rotten-egg smell. Place one near each gas line, usually somewhere in the kitchen and possibly in other locations, such as near your water heater or furnace if it runs on gas. If you're signed up with a security monitoring company, gas monitoring often can be added to the system.

Also important: Regularly check, test and replace the batteries for your existing smoke and carbon monoxide detectors. Check them at least twice a year, if not more often.

●**Take steps to avoid eating spoiled food.** When your nose can't alert you to a food that's turned bad, follow food-safety rules of thumb. Be extra cautious about any food you are not 100% sure about, and throw out leftovers after four days. Check expiration dates on food packages daily—toss them without hesitation.

●**Skip strong household chemicals.** You may not sense how potent strong cleaners are until your eyes start watering—and by then you've most likely already overexposed yourself. And definitely take care not to mix common yet volatile products, such as bleach and ammonia or bleach and vinegar, which can create toxic fumes.

GETTING YOUR NOSE IN GEAR

Since anosmia is caused by injury to the supporting cells around the olfactory or smell nerves, it may be possible to jump-start your recovery with olfactory training.

Choose three or four of your favorite essential oils, and sniff each one deeply for 10 seconds twice a day.

You might also try mindfully smelling things that you encounter during your day, from your morning coffee to a bottle of perfume or the piece of salmon you broiled for dinner.

Another helpful step may be to maintain good nasal hygiene with a neti pot—use it daily with a saline rinse to keep your nose healthy. This will keep your nasal passages clean and may help to reduce inflammation that can prolong or prevent the recovery of your sense of smell.

Portable Locks and Alarms Provide Vacation-Rental Peace of Mind

Earlier guests at Airbnb rentals could have made copies of keys. Portable locks can prevent inward-swinging doors from opening even with a key.

Options: Vincrey Portable Door Lock ($12.99) or DoorJammer ($24.99). Or point AllAbout Adapters' Portable Alarm System ($16) toward a door or window—it will sound if anything moves within its 100-degree field of vision.

Detective Kevin Coffey is a travel-risk consultant retired from the Los Angeles Police Department after 35 years. CorporateTravelSafety.com

Monitor Crime in Your Neighborhood

Detective Kevin Coffey, travel and personal risk consultant and corporate trainer who is CEO of Los Angeles–based Corporate Travel Safety, LLC. He recently retired from the Los Angeles Police Department after 35 years of service. CorporateTravelSafety.com

Is your neighborhood as safe as you think it is? *These free websites and apps* can help you understand the actual risks,*

*All apps and websites are free unless otherwise noted.

whether it's nuisances such as front-porch package thieves or more serious threats...

•**Nextdoor** is a website and app where people post messages to others in their area on a range of topics including local crime. It's a good way to keep up on local chatter and keep tabs on crime-related matters that are too minor to receive attention in local newspapers, such as strangers seen lurking or possessions going missing from unlocked parked cars. Non-crime-related matters covered often include items for sale, lost pets and requests for assistance...plus the inevitable complaints about loud lawnmowers and people who don't clean up after their dogs. Nextdoor's usefulness depends on how many people use it in your neighborhood.

Similar: **Citizen,** available for about 30 US cities, is an app that can send you notifications of nearby 911 emergencies in real time—it's like having access to a police scanner only in app form and curated to focus on the incidents most likely to be of interest.

Examples: You might receive a notice when a dementia sufferer or child goes missing in your neighborhood...a warning when there's an active shooter within miles of your home...or an explanation why there's a police helicopter hovering overhead.

•**Neighbors by Ring.** You might have heard of the Ring Video Doorbell, the digital doorbell and security device that contains a motion-activated camera featuring night vision. When Ring's motion detector records digital video of a crime or suspicious activity, the doorbell's owner often will share that footage through Ring's *Neighbors* app, alerting people who live nearby to the potential threat. You can download this app and view these videos for free even if you don't buy a Ring doorbell.

•**National Sex Offender Public Website** is a US Department of Justice site that can be searched to identify any registered sex offenders living near your address (NSOPW.gov).

Similar: States maintain searchable sex offender databases, too, which sometimes offer better search features than the federal site and typically are updated faster. To find a state's

site, visit FBI.gov, choose "Scams and Safety" from the "More" menu, then click "Sex Offender Registry Websites."

•**SpotCrime** is a website and app that provides local crime stats and crime reports for more than 500 US cities and towns using data gathered mostly from law-enforcement agencies. Crimes are displayed on a local street map to show where danger lies. SpotCrime is especially useful if you're moving to or visiting an unfamiliar area. Crimes are not reported in real time, however—it can take several days for them to appear—and many small towns and rural areas are not covered well or at all.

Tip: If the area you want to see is not well-covered on SpotCrime, visit the town or county website or contact the local law-enforcement agency to see if area crime reports and data are made available directly to the public. Your local law-enforcement agency may maintain a website for crime reports or let you sign up for regular e-mail alerts on local crime.

Dealing with a Burglary

Robert Siciliano, CEO of the security-awareness training firm Protect Now LLC and author of *Identity Theft Privacy: Security Protection and Fraud Prevention.* ProtectNowLLC.com

Y ou arrive home after a vacation, a dinner out with friends, even just from grocery shopping...and find that your home has been broken into. *Here are the things to do—and* not *to do...*

•**Do not go inside.** Break-ins often are committed by desperate people with drug addictions and/or mental-health problems who will stop at nothing to get what they want. Back away, and use your cell or a neighbor's phone to call 911. Wait in your vehicle or other safe place until the police arrive and secure the home.

•**Inventory your belongings.** After the police have made sure the house is empty, walk through and write down missing items—electronics, cash, jewelry, keys, checkbooks, etc.

Sometimes it's days or weeks before people realize something is missing. That's OK. Just file an update with the police in case your insurance company needs an official record.

• **Call your homeowner's insurance** to file a claim.

• **Mitigate identity-theft risk.** Even if the criminals didn't steal personal documents, they may have taken pictures of sensitive information. Freeze your credit. Purchase an identity-theft plan, such as one from my company, Protect Now Pro at ProtectNowLLC.com/id-protection.

• **Look after your mental health.** Break-ins are more traumatic than people would expect. Your sanctuary has been violated. It is not uncommon for a lingering, almost unnoticed malaise to develop into depression. Be on the lookout for a loss of morale or unusual irritability. If you're struggling to come to grips with the crime, seek counseling.

• **Don't let it happen again...**

• Replace the locks if they have been picked or opened with a key.

• Invest in a home-security system or at least in some security-company signs.

• Put up a "Beware of Dog" sign even if you don't have a dog.

• Purchase and install doorjamb reinforcements (look online for "door reinforcement technology") to make it impossible to kick in your doors. *Example:* Door Devil (DoorDevil.com).

• Password-protect every device, even if it never leaves the house.

• Invest in a fireproof safe that can be bolted to the floor for your valuables.

• Take an inventory of your belongings. Periodically walk through your house with your phone's video camera, then e-mail the video to yourself. That will make it easier for you and the insurance company to sort things out if the place is ever broken into again.

Beware of Dog Thieves

Two million dogs are stolen each year in the US, with California and the Midwest being hot spots. Thieves target valuable, sought-after breeds such as French Bulldogs, Pomeranians, Yorkshire Terriers and Maltese—not to keep them for themselves but to resell them to unsuspecting buyers for up to $3,000 apiece. Some are sold to backyard puppy mills as breeding stock. Less-valuable breeds also get stolen, sometimes to be used as bait in dog-fighting operations. Pet thefts typically take place after the crooks have surveilled your property and routines. Installing security cameras is a good idea, but the best advice is never to leave your dog unattended. That means keeping a watchful eye on your pets even on your own property.

Money.com

Items Not to Leave in Parked Cars

Prescription medicines—heat and cold can damage them. *Sunscreen*—heat lowers its effectiveness. *Aerosol cans*—they are heat-sensitive and could explode. *Cell phones*—heat and cold can damage them, and a thief seeing a phone might break into the car to steal it. *Important documents*—thieves could steal them, exposing you to identity theft. *Wooden musical instruments*—cold can crack them, and both heat and cold can cause failure of the glue that holds wooden instruments together. *Canned foods*—temperatures above 100°F can cause spoilage...even at temperatures above 75°F, nutrients can be lost.

Roundup of experts reported at MoneyTalksNews.com. ConsumerAffairs.com and University of Minnesota Extension (Extension.UMN.edu).

Winter-Driving Safety

Keep a 20-pound bag of clay kitty litter in the trunk of your vehicle—the added weight helps stabilize your car, so you'll skid less on icy roads, whether or not you have rear-wheel drive. And spreading some of the litter around each tire can give you some extra traction if you get stuck in snow.

Farmers' Almanac. FarmersAlmanac.com

Is Your Car's Airbag Safe?

Potentially lethal airbags are in at least 14 million US vehicles.

Tens of millions of 2001 to 2015 model-year vehicles were recalled because their Takata airbags could propel metal shrapnel at drivers and passengers—but many of those airbags were never replaced, though the recall dates back a decade and dozens of people have died.

To find out if your vehicle has been recalled: Enter the VIN into the search box at NHTSA.gov/recalls. Check often as models continue to be added. Automakers are required to repair recalls for free for at least 15 years from when the recall was issued.

Rosemary Shahan is founder and president of the nonprofit Consumers for Auto Reliability and Safety, Sacramento, California. CarConsumers.org

Be Cautious When Buying a Used Car

According to an investigation of 10 popular models with previous recalls (including Ford Escape, Honda Accord, Toyota Corolla and Volvo S60), nearly 40% that were for sale had unaddressed safety problems. Under federal law, sellers do not have to disclose safety-recall issues.

Self-defense: Check any used car for unrepaired recall defects by entering its VIN at NHTSA.gov/recalls.

Kevin Brasler is executive editor of *Consumers' Checkbook*, a Washington, DC–based nonprofit consumer-rights organization. See the full report at Checkbook.org/recalls.

TAKE NOTE...

Danger Alerts

Stay up to date on recalls from the Consumer Product Safety Commission by signing up for emails at CPSC.gov/Recalls. Find out about each recall as it occurs—or sign up for alerts in specific categories (household products, sports and recreation, etc.).

CPSC.gov/Recalls

Dangerous Clothes and Furniture

Stain- and water-resistant materials, such as used for rain jackets, hiking clothes, mattress pads, comforters, napkins and tablecloths, have been found to contain *perfluoroalkyl* and *polyfluoroalkyl* (PFAS) chemicals. PFAS are sometimes called "forever chemicals" because they do not degrade. They are linked to heart and liver damage as well as cancer and hormone disruption.

Self-defense: Don't purchase items marked "stain-resistant" and "water-resistant"...and choose rainwear that repels water with fabrics made of tighter weave or coated with paraffin wax.

Results of chemical tests run on 60 products by research company Toxic-Free Future, Seattle. ToxicFreeFuture.org

Potential Risks from Popular Cookware

Andrew Rubman, ND, FABNE, medical director of Southbury Clinic for Traditional Medicines in Southbury, Connecticut. He is a founding member of the American Association of Naturopathic Physicians. SouthburyClinic.com

"Cooking healthy" isn't only about nutritious ingredients—the cookware you choose can have medical consequences as well...

•**Stainless steel cookware can create trans fats**—the least healthy fats, raising bad cholesterol and lowering good cholesterol. The FDA has largely banned food manufacturers from adding trans fats to foods sold in the US—but some people accidentally add trans fats when they cook in stainless steel. Stainless steel cookware contains nickel, a catalyst in a "hydrogenation" process that can create trans fats from cooking oils.

Self-defense: When cooking in stainless steel, keep oils below their smoke point. Oils with high smoke points—and thus lower trans-fat risk—include avocado, peanut and grapeseed oils. Or switch to enamel-coated cast-iron pots and pans, such as Le Creuset cookware.

•**Uncoated cast-iron cookware can increase the iron level in your blood.** The more acidic the food you are cooking, the more iron that is shed by the pan. That's not a problem for most people, but when iron levels get too high, it can lead to serious health consequences such as liver damage, heart disease or cancer.

Self-defense: Replace uncoated cast-iron cookware with enamel-coated, as above, if a blood test suggests that you have elevated iron levels and/or you have been diagnosed with hereditary hemochromatosis, which leads to high iron levels. Symptoms can include joint pain, abdominal pain, fatigue, weakness and loss of sex drive. An enamel coating prevents the iron from leaching into food.

If you prefer to keep using your non-enamel cast-iron pans, the best way to avoid undue shedding is by "seasoning" the cookware to give it a protective, nonstick-type coat…and using hot water and a "chainmail" stainless steel scrubber to clean it. Soap is not recommended for cleaning cast iron, as it can leave residue and remove the protective seasoning coating.

Also helpful: Ask your doctor to run an "iron panel" blood test for guidance on your personal use of uncoated cast iron.

•**Nonstick cookware can release toxic chemicals.** Cancer-causing chemicals in non-stick Teflon coatings can flake into food if the cooking surface gets scratched…and toxic fumes can be released into kitchen air if this cookware is overheated.

Self-defense: Switch to "nonstick stoneware" or ceramic nonstick cookware, which has a natural nonstick surface but does not come with these cancer risks. It's extremely durable, too. Choose brands described in marketing materials as being completely free of *alkylphenol ethoxylates* (APEOs) and *perfluorooctanoic acid* (PFOA). These compounds undercut stoneware's safety advantage.

Good Fish/Bad Fish… How to Tell What's Safe

The US Food and Drug Administration and the Environmental Protection Agency have jointly created a chart that ranks the safety of more than 60 fish and shellfish based on their mercury levels. The chart, which is divided into Best Choices, Good Choices and Choices to Avoid, was developed as a guide for women who are or might become pregnant or are breastfeeding and for children ages one to 11. It gives recommended serving sizes as well as suggested frequency of consumption.

More information: A PDF of the chart is available at https://bit.ly/3H3T6Ui.

TAKE NOTE…

Are Eggs with Cracked Shells Safe to Eat?

Not if you bought them that way. Visible cracks are wide enough to let in salmonella, which could make you sick, so check eggs carefully before you buy. But if an egg cracks while in your custody, just remove it from its shell, seal it in a clean container, refrigerate it and use it within the next few days.

Lynne Ausman, DSc, director of the Master of Nutrition Science and Policy program, Tufts University, Boston.

Everyday BPA Dangers

Chris Iliades, MD, retired ear, nose, throat, head, and neck surgeon who now dedicates his time to educating patients through his medical writing.

B isphenol A (BPA) is an industrial chemical that's used in plastic bottles, inside metal cans, and in the lining of bottle caps.

When it became widely known that BPA was leaching into the foods and drinks inside those containers, many people ditched the cans and bottles, and the U.S. Food and Drug Administration banned the use of BPA in baby products.

A MUCH BIGGER PROBLEM

New research, however, shows that another common product exposes people to up to 1,000 times more BPA than what you might get from food or drink packaged in BPA polycarbonate: thermal paper. That's the thin paper that many receipts, boarding passes, and theater tickets are printed on. A 2016 study found that BPA levels in urine were almost three times higher in cashiers who handled thermal paper receipts than people in a control group.

Not all receipts are printed on thermal paper. The Environmental Working Group found that while McDonald's, CVS, KFC, Whole Foods, Walmart, Safeway, and the U.S. Postal Service use thermal paper, Target, Starbucks, and Bank of America automated teller machines do not. You can easily check if paper is thermally treated by rubbing it with a coin. Thermal paper will discolor when rubbed.

WHY IT MATTERS

Many animal studies have warned that BPA can interfere with hormone signals. Hormones are chemical messengers that help control body functions. Studies suggest a link with cancer, diabetes, high blood pressure, infertility, and behavioral problems in children.

The FDA's current stance on BPA was based on a four-year review of more than 300 research studies that was completed in 2014. Since then, new research has emerged. A 2019 study presented to the European Respiratory

Have You Been Exposed to BPA?

Almost every American adult has been exposed to BPA. Even if you avoid it in food packaging and thermal paper, it has been used in water pipes and has been deposited in enough dump sites to leave trace amounts in air, dirt, and water samples. As a result, BPA has been found in 90% to 93% of U.S. urine samples. A 2019 study from Washington State University found levels to be more than 40 times higher than what the FDA deems very low and safe. It has also been measured in blood and breast milk.

Society found that pregnant women with high levels of BPA in their urine had children that were at higher risk for poor lung capacity and wheezing. There were more than 2,500 women in the study, and close to 80% of them had detectable levels of BPA in their urine. Those with the highest levels gave birth to children with a 23% higher risk of asthma.

REDUCE YOUR EXPOSURE

Lowering your exposure to BPA can be simple with these steps…

• **Avoid plastic when possible.** Glass and metal food storage containers and water bottles are now widely available.

• **When you do need plastic, check for the recycle code** and don't use anything with a 3 or 7. Those types of plastic are likely to contain BPA.

• **Don't put any food containers that may have BPA in the dishwasher or microwave.** Heating increases the risk of BPA leaking out.

• **Throw away old plastic containers.** Age breaks down the plastic, releasing BPA.

• **Use plastic containers marked BPA-free with caution.** Studies show that these replacements can also interfere with the body's hormones.

• **Avoid canned foods and metal bottle caps when possible.** Use fresh, frozen, or dried food instead of canned.

• **If you can't avoid foods in BPA-lined cans, rinse the food in water before eating.**

• **Never heat food in a can.**

• **If you don't need a receipt, don't take it.** If you need a record, ask for an email or text receipt instead.

• **If you save your receipts,** wash your hands when you get home and save your receipts inside a bag or envelope.

• **Do not let children handle thermal paper.**

• **Don't put thermal paper into your recycling.** BPA residue from receipts will contaminate recycled paper.

Wildfire Smoke Damages Skin

Recent finding: Exposure—even short term—to hazardous air quality from wildfire smoke can damage skin, causing eczema, itching and other conditions. The smoke already is known to cause respiratory and cardiovascular symptoms, from runny noses and coughs to stroke and heart attack.

Self-defense: During wildfire season in areas where the fires occur, stay indoors as much as possible, and wear clothing that covers skin when outside. Also use creams, lotions or ointments that soften skin and can strengthen its ability to act as a barrier to environmental toxins.

Study by researchers at University of California, San Francisco, published in *JAMA Dermatology.*

Mobile Health Apps: Proceed with Caution

Mobile health apps may compromise your privacy.

Recent study: As many as 88% of free health apps have the potential to share your personal information with companies such as Google and Facebook…about one-third don't

post their privacy policies (even though it is required by law)…and about 25% violate their own stated privacy policies. Before you use a health app, check it out—look in the app's description under "about this app" or "app permission" for details of what it intends to share. If you're unsure, don't download it.

Study of 16,000 free health apps by researchers at University of Toronto, Canada, published in *The BMJ.*

Guard Against Theft of Delivered Packages

Use in-store pickup…choose the "signature required" option…sign up for a delivery alert…have packages delivered to your workplace or a stay-at-home neighbor…install outdoor security cameras or a lockable package delivery box. Going out of town? Request a free "vacation hold" at a local post office or USPS.com.

Free Amazon option: Have purchases sent to a Hub locker at a nearby store or other location.

Bottom Line Personal.

Fake Amazon Phishing Scams

When shoppers are already getting loads of e-mails from retailers about legitimate shopping deals and items they've ordered, scammers are quick to take advantage.

Typical scams: You receive an e-mail that looks like it comes from Amazon saying that your account has been locked and asking you to click on a link to verify your account.

Or: You receive an e-mail purportedly from Amazon that offers a "$50-bonus voucher" or other free bonus if you "quickly review your product." The scammers count on the fact that people who have purchased something on Amazon will click on the link expecting to review something they purchased and get a "reward."

Self-defense: When you get an e-mail that says it comes from Amazon—or any retailer—don't click on any links in the message. Instead, check on the retailer's website using a separate browser.

Better Busines Bureau, BBB.org and Komando.com.

BEWARE...

Package-Delivery Scams Use Fear

Thieves impersonate US Customs and Border Protection agents with a call, e-mail or text—and even make threats, such as that a warrant will be issued for your arrest if you do not provide personal information. Or they may say a package is valuable and that you must pay for special shipping labels. Such claims are scams—file a report at ReportFraud.FTC.gov.

Federal Trade Commission. FTC.gov

Financial Fraud Against Seniors

Financial fraud against seniors rose 186% from 2014 to 2020—more than the overall 125% increase in fraud affecting people of all ages.

If you or a loved one are a victim of fraud: Call the National Elder Fraud Hotline, 833-372-8311. And contact state authorities as well—get information at https://bit.ly/3yKDPmx.

Study by SeniorHousingNet.com.

Protect Yourself from a Legal Nightmare

Rebecca Strub, JD, LLM (Tax), a personal family lawyer and the owner of Strub Law LLC. She is licensed in New Jersey, New York, and Pennsylvania.

For many people, retirement is a time of long-awaited freedom. Gone are the constraints of bosses and the needs of children, and a lifetime of careful savings provides a passport to travel, fun with friends, and limitless choices.

Sure, retirement age often comes with some aches and pains or more significant health conditions, but each person is free to choose how to accommodate those conditions in the way they best see fit.

At least that's what hundreds of people believed before they met April Parks, professional guardian and master con artist. It turns out there is a terrifying loophole in the legal system that allows a complete stranger to take control over every aspect of your life if you're deemed to be unable to care for yourself. If you think that means something as serious as being in a coma, think again. Parks's victims lost everything—from their life savings to their very freedom—for issues as simple as being falsely accused of having dementia.

We spoke with Rebecca Strub, Esq., to find out how you can make sure this never happens to you or your loved ones.

APRIL PARKS CASE

First, let's take a look at how April Parks took advantage of people who didn't have some simple legal documents in place. Parks and her accomplices sought out seniors who had both a history of some kind of medical condition, not necessarily a severe one, and assets that she could seize. She then used a legal maneuver called ex parte that allowed her to go before a judge and request emergency temporary guardianship over a person—without informing that person or his or her family. Her medical claims were dubious, but she always won, and temporary guardianship invariably became permanent.

Parks and her associates would promptly show up at her new ward's home, with no advance notice, and force the unwitting person to hastily pack so she could move him or her to an assisted living facility. She would then plunder the home, seizing personal belongings and assets, and selling everything of value her ward owned.

Parks prevented her wards from seeing or speaking to their families, and billed the estates outlandish fees—enriching herself while providing the bare minimum for her wards.

Act Now!

No matter how old you are, these tools should be implemented immediately. It's important to note that any adult could face court-ordered guardianship if they become incapacitated by illness or injury. So it's critical that every person over age 18—not just seniors—puts these estate planning tools in place to prepare for potential incapacity.

The high-profile case of Terry Schiavo was a heartbreaking example of the need for planning ahead. In 1990, the 26-year-old went into cardiac arrest and entered a persistent vegetative state. Eight years later, her husband petitioned for her feeding tube to be removed, insisting that she would not have wanted to continue life-prolonging measures with no hope of recovering, while her parents argued that she would, in fact, want to be kept alive by any means necessary.

Because Mrs. Schiavo did not have a living will, her loved ones engaged in a high-profile legal battle that dragged on for seven years. The governor of Florida, Congress, and the U.S. president all got involved—as did the court of public opinion. Mrs. Schiavo's feeding tube was removed and replaced multiple times before her death.

—Rebecca Strub

Assisted-living workers reported that they could always tell which residents were under her care because of how poorly they were dressed. She refused to give them their own clothes or release their funds to buy new ones. Parks defrauded and terrorized more than 150 people before she was finally stopped and sentenced to prison in 2017.

WHAT GUARDIANS CAN LEGALLY DO

While Parks's extreme abuses and self-enrichment led to her downfall, much of what she was doing was perfectly legal. *A court-appointed guardian has the legal authority to control every aspect of your life...*

- **Determining where you live,** including moving you into assisted living or a nursing home of their choice
- **Controlling your finances,** real estate, and other assets
- **Making all of your health-care decisions and providing consent for medical treatments**
- **Placing restrictions on your communications and interactions with others, including family members**
- **Making decisions about your daily life,** such as recreational activities, clothing, and food choices
- **Making end-of-life and other palliative-care decisions**

Perhaps one of the most disturbing aspects of guardianship cases is that once a person has been assigned a guardian, it's extremely difficult to have the guardian removed—even if an illness was temporary or a family member tries to intervene. A study by the American Bar Association found that family members who try to fight against court-appointed guardians incur vast costs, even going bankrupt, and still often lose.

While the April Parks case has brought attention to the abuses in the guardian system, it hasn't eliminated them. In fact, as the population ages and the court system struggles to keep up with its current load, it will only grow harder to provide proper oversight of the professional guardian profession, Strub warns.

PROTECT YOURSELF NOW

Fortunately, you can protect yourself from falling prey to this broken system by creating a plan where you choose who will take care of you. *An "incapacity plan" or a "care-and-protection plan" will include some, or all, of the following documents...*

- **Health-care power of attorney.** This document grants an individual of your choice the immediate legal authority to make decisions about your medical treatment in the event of your incapacity.
- **Living will/advance directive for health care.** This provides specific guidance about how your medical decisions should be made during your incapacity.

- **Durable financial power of attorney.** Use this document to choose who will have the immediate authority to make decisions related to the management of your financial and legal interests.

- **A revocable living trust** transfers control of all assets held by the trust to a person of your choosing to be used for your benefit in the event of your incapacity. The trust can include legally binding instructions for how your care should be managed and even spell out specific conditions that must be met for you to be deemed incapacitated.

- **Family/friends meeting.** Even more important than all of the documents listed here, the very best protection for you and the people you love is to ensure that everyone is on the same page. Set up a meeting with the attorney that you hire to prepare your documents and any people affected by your plan to explain to them the plans you've made, why you've made them, and what to do when something happens to you.

It could be a good idea (though not necessary) to name different people for each of the roles in your planning documents. In this way, not only will you spread out the responsibility among multiple individuals, but you'll ensure that you have more than just one person invested in your care and supervision.

HOW TO GET THE DOCUMENTS

An experienced estate planning attorney who focuses his or her practice in this area can help you choose the plan that will work the best for your unique circumstances and prepare the needed legal documents. But this isn't a once-and-done process. You'll need to regularly review and update these planning tools to keep pace with changes in your assets, your life and relationships, and federal and state tax laws.

While you can't eliminate the risk of incapacity, you can use estate planning to ensure that you have some control over how your life and assets will be managed if it ever does occur.

Never Unsubscribe from Spam E-Mails

We're not talking about an unwelcome newsletter or sales pitch from a legitimate company with which you have a relationship. We mean random illicit messages sending you malware links or fake insurance rates. Clicking the "Unsubscribe" link might seem like a good idea, but it actually could make your situation worse. Spammers blast out millions of such messages, and a click from you is like a ping back to them from out of the void—it marks you as a live one, and now you'll be more specifically targeted. Instead, simply mark the message as spam and delete it.

LifeHacker.com

GOOD TO KNOW...

Work-from-Home Security Tips

Secure your network—change the password and username from the factory-set ones on your Wi-Fi router, which can be an entry point for cybercriminals. ***Best password***—eight characters or more, combining special characters, lower- and uppercase letters and numbers. ***Don't use identifying information,*** such as a pet's name, birthday, etc. ***Enable two-factor authentication*** so the password and another means of verification—such as a code from a text message—will be required when logging into an account. ***Keep software up to date***—that often fixes security issues and bugs and improves performance. ***Use a VPN*** (virtual private network) to create a secure "tunnel" between you and any site you're connecting to. ***Separate your devices***—using a business computer for Facebook or Twitter can be a security risk. If possible, have a separate computer for business and one for personal use.

Pentagon Federal Credit Union. PenFed.org

Protect Yourself Online with a Burner Identity

Cybersecurity expert and keynote speaker John Sileo, CEO of The Sileo Group, a Denver-based data security think tank whose clients include the US Department of Defense and Amazon. Sileo.com

In the movies, spies often use "burners"—disposable cell phones—to protect their identities and information. The same concept can help you avoid spam, junk calls and fraudulent charges.

By 2022, the average Internet user will have signed up for 300 online accounts, from delivery services to apps to shopping websites. Many websites sell your sign-up information to marketers or it gets leaked if their databases are hacked. These sites often allow you to opt out of having your data shared, but it's easy to forget to choose that option.

Alternative: Maintain your current e-mail, phone and credit card numbers for only family, friends, coworkers and websites that you trust. For everything else, consider using burner tools.

E-MAIL

• **Sign up for a temporary e-mail address that expires in a few minutes.** 10MinuteMail.com generates an e-mail address for free that lasts only 10 minutes, then deletes all records of that e-mail address. It's very useful when you want to get a discount code or read an article on a site that requires e-mail verification but that you may never visit again.

• **Create a free, permanent e-mail address at Gmail or Yahoo mail.** You can generate multiple additional e-mail addresses. If you want anonymity, make sure your new username and address aren't similar to ones you already have.

PHONE NUMBERS

• **Check if your mobile phone service carrier offers a way to add a new number to your account.** Verizon charges $15/month/number for its My Numbers program and T-Mobile charges $5/month/number for its DIGITS program.

Cell Phone Self-Defense

Your Phone Could Be Infected with Spyware

Certain governments have used the spyware tool Pegasus to monitor the phones of journalists and activists remotely. While Pegasus is a small threat to most people, other kinds of spyware—called "stalkerware"—are disturbingly common. Anyone with physical access to your smartphone could install software that monitors your activities and even controls your camera.

Self-defense: Always update your software, install a screen lock, and run a malware scanner regularly.

David Ruiz is an online privacy advocate at Malwarebytes Labs, San Francisco. Malwarebytes.com

QR Codes Can Download Malware onto Your Cell Phone

QR codes (those matrix barcodes that your phone scans) are everywhere—even being used by diners at restaurants to obtain menus. But scammers are creating fake codes to steal sensitive data, such as account passwords.

Self-defense: Don't scan codes printed on stickers—scammers sometimes stick fake codes over legitimate ones. Don't scan codes found online or in e-mails unless you're certain the site or sender is legitimate. Download the free app Kaspersky QR Scanner, which warns when a QR code is dangerous.

Steven J. J. Weisman, Esq., an attorney, is founder of the scam-information website Scamicide.com

• **Get Google Voice.** If you have a Google account, you get one phone number via Google Voice, a voice-over-the-Internet phone service that works on smartphones and mobile devices and that allows you to place and receive free calls and texts within the US and Canada. The number comes with call-forwarding and a voicemail in-box. Sign up at Voice.Google.com.

• **Download the Burner app.** This is best if you want a secondary phone number that connects to your real phone number and that can be replaced whenever you want. The app lets you control who can call you on your burner number. When you're done with a number, just eliminate it at the press of a button.

Caution: Phone calls and texts made through your burner number count as minutes and data on your regular mobile phone account.

Cost: $4.99 per burner number per month.

CREDIT CARD NUMBERS

•**Ask your bank about virtual credit card numbers.** These substitute a unique replacement number generated by software for your real credit card number.

•**Try a virtual credit card service.** The Privacy app (Privacy.com) allows you to create up to 12 virtual credit cards per month for free. The virtual numbers are useless to scammers and hackers because you tie them to specific retailers, designate the numbers for onetime use or limit the amount that can be purchased.

•**Use popular mobile-pay and digital-wallet services such as PayPal, Apple Pay and Google Pay.** These services create a random, temporary card number for every transaction, so retailers never get your real credit card number.

Criminals Are Using AirTags to Stalk You

Apple's AirTags are meant to help you keep track of items you often misplace.

Example: You can attach an AirTag to your keys so you can use your iPhone to find them.

Downside: Crooks have been sticking Air Tags on bags, cars and other items to stalk people or track cars they want to steal. Apple is supposed to alert you if you are being tracked, but this doesn't always happen. If you get an alert about an unfamiliar AirTag, tap the notification…then "Continue"…"Play Sound" to locate the AirTag…"Instructions to Disable AirTag." You will not get a notification if you have an Android phone, but you can download the Tracker Detect app available at Google Play. Meanwhile, Apple is working on security improvements.

Komando.com

ID Theft from Yearbook Photos

Scammers search social media to look for photos posted by recent high school graduates and get the victims' high school name and graduation year, information often used in online security questions. More searching can give scammers a victim's birth date, hometown and family members' names.

Self-defense: Be careful about posting personal info…change security settings regularly.

Better Business Bureau. BBB.org

Google Ups Security

Google has rolled out required two-factor authentication.

"2FA" or "2SV" (two-step verification) is a simple cybersecurity measure already in use in many places, such as for online banking. When logging into your Google account, you will be required to confirm from your cell phone that it's you trying to log in.

ReviewGeek.com

Index